I0027438

Current and Future Developments in Hypertension
(Volume 1)

(Novel Strategies and Approaches in Hypertension Therapy)

Edited by
Hafize Uzun & Pınar Atukeren
Department of Medical Biochemistry, Cerrahpaşa Faculty of Medicine,
Istanbul University-Cerrahpasa, Istanbul, Turkey

Current and Future Developments in Hypertension

Volume # 1

Novel Strategies and Approaches in Hypertension Therapy

Editors: Hafize Uzun & Pınar Atukeren

ISBN (Online): 9789811422720

ISBN (Print): 9789811422713

need for a court order if at any point you breach any terms of this License Agreement. In no event will any delay or failure by Bentham Science Publishers in enforcing your compliance with this License Agreement constitute a waiver of any of its rights.

3. You acknowledge that you have read this License Agreement, and agree to be bound by its terms and conditions. To the extent that any other terms and conditions presented on any website of Bentham Science Publishers conflict with, or are inconsistent with, the terms and conditions set out in this License Agreement, you acknowledge that the terms and conditions set out in this License Agreement shall prevail.

Bentham Science Publishers Pte. Ltd.
80 Robinson Road #02-00
Singapore 068898
Singapore
Email: subscriptions@benthamscience.net

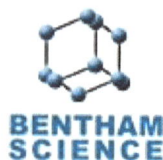

BENTHAM
SCIENCE

CONTENTS

PREFACE

Hypertension has become a major public health problem and highly prevalent in the last decades in worldwide. High blood pressure is a serious risk factor for not only premature cardiovascular disease but also for end-organ damage, including left ventricular hypertrophy and congestive heart failure, which in turn increases the risk of cardiovascular morbidity and mortality. Also, peripheral arterial disease, aortic aneurysms, kidney disease and vascular dementia emerges with persistent high blood pressure as potentially life-threatening conditions. Studies of hypertension have been performed in a variety of epidemiological settings such as diabetes, renal function, obesity, thyroid disorders. Novel treatment strategies should also be clarified comprising traditional medicine, drug interactions involving psychopharmacological agents, diuretics etc. correlated with molecular genetics. Effective treatment targets are changing and debated. Biochemical testing serves to identify hypertensive individuals who are at higher risk based on co-morbidities such as dysglycaemia, dyslipidaemia or renal impairment and supports risk stratification of patients facilitating tailored management and treatment. With this book we aim to evaluate hypertension in all aspects; in practice, in prescribing, in setting up a treatment program and in guiding patients clarifying the basic molecular and biochemical mechanisms with a considerable amount of new information providing enough pathophysiology to permit clinical judgment presented in a manner enabling the readers to grasp its significance. We believe that this textbook will provide grounding pointing the way to new disciplines that will contribute to the evolution of strategies for creating, analyzing and presenting medical information in the future stimulating our colleagues at all multidisciplinary levels.

Dr. Hafize Uzun & Dr. Pınar Atukeren
Department of Medical Biochemistry,
Cerrahpaşa Faculty of Medicine,
Istanbul University-Cerrahpasa,
Istanbul,
Turkey

DEDICATION

To hypertension patients.. we hope this will be a useful book on clinical hypertension both in basic knowledge and novel therapeutic approaches....

List of Contributors

Abdulhalim Senyigit	Department of Internal Medicine, Istanbul Biruni University, Istanbul, Turkey
Aykut Oruc	Department of Physiology, Istanbul University-Cerrahpaşa, Cerrahpasa Faculty of Medicine Istanbul, Istanbul, Turkey
Berrin Papila Kundaktepe	Department of General Surgery, Cerrahpaşa Faculty of Medicine Istanbul, Istanbul, Turkey
Bahadir Simsek	Department of Medical Biochemistry, Istanbul University – Cerrahpaşa, Cerrahpaşa Faculty of Medicine Istanbul, Istanbul, Turkey
Cigdem Usul Afsar	Department of Internal Medicine and Medical Oncology, Acıbadem Mehmet Ali Aydınlar University Medical Faculty, Istanbul, Turkey
Dildar Konukoglu	Department of Biochemistry, Istanbul University-Cerrahpasa, Cerrahpasa Faculty of Medicine, Istanbul, Turkey
Gonul Simsek	Department of Physiology, Istanbul University-Cerrahpaşa, Cerrahpasa Faculty of Medicine Istanbul, Istanbul, Turkey
Hafize Uzun	Department of Medical Biochemistry, Cerrahpaşa Faculty of Medicine, Istanbul University-Cerrahpasa, Istanbul, Turkey
Karolin Yanar	Department of Medical Biochemistry, Cerrahpaşa Faculty of Medicine, Istanbul University-Cerrahpaşa, İstanbul, Turkey
Lebriz Uslu-Beşli	Department of Nuclear Medicine, Cerrahpaşa Faculty of Medicine, Istanbul University-Cerrahpasa, Istanbul, Turkey
Mustafa Kanat	Division of Diabetes, Department of Internal Medicine, University of Istanbul Medeniyet, Goztepe Training and Research Hospital, Istanbul, Turkey
Mustafa Erinç Sitar	Department of Medical Biochemistry, Faculty of Medicine, Maltepe University, Istanbul, Turkey
Muhammad A. Abdul-Ghani	Division of Diabetes, University of Texas Health Science Center at San Antonio, San Antonio, TX, USA
M. Emel Tüfekçi Alphan	Okan University, Institute of Health Sciences, Department of Nutrition and Dietetics, Istanbul, Turkey
Pelin Uysal	Department of Chest Diseases, Faculty of Medicine, Mehmet Ali Aydınlar University, Atakent Hospital, Istanbul, Turkey
Pınar Atukeren	Department of Medical Biochemistry, Cerrahpaşa Faculty of Medicine, Istanbul University-Cerrahpasa, Istanbul, Turkey
Sibel Ozyazgan	Department of Pharmacology and Clinical Pharmacology, Istanbul University, Cerrahpasa Medical Faculty, İstanbul, Turkey
Sinem Durmus	Department of Biochemistry, Cerrahpasa Faculty of Medicine, Istanbul University-Cerrahpasa, Istanbul, Turkey
Suranjith L. Seneviratne	Institute of Immunity and Transplantation, Royal Free Hospital and University College London, London, UK
Ufuk Çakatay	Department of Medical Biochemistry, Istanbul University – Cerrahpaşa, Cerrahpaşa Faculty of Medicine Istanbul, Istanbul, Turkey

Umesh Jayarajah   Professorial Medical Unit, National Hospital of Sri Lanka, Colombo, Sri Lanka

CHAPTER 1

Environmental Aspects of Hypertension

Umesh Jayarajah[1,3] and **Suranjith L. Seneviratne**[2,3,*]

¹ Professorial Medical Unit, National Hospital of Sri Lanka, Colombo, Sri Lanka

² Institute of Immunity and Transplantation, Royal Free Hospital and University College London, London, UK

³ Department of Surgery, Faculty of Medicine, University of Colombo, Sri Lanka

Abstract: Environmental factors are an important cause of poor health globally. Hypertension is known to occur due to complex interactions between adverse lifestyles and environmental factors on a background of polygenic inheritance. Although pharmacological interventions have taken a prominent place, environmental factors and interventions have generally received less consideration. The short-term and long term impact of several environmental factors on blood pressure changes such as cold ambient temperature, exposure to loud noise, air pollution, high altitude, certain organic pollutants, and heavy metals have been recently reported. In this chapter, the current evidence on the effect of such environmental risk factors on blood pressure with its pathophysiological mechanisms and clinical relevance have been described in detail. As some of these effects are clinically relevant, clinicians, patients with hypertension or cardiovascular disease and individuals at high risk for cardiovascular disease would need to be aware of these environmental factors. Furthermore, close attention to monitoring blood pressure during such exposures is necessary and in individuals with hypertension, treatment schedules may need adjustment to ensure more optimal blood pressure control.

Keywords: Air pollution, Aircraft noise, Ambient temperature, Blood pressure, Cardiovascular diseases, Diastolic hypertension, Environmental factors, Heart disease, Heavy metals, High altitude, Hypertension, Lifestyle, Loud noise, Noise pollution, Organic pollutants, Pathophysiology, Risk factors, Sleep apnoea, Systolic hypertension, Work environment.

INTRODUCTION

Hypertension occurs due to complex interactions between adverse lifestyles and environmental factors on a background of polygenic inheritance [1]. Recently, there has been a pandemic of metabolic disorders such as hypertension. Several

*Corresponding author Suranjith L. Seneviratne: Institute of Immunity and Transplantation, Royal Free Hospital and University College London, London, UK; Tel: 00442078302141; E-mail: s.seneviratne@ucl.ac.uk

Hafize Uzun & Pınar Atukeren (Eds.)

behavioural interventions and medications have been found to be effective in lowering blood pressure and reducing cardiovascular complications [1]. In clinical practice, although pharmacological interventions have taken a prominent place, environmental factors and interventions have generally received less consideration [2]. There is published evidence on the effects of environmental factors such as cold temperatures, high altitudes, loud noise, air pollution and heavy metal exposure in the causation of hypertension [2]. According to the report of the 'Environmental Burden of Disease in European Countries' project, particulate matter air pollution and noise pollution, result in >75% of the burden of disease attributable to environmental factors [3]. As they primarily affect cardiovascular diseases and risk factors, they in turn contribute significantly to an increase in disability adjusted life years [4]. Although the effect on blood pressure is generally small, owing to the global presence of hypertension, the overall effect is fairly significant. Thus, early identification of relevant environmental factors and their correction may have important clinical implications in the control of hypertension [2]. We have discussed the clinical effects and pathophysiological mechanisms of a range of environmental factors on blood pressure.

COLD AMBIENT TEMPERATURE RELATED HYPERTENSION

The association between seasonality/outdoor temperatures and cardiovascular disorders has been extensively studied [5 - 10] (Table **1**). Several studies have described associations between changes in outdoor temperature during the year and morbidity and mortality rates from cardiovascular disease. An increased incidence of acute coronary events and stroke has been reported during winter [6]. This seasonal pattern in cardiovascular diseases may be explained by seasonal changes in blood pressure [9]. A number of studies done in several countries and varying climates have found an inverse relationship between ambient temperature and blood pressure. Yang *et al.,* explored the relationship between blood pressure, outdoor temperature, and cardiovascular mortality in around 500,000 Chinese adults from both urban and rural regions prospectively followed up for seven years [9]. They found a strong relationship between monthly outdoor temperatures and blood pressure. The mean systolic blood pressure was 9 mm Hg higher in winter compared to summer. Above an outdoor temperature of 5°C, each 10°C decrease in temperature caused an increase in systolic blood pressure of 6.2mm Hg. Overall, there was a 41% increase in cardiovascular mortality during winter. The authors suggested the increase in cardiovascular events may at least partly be explained by an increase in blood pressure [11].

In a cross-sectional study of 1395 patients (89.3% of whom were hypertensive), Fedecostante *et al.,* compared blood pressure measurements taken in the two hottest and two coldest months. Mean daytime systolic and diastolic blood pressure was significantly higher in winter [12]. Modesti *et al.,* confirmed these findings when ambulatory blood pressure monitoring and temperature measurement were done in nearly 1900 patients referred to two Hypertension Units [13]. Temperature and seasonality were found to independently affect blood pressure, where the temperature had an inverse relationship with daytime systolic blood pressure and seasonality (expressed as the number of daylight hours), mainly affected night-time systolic blood pressure. An increase in daylight hours was associated with higher night-time blood pressure and could at least be partly due to a reduction in sleep quality [13]. A study on 2078 cardiac rehabilitation patients from Michigan, found a similar inverse association. A reduction in outdoor temperatures by 10.4° C during the prior 1 to 7 days was associated with a 3.6mm Hg increase in systolic blood pressure [14]. However, some studies have found nocturnal blood pressure to be higher during summer than winter months [12, 13, 15, 16]. Variations have also been observed in relation to indoor versus outdoor temperature exposures [13, 16, 17].

Table 1. Summary of studies on the effects of cold ambient environmental temperature on blood pressure.

Author	Year	Country/Place	Study Type	Study Population	Methods	Main Findings
Woodhouse PR [24]	1993	Cambridge, UK	Prospective study	96 participants aged 65-74	Seasonal variations of blood pressure, ambient temperature and body mass index were measured	Both systolic and diastolic blood pressure were highest during winter across the whole distribution of blood pressures. There was a fourfold increase in the proportion of subjects with blood pressures > 160/90 mmHg in winter compared with summer. A 1 degree C decrease in living-room temperature was associated with a rise of 1.3/0.6 mmHg in systolic/diastolic blood pressure

(Table 1) cont.....

Author	Year	Country/Place	Study Type	Study Population	Methods	Main Findings
Minami J [23]	1996	Japan	Prospective study	50 outpatients with essential hypertension	Monitoring of blood pressure was done. The daytime and night-time blood pressures were calculated according to the true waking and sleeping times of individual patients.	In patients with essential hypertension, office, home and daytime ambulatory blood pressure levels were higher in winter than in summer. However, the seasonal variations in average 24 h blood pressure may be small because of the lack of changes in night-time blood pressure.
Danet S [7]	1999	France	Prospective study	3616 cardiovascular events	Percentages of variation of event rates according to meteorological variations were derived from the relative risks estimated with a Poisson regression model.	A 10 degrees C decrease was associated with a statistically significant 13% increase in event rates.
Charach G [42]	2004	Israel	Prospective study	182 patients aged 65-91	Seasonal variation in blood pressure and the variables age, gender, body mass index and related complications were analysed in elderly patients with essential hypertension	Both systolic and diastolic mean blood pressures were significantly higher during winter compared to summer. Patients aged 65-75 years were unexpectedly more sensitive to winter-summer changes than older patients.

(Table 1) cont.....

Author	Year	Country/Place	Study Type	Study Population	Methods	Main Findings
						Complications such as myocardial infarctions and strokes occurred twice as frequently in winter than during any other season.
Madsen C [43]	2006	Oslo, Norway	Population based study	8,770 Oslo citizens	Associations between blood pressure and environmental conditions including season, smoking, outdoor temperature and air pollution were assessed	Blood pressure was higher during the winter season, but the association disappeared when adjusted for temperature. A 10 degrees C reduction in outdoor temperature on the day blood pressure was measured was related to an increase in blood pressure for both men and women.
Modesti PA [15]	2006	Italy	Retrospective analysis	6404 subjects	The combined effects of aging, treatment, and daily mean temperature on clinic and ambulatory blood pressure were investigated	Office and mean 24-hour systolic blood pressure, as well as morning pressure surge, were significantly lower in hot, and higher in cold days when compared with intermediate temperature days. No significant relationship was found between air temperature and heart rate.

(Table 1) cont.....

Author	Year	Country/Place	Study Type	Study Population	Methods	Main Findings
Alpérovitch A [25]	2009	France	Prospective study	8801 subjects 65 years or older	Blood pressure was measured at baseline and 2-year follow-up examinations. Daily outdoor temperature measured at 11 am was provided by the local meteorological offices.	Both systolic and diastolic blood pressures differed significantly with outdoor temperature. Systolic blood pressure decreased with increasing temperature, with an 8.0-mm Hg decrease between the lowest and the highest temperature quintile. Outdoor temperature and blood pressure are strongly correlated in the elderly, especially in those 80 years or older.
Brook MD [6]	2011	Michigan, USA	Prospective study	51 non-smoking patients	24-hour personal-level environmental temperature monitoring along with daily cardiovascular measurements, during summer and/or winter periods	Systolic and diastolic blood pressures were positively associated with several hour-long personal-level environmental temperature measurements.
Fedecostante M [12]	2012	Italy	Retrospective analysis	1395 patients referred to hypertension centre	Ambulatory pressure measurements were correlated with seasonal variations in temperature.	The hottest summer months were associated with lower daytime blood pressure and lower 24-h diastolic blood pressure.

(Table 1) cont.....

Author	Year	Country/Place	Study Type	Study Population	Methods	Main Findings
Lewington S [17]	2012	China	Cross-sectional study	506,673 adults aged 30-79 years	Analyses related mean blood pressure - overall and in various subgroups - to mean local outdoor temperature.	Blood pressure was inversely associated with outdoor temperature in Chinese adults across a range of climatic conditions. Access to home central heating appeared to remove much of the association during the winter months.
Chen Q [10]	2013	China	Prospective study	1,831 hypertensive patients	Patients were followed up for three years, in two or four weekly check-ups, accumulating 62,452 follow-up records.	Both baseline and follow-up blood pressure showed a significant inverse association with ambient temperature, which explained 32.4% and 65.6% of variation of systolic blood pressure and diastolic blood pressure respectively. Gender, drinking behaviour and body mass index were also found to modify the association between temperature and diastolic blood pressure.

(Table 1) cont.....

Author	Year	Country/Place	Study Type	Study Population	Methods	Main Findings
Ke L [32]	2014	Macau	Cross-sectional study	1410 residents aged ≥18 years	Anthropometry and blood pressure were measured and demographic, exercise and dietary data were collected. Sunlight exposure on weekdays and weekends (in winter and summer) were estimated.	Modifiable predictors of hypertension were lack of sunlight exposure, low intake of fish, smoking, obesity and lack of exercise.
Su D [40]	2014	China	Cross-sectional study	57 375 participants aged 30-79 years	Analyses related daily mean outdoor temperature obtained from local Meteorological Bureau, to mean systolic and diastolic blood pressure.	Each 10°C lowering of ambient temperature was associated with a 6.9/2.9 mmHg higher systolic/diastolic blood pressure. There was a 14.1% higher prevalence of newly detected hypertension and 13.0% lower rate of hypertension control.
Giorgini P [14]	2015	Michigan, USA	Prospective study	2078 cardiac rehabilitation patients	Multiple linear regression analyses adjusting for age, sex, BMI, ozone and the same-day alternate environmental factor (*i.e.* PM2.5 or temperature).	Higher temperature levels (per 10.4°C) during lag days 4-6, were associated with reductions in both systolic (-3.6 to -2.3 mmHg) and diastolic blood pressures (-2.5 to -1.8 mmHg).

(Table 1) cont.....

Author	Year	Country/Place	Study Type	Study Population	Methods	Main Findings
Yang L [9]	2015	China	Prospective study	23 000 individuals with prior cardiovascular disease	Baseline survey data were used to assess seasonal variation in systolic blood pressure (SBP) and its association with outdoor temperature.	Mean systolic blood pressure was significantly higher in winter than in summer (145 vs. 136 mmHg), especially among those without central heating. Systolic blood pressure predicted subsequent cardiovascular disease mortality, with each 10 mmHg higher usual systolic blood pressure associated with 21% increased risk.

Pathophysiology of Cold Ambient Temperature Related Hypertension

Cold weather leads to compensatory activation of the sympathetic nervous system and hypothalamic-pituitary-adrenal axis so as to increase the body temperature. Increased sympathetic activity leads to stimulation of the juxtaglomerular apparatus and increased activity of the renin-angiotensin-aldosterone system causing sodium and water retention [18]. Due to poorly understood mechanisms, atherosclerotic coronary arteries undergo a higher degree of vasoconstriction in response to cold, leading to an imbalance in the myocardial oxygen demand and supply [19]. The cold pressor test evaluates sympathetic cardiovascular reactivity. Cold induced sympathetic responses lead to acute peripheral arteriolar vasoconstriction and affect the diastolic blood pressure, heart rate and cardiac load [20]. In addition, colder temperatures increase blood viscosity, red cell counts, plasma cholesterol, and plasma fibrinogen and promote platelet aggregation [21]. Increased cardiac load and hypercoagulability, may lead to acute coronary events, especially in those with pre-existing coronary vascular disease, atherosclerotic plaques and hypertension [22, 23].

Variations in systolic and diastolic blood pressure with outdoor temperature depend on the age [24]. Elderly people are more susceptible to seasonal blood pressure variations.

The Three-City Study was a prospective study conducted in 8801 participants 65 years or older, where oscillations in blood pressures in relation to temperature were analyzed [25]. An inverse relationship between environmental temperature and blood pressure was observed, with higher changes in blood pressure noted in older participants. In those aged between 65 - 74 years and older than 80 years, a 15°C decrease in outdoor temperature led to an increase in systolic blood pressure by 0.8 and 5.1mm Hg, respectively. The exact reasons for this observation are poorly understood, but may at least be partly due to reduced homeostatic responses due to impaired baroreflexes [26, 27]. Furthermore, increased atherosclerosis in the elderly may give result in an increased vasoconstrictor response. Such findings may explain greater cardiovascular mortality among the elderly during winter.

Outdoor temperature is only one of the environmental factors affecting the seasonality of hypertension and cardiovascular disease. Other known environmental factors include sunlight exposure, cold perception, changes in dietary and exercise habits, air pollution, disturbance in the circadian rhythm and sleep alterations [13, 28 - 31]. Studies have found longer life expectancy amongst women with active sun exposure. Thus lower sunlight exposure may be contributing to a higher incidence of cardiovascular diseases in winter [28]. In a random household survey of 1410 Chinese residents, more than half an hour's sun exposure daily (compared to none) was associated with a lower prevalence of hypertension [32]. Stephen *et al* analyzed relationships between blood pressure, sunlight exposure and plasma vitamin D concentrations in 1104 participants of the Reasons for Racial and Geographic Differences in Stroke (REGARDS) study. A significant inverse association between hypertension and Vitamin D levels and solar insolation was found. Adjusting for vitamin D levels, had no effect on the significant inverse association of solar insolation with blood pressure suggesting that the blood pressure lowering effect of sun exposure seems to be independent of Vitamin D levels [33]. This direct effect may be explained by the vasodilator effect of nitric oxide (NO). The skin contains considerable stores of nitrogen oxides, which are converted to NO by ultraviolet radiation and then transported to the systemic circulation. Human studies have shown NO to cause arterial vasodilatation and thus lower blood pressure. Furthermore, murine studies suggest similar mechanisms may lead to a reduction in the metabolic syndrome [34]. Additionally, increased sunlight exposure may lead to increased body temperatures, which then cause cutaneous vasodilatation, lower peripheral resistance and blood pressure [35].

Seasonal fluctuations in air pollution may contribute to variations in blood pressure. This is more relevant in urban areas, where air pollution is more commonly seen and characterized by both seasonal and daily fluctuations. For example, sulfur dioxide (SO_2) levels that are known to have a blood pressure increasing effect, peaks during winter. SO_2 is mainly derived from heating systems in buildings. Ozone (O_3), linked to photochemical smog has a blood pressure lowering effect. It reaches a peak during the summer months and the central hours of a day [36].

Seasonal variations in sleep onset, duration and quality may influence blood pressure and cardiovascular disease. Obstructive sleep apnoea (OSA) is characterized by repetitive interruptions of pulmonary ventilation during sleep. It is commonly seen in obese individuals and known to be associated with increased cardiovascular morbidity and mortality [37]. Recent evidence points to OSA being the most prevalent secondary contributor to hypertension. It can cause or worsen hypertension in susceptible individuals [11]. The severity of OSA is inversely related to ambient temperature and directly related to atmospheric pressure, carbon monoxide levels and relative air humidity [31]. The seasonality of OSA remained significant even after adjustment for sex, age, body mass index, neck circumference, and relative air humidity.

Lifestyle factors such as increased food and salt intake, cause a seasonal change in blood pressure [38]. Lack of physical activity is a risk factor for hypertension and cardiovascular disease. As physical activity may be reduced in winter, it may contribute to the seasonality of hypertension [39]. There is some evidence to suggest that close monitoring of blood pressure during winter may be beneficial in hypertensive patients [17, 40, 41]. Some patients may require anti-hypertensive medication dose adjustments for optimal blood pressure control [42]. Although improved residential heating might be helpful in combating the hypertensive effects of cold, further large scale prospective studies are needed before implementing such findings into clinical practice [17, 43]. The use of practical lifestyle modifications (such as using space heaters, wearing warmer clothes and reducing cold outdoor exposures) may be beneficial.

NOISE EXPOSURE-RELATED HYPERTENSION

Loud noise and noise pollution have been associated with raised blood pressure and increased cardiovascular disease [44]. Exposure to loud noise even for brief periods may increase blood pressure within minutes [45, 46]. Chronic exposure to loud noise may increase the risk of overt hypertension [47 - 49]. Whether these are due to specific types of exposure or the timing of exposure needs further study. Increases in blood pressure are higher following nocturnal than day time exposure to loud noise [46]. Several studies have attempted to describe the relationship between noise exposure and hypertension (Table **2**). Andren *et al* found a statistically significant increase in diastolic blood pressure at 95 decibels (dB) and proposed that repetitive loud noise could contribute to the development of hypertension [50]. Chronic noise exposure has been found to associate with raised urinary epinephrine and norepinephrine levels, increases in pulse rate and cholesterol levels, all of which may, in turn, contribute to increased blood pressure [51].

Table 2. Summary of studies on the effects of environmental noise exposure on blood pressure.

Author	Year	Country/Place	Study Type	Study Population	Methods	Main Findings
Green MS [56]	1991	Israel	Cross-sectional study	85 workers aged 25-44 and 77 workers aged 45-65 years	Ambulatory blood pressure and heart rate were monitored simultaneously with noise exposure in normotensive male industrial workers.	Industrial noise exposure is associated with higher ambulatory blood pressure and heart rates in men under 45 years old, but the effect on blood pressure appears to diminish considerably with age.
Lang T [59]	1992	Paris	Cross-sectional study	7901 participants	Noise was measured by the worksite physicians, and length of exposure was collected through interview	Blood pressure and the prevalence of hypertension increased for exposure of durations >25 years. This relationship was still significant after adjustment for age, body mass index and alcohol intake.
Lercher P [55]	1993	Austria	Cross-sectional study	174 participants	Effect on blood pressure of occupational noise annoyance and its combined effect with social support at work, nightshift work, and work satisfaction were assessed	In a multivariate analysis, the effect of noise annoyance alone was 2.1 (−3.0, 7.3) mmHg for systolic and 3.5 (0.3, 7.4) mmHg for diastolic blood pressure.

(Table 2) cont.....

Author	Year	Country/Place	Study Type	Study Population	Methods	Main Findings
Kristal-Boneh E [58]	1994	Israel	Cross-sectional study	3,105 blue-collar workers	Heart rate and blood pressure were measured in different workers at various times during the workday. Analysis was done after controlling for several possible confounders.	Although the resting heart rate was associated with noise intensity, no such associations were found for blood pressure in either sex.
Tomei F [57]	2000	Italy	Case control study	52 workers exposed to chronic noise and two control groups	Blood pressure was measured for each person in the supine and standing positions, and an electrocardiogram was also performed. Sound-level measurements were taken in the workplaces.	Mean systolic and diastolic blood pressures and diastolic blood pressure distributions were significantly higher in the noise-exposed group than in both control groups. Among the three groups, there were significantly different frequencies of hypertension, drops in blood pressure, and electrocardiogram anomalies.
Lusk SL [85]	2004	USA	Cross-sectional study	46 workers	Workers wore ambulatory blood pressure monitors and personal noise dosimeters during one work shift.	After adjustment for covariates of cardiovascular function, systolic and diastolic blood pressure, along with heart rate, were shown to be significantly positively associated with noise exposure.
van Kempen E [71]	2006	Netherland and England	Cross-sectional study	1283 children (age 9-11 years)	Data were pooled and analysed using multilevel modelling.	Aircraft noise exposure at home was related to a statistically significant increase in blood pressure.

(Table 2) cont.....

Author	Year	Country/Place	Study Type	Study Population	Methods	Main Findings
					Adjustments were made for a range of socioeconomic and lifestyle factors	Aircraft noise exposure at home was related to a statistically significant increase in blood pressure.
Aydin Y [70]	2007	Frankfurt	Prospective study	53 volunteers	Blood pressure and heart rate was monitored over a period of three months by using an automatic device with digitized readings. Subjective perception of noise and sleep quality were taken.	Those exposed to a nocturnal equivalent continuous air traffic noise level for three quarters of a given time had a higher average blood pressure compared to a population exposed to the same equal energy noise level for only one quarter of the time.
De Kluizenaar Y [65]	2007	Groningen City, Netherlands	Cross-sectional study	40856 participants	Cross-sectional analyses in a large random sample (N=40,856) of inhabitants of Groningen City, and in a subsample. Adjustment for confounders.	Before adjustment for confounders, road traffic noise exposure was associated with self-reported use of antihypertensive. Adjusted odds ratios were significant for those aged 45-55 years old in the full model when adjusted for PM10 and at higher exposure only.
Haralabidis AS [45]	2008	Greece	Prospective study	140 subjects living near airports	Non-invasive ambulatory BP measurements at 15 min intervals were performed. Noise was measured during the night sleeping period	An increase in blood pressure (6.2 mmHg (0.63-12) for systolic and 7.4 mmHg (3.1-12) for diastolic was observed

(Table 2) cont.....

Author	Year	Country/Place	Study Type	Study Population	Methods	Main Findings
					and recorded digitally for the identification of the source of a noise event.	over 15 min intervals in which an aircraft event occurred.
Jarup L [47]	2008	six major European airports	Cross-sectional study	4,861 persons 45-70 years of age	Blood pressure measurement with assessment of risk factors. Noise exposure assessed using detailed models	Significant exposure-response relationships was seen between night-time aircraft and average daily road traffic noise exposure and risk of hypertension after adjustment for major confounders. For night-time aircraft noise, a 10-dB increase in exposure was associated with an odds ratio of 1.14 [1.01-1.29].
Barregard L [48]	2009	Sweden	Cross-sectional study	1953 individuals	A-weighed 24 h average sound levels from road and railway traffic were calculated at each residential building using a geographical information system and a validated model.	When road traffic noise, age, sex, heredity and body mass index were included in logistic regression models, and allowing for >10 years of latency, the odds ratio for hypertension was 1.9 (1.1- 3.5) in the highest noise category and 3.8 (1.6 -9.0) in men.
Chang TY [44]	2009	China	Prospective study	60 adults aged 18-32 years	Individual noise exposure and personal blood pressure were measured simultaneously for 30 males	Total subjects had transient elevations of 1.15 mmHg systolic and 1.16mmHg diastolic blood pressure at daytime,

(Table 2) cont.....

Author	Year	Country/Place	Study Type	Study Population	Methods	Main Findings
				and 30 females. Linear mixed-effects regression models were applied to estimate effects.		as well as 0.74mmHg SBP and 0.77 mmHg diastolic blood pressure at night-time, significantly associated with a 5-dBA increase in noise exposure which persisted at the 30- and 60-min time-lagged noise exposure. Young females are more susceptible to noise exposure than males.
Singhal S [54]	2009	India	Case control study	114 workers exposed to noise and a control group	Workers employed in lock factories exposed to industrial noise levels exceeding 80 dB were compared with a control group consisted 30 people who never lived or worked in a noisy environment.	Significant increase in systolic blood pressure, diastolic blood pressure, mean arterial pressure, pulse pressure and heart rate in the workers of lock factories.
Eriksson C [74]	2010	Stockholm, Sweden	Prospective study	4721 subjects, aged 35-56 at baseline	The exposure assessment was performed by geographical information systems and based on residential history during the period of follow-up. Blood pressure was measured at baseline and at the end of follow-up after 8-10 years.	In the overall population, no increased risk for hypertension was found. Significant increase in blood pressure with noise exposure was seen in smoking men. In both sexes combined, an increased risk of hypertension related to aircraft noise exposure was seen among those reporting annoyance to aircraft noise.

(Table 2) cont.....

Author	Year	Country/Place	Study Type	Study Population	Methods	Main Findings
Bendokiene I [68]	2011	Lithuania	Cross-sectional study	3,121 pregnant women, 20-45 years old	Geographic information system was used to assess the average road noise at the current residential address were used. Effects on physician-diagnosed hypertension were estimated by logistic regression with adjustments confounders.	The prevalence of hypertension in lowest, medium and highest exposure category was 13.1%, 13.6% and 18.1% respectively. After making adjustments for confounders, no exposure effects were noted in the medium exposure category. However, a slight increase was noted in the highest exposure category (not statistically significant)
Sørensen M [66]	2011	Denmark	Cross-sectional analysis	57,053 participants aged 50-64 year	Residential long-term road traffic noise was estimated for 1- and 5-year periods preceding enrolment and preceding diagnosis of hypertension. Pre and post exposure assessment.	A 0.26 mm Hg higher systolic blood pressure per 10 dB increase in 1-year mean road traffic noise levels, with stronger associations in men and older participants. Road traffic noise was not associated with diastolic blood pressure or hypertension. Exposure to railway noise above 60 dB was associated with 8% higher risk for hypertension.

(Table 2) cont.....

Author	Year	Country/Place	Study Type	Study Population	Methods	Main Findings
Dratva J [84]	2012	Switzerland	Retrospective design	6,450 participants	Noise data were provided by the Federal Office for the Environment. Stratified analyses by self-reported hypertension, cardiovascular disease (CVD), and diabetes were performed.	Adjusted regression models yielded Significant positive association with increase in railway noise during the night with systolic and diastolic pressures and during day with systolic blood pressure.
van Kempen E [60]	2012	Multiple	Meta-analysis	24 observational studies	Meta-analysis of pooled data	Road traffic noise was positively and significantly associated with hypertension: odds ratio: 1.034 [95% CI: 1.011-1.056] per 5 dB increase of the 16 h average road traffic noise level.
Babisch W [64]	2014	Germany	Cross-sectional study	4,166 participants 25-74 years of age	Annual average $PM2.5$ at residential addresses were estimated by land-use regression.	Traffic noise and $PM2.5$ were both associated with a higher prevalence of hypertension. Mutually adjusted associations with hypertension were positive but no longer statistically significant
Foraster M [62]	2014	Spain	Cross-sectional study	1926 participants	Outdoor annual average levels of night-time traffic noise and NO_2 were estimated at postal addresses with a traffic noise model and land-use regression model.	Long-term exposure to indoor traffic noise was associated with prevalent hypertension and systolic blood pressure, independently of NO_2. Associations were less consistent for outdoor traffic.

(Table 2) cont.....

Author	Year	Country/Place	Study Type	Study Population	Methods	Main Findings
Fuks KB [69]	2014	Europe	Cross-sectional study	113,926 participants	Residential exposure to particulate matter and nitrogen oxides was modelled with land use regression using a uniform protocol.	Traffic load on major roads within 100 m of the residence was associated with increased systolic and diastolic BP in no medicated participants. Modelled air pollutants and BP were not clearly associated.
Ismaila SO [53]	2014	Nigeria	Prospective study	62 participants	The noise emitted by the machines was obtained using a digital sound level meter. The blood pressures (systolic and diastolic) were obtained using a digital sphygmomanometer.	Exposure to noise significantly increased systolic blood pressure but had no significant increase in the diastolic pressure of the workers.
Kalantary S [52]	2015	Iran	Case control study	26 cases exposed to noise and control group	Sound pressure level was measured at different units of the factory with a calibrated instrument. Risk factor assessment. Heart rate and blood pressure were measured serially.	Significant differences between the mean changes of heart rate, systolic and diastolic blood pressures of workers in the case and control groups
Kingsly SL [61]	2015	USA	Cross-sectional study	38,360 post-menopausal women	Using Cox proportional hazards models the residential proximity to major roadways and incident hypertension was analysed	After adjusting for confounders, the hazard ratios for incident hypertension were 1.13, 1.03, 1.05, and 1.05 for participants living ≤50, >50-200, >200-400, and >400-1000 m vs >1000 m from the nearest major roadway, respectively in selected regions.

(Table 2) cont.....

Author	Year	Country/Place	Study Type	Study Population	Methods	Main Findings
Schmidt F [82]	2015	Germany	Randomised trial	60 Patients were randomised to aircraft noise and no noise.	Noise was simulated in the patients' bedroom. Polygraphy was recorded, questionnaires and blood sampling were performed on the morning after each study night.	Significant positive association with noise and systolic blood pressure was found.
Evrard AS [73]	2016	France	Cross-sectional study	1244 participants older than 18 years of age	Information about health, socioeconomic and lifestyle factors were collected. Aircraft noise exposure was assessed for each participant's home address using noise maps.	After adjustment for confounders, an exposure-response relationship was evidenced between the risk of hypertension and aircraft noise exposure at night for men only
Pedersen M [67]	2017	Denmark	Retrospective study	72,745 singleton pregnancies	Birth Cohort with complete covariate data and residential address history from conception until live born birth was obtained. Noise exposure was modelled at all addresses. Outcome was derived from registries, hospital records, and questionnaires	A 10-μg/m^3 increase in NO$_2$ exposure and 10 dB higher road traffic noise was associated with increased risk of pre-eclampsia and pregnancy-induced hypertensive disorders.

Industrial Noise Exposure and Hypertension

Several studies have looked at the association between industrial noise exposure and hypertension [52 - 57]. A case-control study that analyzed the effect of noise exposure after eliminating known confounding factors, found a significant positive association of hypertension with high amplitude noise exposure [57]. However, one needs to remember that confounding factors associated with noise exposure may themselves contribute to hypertension. For instance, Lercher *et al.,* found that workers with increased noise exposure had significantly higher body mass index and alcohol consumption and did more night shifts, all factors that may independently contribute to raised blood pressure [55]. A large scale prospective study on 3106 employees in 21 Israeli industrial plants, did not find a clear relationship between noise exposure and either systolic or diastolic blood pressure, after following correction of confounding factors [58]. Another large study in 7,679 French workers, failed to show a significant association between blood pressure and noise exposure after adjusting for confounding factors such as age, body mass index, alcohol consumption and occupational category [59].

Road Traffic Noise Exposure and Hypertension

Chronic exposure to road traffic and/or railway or aircraft noise is known to increase blood pressure. Several studies have found adverse short-and long-term effects of noise on blood pressure [44]. A meta-analysis of 24 cross-sectional studies, found a 7% increase in the prevalence of hypertension for each 10dB increase in average traffic noise exposure [60]. Residing near roadways has been associated with raised blood pressure. Among more than 38,000 US women, residing within 50m of a major roadway was independently associated with a 13% higher incidence of hypertension [61]. An independent contribution of noise to increasing blood pressure has been supported by some but not all studies [62 - 64]. Considerable heterogeneity was noted among the studies, with respect to age, gender and study methodology and this may account for some of the conflicting findings. In the large HYENA study, road traffic noise was associated with hypertension in men but not in women [47]. Furthermore, in the Groningen study, road traffic noise was significantly associated with hypertension only in a subset of people aged between 45 and 55 years [65]. A large Danish cohort study in middle-aged subjects found a significant increase in systolic blood pressure for each 10dB increase in road traffic noise. This association was more significant in men and older subjects [66]. Similarly, a Spanish cohort study found road traffic noise to be significantly associated with systolic blood pressure [62]. In this study, indoor night-time noise levels were more consistently associated with systolic hypertension. A meta-analysis of 14 studies (n= 8,770 kindergarten and school children) found a relationship between road traffic noise and blood pressure [67]. A 5dB rise in road traffic noise at kindergarten/school was associated with a 0.48mmHg higher systolic blood pressure and a 0.22 mmHg higher diastolic blood pressure. One needs to be aware that these studies varied in the methodology used and most were cross-sectional. A prospective study that evaluated the association between road traffic/railway noise and hypertension found no association between chronic exposure to road traffic noise and hypertension but found a significant association with railway noise. The main limitation of this study was that hypertension was self-reported and thus may have been underestimated [66].

Several studies have analyzed the effect of noise exposure on pregnancy-induced hypertension. A large study of almost 77,000 Danish pregnant women found road traffic noise to be significantly associated with hypertension. A 10dB higher exposure to residential road traffic noise during the first trimester of pregnancy was associated with an increased risk of pre-eclampsia and pregnancy-induced hypertension. Adjusting for air pollution, slightly lowered the risk estimate [67]. A Lithuanian study on around 3,000 women, found a non- significant association between road traffic noise and gestational hypertension [68]. The concomitant exposure to air pollution (which is independently associated with hypertension), is a potential confounder in such studies [69].

Aircraft Noise Exposure and Hypertension

A relationship between aircraft noise and early-morning blood pressure was observed even within the physiological blood pressure range [70]. A prospective study was done in two groups of individuals near the Frankfurt airport exposed to night-time outdoor aircraft noise of 50 dB. One group was exposed for 75% and the other for 25% of the time and then followed up for three months. A statistically significant higher blood pressure (of 10/8 mm Hg) was seen in the group exposed for 75% of the time. The HYENA study, conducted in 4861 individuals residing near six major European airports for at least 5 years, found a dose-response association between night-time aircraft noise and prevalence of hypertension [47].

The RANCH study, conducted among 9-10-year-old children, reported an association between both daytime and nocturnal home noise exposure and blood pressure [71]. A meta-analysis of 4 cross-sectional and 1 cohort study examined the relationship between aircraft traffic noise and the prevalence of hypertension [72]. A significant association for each 10dB increase in day-night weighted noise level was seen [72]. This was further confirmed by a French study, in which a 10dB higher night-time aircraft noise was associated with a 34% higher prevalence of hypertension among men [73]. A large prospective cohort of around 5,000 individuals living around the Stockholm Arlanda airport found a 5dB increase in long-term exposure to aircraft noise was associated with an 8% increased risk for developing hypertension among men. Interestingly, the percentage rose to 21% after smokers were excluded. No association was found among women [74].

Pathophysiology of Noise Exposure Related Hypertension

Several animal studies have found noise to modify the function of multiple organs and systems. Following acute noise exposure, both hypertensive and normotensive rabbits show a significant increase in blood pressure and renal sympathetic nerve activity [75]. Furthermore, among borderline hypertensive rats, chronic noise exposure and a high sodium diet have an additive effect in increasing blood pressure [76]. Acute noise exposure, in both laboratory settings (where traffic noise was simulated) and in real-life working environments, can cause increases in blood pressure, heart rate, and cardiac output. Allostasis is the process of achieving homeostasis through physiological or behavioral change [77]. During environmental or physiological challenges, acute activation of the hypothalamic-pituitary-adrenal axis and sympathetic nervous system are important for achieving biological homeostasis. Although such mechanisms are useful for restoring homeostasis and thus increasing the chance of survival, repetitive exposure to stressful conditions may produce potentially harmful cardiovascular effects [78]. For example, chronic activation of the hypothalamic-pituitary-adrenal axis and the sympathetic nervous system may lead to endothelial dysfunction, hypertension and early atherosclerosis [77, 79]. Chronic noise exposure is perceived by the body as a stressful event and leads to increased cortisol and catecholamine levels [80]. Such stress hormones may produce both cardiovascular (rise in blood pressure, increases in heart rate and cardiac output) and metabolic (increases in blood lipids and glucose, activation of coagulation cascade) changes that lead to adverse cardiovascular events in the long run [81].

In one study, where nocturnal aircraft noise was played-back with loudspeakers in the participants' bedrooms, dose-dependent endothelial dysfunction (measured by flow-mediated dilation) was seen in both healthy subjects and those with established coronary artery disease [82, 83]. The decrease in endothelial function was associated with increased catecholamine production and poor sleep quality [83]. No habituation was seen in relation to noise and cardiovascular effects. Thus, chronic exposure to noise would continue to exert its harmful effects on the cardiovascular system. Nocturnal noise exposure has a more damaging effect on the cardiovascular system compared to day time noise exposure [45]. The previously mentioned HYENA study found no significant association of daytime noise with hypertension, but a 10dB increase in night-time noise exposure to be significantly associated with hypertension [47]. A similar study that analyzed the effect of railway noise, found blood pressure to be more strongly associated with night-time noise exposure [84]. Following night-time noise exposure, hormonal, inflammatory and autonomic pathways [46, 85, 86] get activated by both direct (noise induced stress) and indirect mechanisms (sleep fragmentation and deprivation) [87]. Repeated night-time autonomic arousal would impair the normal sustained decrease in blood pressure seen at night [88]. Such an effect is seen even if the individual is not aroused from sleep [44, 82, 89]. Importantly, both noise exposure and air pollution may coexist. Both are independent environmental factors in the causation of hypertension and share similar pathophysiological mechanisms (such as immune effects, endothelial dysfunction and dyslipidaemia) in relation to cardiovascular disease [90]. Recently, there has been increased awareness about the damaging effects of excess noise exposure.

Proper urban planning and local noise ordinances are some of the methods that may help in lessening this effect [91, 92]. Several other individual measures may be taken such as avoiding continuous exposure to high amplitude sounds and the use of personal noise protection devices. Further well designed studies would be needed to ascertain the true beneficial effect of such measures. Maximal noise intensity thresholds from a cardiovascular risk and blood pressure perspective need to be better defined. Measures should be taken within the community or at places of work, for controlling noise intensity and the long term noise exposure.

AIR POLLUTION-RELATED HYPERTENSION

Air pollution and hypertension are considered as major independent risk factors for premature mortality worldwide. The pattern of air pollution and its impact on global health has changed over the past few decades. The use of solid fossil fuels appears to be declining at household level. Although the impact of ambient matter pollution is decreasing in Western countries, an abrupt increase has been seen in low income countries [93]. Several mechanisms have been put forward about the pathophysiological basis of air pollution and hypertension, atherosclerosis, myocardial infarction, stroke, and heart failure. These include dysregulation of the autonomic nervous system and/or sympathoadrenal activation, accompanied by the release of pro-inflammatory mediators. These in turn lead to leucocyte activation, lipid modification, endothelial dysfunction due to oxidative stress and activation of prothrombotic pathways [90, 94]. Several epidemiological and analytical studies have reported the observed effects of short and long-term exposure to air pollution on blood pressure and other cardiovascular measurements (Table **3**). Exposure to air pollution was made using data from pollution monitoring stations, complex dispersion models or land use regression models [36, 95, 96]. Tackling the presence of confounding factors such as noise pollution that may be closely associated with air pollution was an important challenge in these studies.

Table 3. Summary of studies on the effects of air pollution on blood pressure.

Author	Year	Country/Place	Study Type	Study Population	Methods	Main Findings
Brook RD [131]	2002	USA	Randomized double-blind crossover study	Twenty-nine healthy adults randomised to concentrated ambient	High-resolution vascular ultrasonography was used to measure alterations in brachial artery diameter,	Exposure to PM plus ozone caused a significant brachial artery vasoconstriction compared with filtered air inhalation.

(Table 3) cont.....

Author	Year	Country/Place	Study Type	Study Population	Methods	Main Findings
				fine particulate matter (PM) and ozone versus filtered air	endothelial-dependent flow-mediated dilatation and endothelial-independent nitroglycerin-mediated dilatation.	There were no significant differences blood pressure responses between exposures.
Beelen R [127]	2008	Netherland	Prospective cohort study	120,852 subjects who were followed from 1987 to 1996	Exposure to black smoke, nitrogen dioxide, sulphur dioxide, and particulate matter, as well as various exposure variables related to traffic, were estimated at the home address	Relative risk for cardiovascular mortality was 1.22 (0.99-1.50).
Makris TK [119]	2009	Greece	Prospective study	254 participants	Echocardiography and routine biochemical profile assessment was performed, followed by ambulatory blood pressure monitoring.	Masked hypertension is associated with passive smoking in a dose-related manner and low physical activity, increased heart rate and postural haemodynamic reaction may represent potential accelerators of that phenomenon
Seki M [121]	2010	Japan	Cross-sectional study	Five hundred and seventy-nine non-smoking women	Variables were compared using analysis of covariance adjusted for age, marital status, body mass index, diabetes mellitus, stroke, heart disease, hyperlipidaemia, alcohol intake, salt intake and activity levels	A positive association between home blood pressure levels and environmental tobacco smoke exposure was confirmed
Guo Y [104]	2010	Beijing, China	Time-stratified case-crossover study	-	time-stratified case-crossover design was conducted to evaluate the relationship between urban gaseous air pollution and emergency hospital visits for hypertension	A 10 $\mu g/m^3$ increase in SO_2 and NO_2 were significantly associated with emergency hospital visits for hypertension.

(Table 3) cont.....

Author	Year	Country/Place	Study Type	Study Population	Methods	Main Findings
Yarlioglues M [120]	2010	Turkey	Prospective study	Thirty healthy non-smoker female	Serial measurements of cardiovascular parameters and risk factor assessment	Passive smoking has positive significant acute effect on heart rate and blood pressure in young healthy females
Fuks [96]	2011	Germany	Cross-sectional study	4,291 participants, 45-75 years of age	Urban background exposure to PM with aerodynamic diameter ≤ 2.5 µm (PM(2.5)) and ≤ 10 µm (PM(10)) was assessed with a dispersion and chemistry transport model	An interquartile increase in PM2.5 was associated with estimated increases in mean systolic and diastolic pressures of 1.4 mmHg and 0.9 mmHg respectively. The observed relationship was independent of long-term exposure to road traffic noise and robust to the inclusion of many potential confounders.
Coogan PF [95]	2012	Los Angeles, USA	Prospective cohort study	59,000 African-American women aged 21 - 69 years	Cox proportional hazards models to assess incidence rate ratios	Incidence rate ratios for hypertension for a 10 µg/m^3 increase in PM2.5 was 1.48 (95% CI 0.95-2.31).
Krishnan RM [133]	2012	USA	Prospective study	3,040 subjects included 50% female patients	Demographic characteristics, medical history, anthropometry, laboratory data, and brachial ultrasound measurements.	Women, non-smokers, younger participants, and those with hypertension seemed to show a greater association of PM2.5 with flow mediated dilation. Long-term PM (2.5) exposure was significantly

(Table 3) cont.....

Author	Year	Country/Place	Study Type	Study Population	Methods	Main Findings
						associated with decreased endothelial function according to brachial ultrasound results.
Foraster M [115]	2014	Spain	Prospective cohort study	3,700 participants, 35-83 years of age	Estimation of home outdoor annual average concentrations of nitrogen dioxide (NO_2) with a land-use regression model. Blood pressure measurement at baseline and after exposure.	A 10-μg/m^3 increase in NO_2 levels was associated with 1.34 mmHg higher systolic pressures in non-medicated individuals, after adjusting for transportation noise. Associations of NO_2 with systolic and diastolic pressures were stronger in participants with cardiovascular disease. The association with systolic pressures was stronger in those exposed to high traffic density and traffic noise levels $\geq$ 55 dB.
Liang R [100]	2014	Multiple	Systematic review and meta-analysis	22 studies	systematic review and meta-analysis of pooled data	Blood pressure was positively related to PM2.5 exposure. Long-term exposure showed the strongest associations with blood pressure. For short-term effect, the largest magnitude was seen at the lag of the previous 5 days average prior to measurement.

(Table 3) cont.....

Author	Year	Country/Place	Study Type	Study Population	Methods	Main Findings
Pedersen M [108]	2014	Multiple	Systematic review and meta-analysis	17 articles	systematic review and meta-analysis of pooled data	Meta-analyses showed increased risks of hypertensive disorders in pregnancy for all pollutants except CO.
Chen H [114]	2015	Ontario, Canada	Prospective cohort study	35 303 non-hypertensive adults	Estimates of long-term exposure to PM2.5 at participants' postal-code residences were derived from satellite observations. Cox proportional hazards models were used.	For every 10-$\mu g/m^3$ increase of PM2.5, the adjusted hazard ratio of incident hypertension was 1.13 (95% CI: 1.05-1.22). Estimated associations were comparable among all sensitivity analyses.
Brook RD [106]	2015	Edmonton and Calgary, Canada	Case-crossover study	6,532 patients	The associations were evaluated using a case-crossover design	Recent exposures to ambient levels of several air pollutants showed elevating blood pressure to a clinically significant extent and leads to emergency department visits for hypertension
Chen SY [114]	2015	Taipei City	Cross-sectional study	27,752 Taipei City residents > 65 years of age	Data obtained from a health examination program in 2009. Land-use regression models were used to estimate exposure to pollutants.	One-year exposures to PM10, PM2.5-10, PM2.5 absorbance, and NOx were associated with higher diastolic BP in elderly residents of Taipei. However, one-year air pollution exposures were not associated with hypertension by definition.

(Table 3) cont.....

Author	Year	Country/Place	Study Type	Study Population	Methods	Main Findings
Li N [125]	2015	Northern China	Cross-sectional study	392 non-smoking women	Data on female passive smoking, and other factors known to influence hypertension, were collected during face-to-face interviews.	118 participants (30.1%) reported exposure to passive smoking, of whom 88.4% were exposed to smoke in the home. After adjusting for possible confounders, passive smoking conferred an approximately two-fold risk increase of hypertension (adjusted odds ratio=1.99, 95% CI: 1.16-3.39).
Olsson D [110]	2015	Sweden	Retrospective study	100, 190 pregnancies	The pregnancy average nitrogen oxide, NOx, levels and annual mean daily vehicles at the home address were used as exposure variables	Strong association was noted between vehicle exhaust levels at the home address and pregnancy-induced hypertensive disorders, after adjustment for important risk factors.
Pope CA [112]	2015	North America	Retrospective study	669 046 participants	Cox proportional hazards regression models were used to estimate adjusted hazards ratios for death from CVD and cardiometabolic diseases based on death-certificate information. Modelled PM2.5 concentrations at geocoded home addresses were used.	Pollution-induced cardiovascular disease mortality risk is observed for those with and without existing cardiometabolic disorders. Deaths linked to hypertension and diabetes mellitus were also associated with PM2.5.

(Table 3) cont.....

Author	Year	Country/Place	Study Type	Study Population	Methods	Main Findings
Zhang H [116]	2015	Multiple	systematic review and meta-analysis	20 articles	systematic review and meta-analysis of pooled data	Significant associations were found between higher blood pressures and higher PM10 levels, but the association with PM2.5 levels was unclear.
Brook RD [98]	2015	Beijing, China	Prospective cohort study	65 non-smoking adults with metabolic syndrome and insulin resistance	Associations between prior 1-7 days exposures to particulate air pollutants with cardio-metabolic responses were studied.	Cumulative fine particulate matter exposure windows across the prior 1 to 7 days were significantly associated with systolic blood pressure elevations, whereas cumulative black carbon exposure during the previous 2 to 5 days were significantly associated with ranges in elevations in diastolic blood pressure.
Savitz DA [109]	2015	New York, USA	Retrospective study	268,601 births	Birth certificates in New York City in 2008-2010 to hospital discharge diagnoses were traced and estimated air pollution exposure based on maternal address was done.	After adjustment for individual covariates, no association was found between PM2.5 or NO_2 in the first or second trimester and any of the outcomes.
Byrd JB [132]	2016	USA	Randomized double-blind crossover study	Twenty-nine healthy adults randomised to concentrated	Cardiovascular outcomes were measured during,	Blood pressure levels were higher throughout coarse PM compared with filtered air exposures by mixed-model analyses.

(Table 3) cont.....

Author	Year	Country/Place	Study Type	Study Population	Methods	Main Findings
Byrd JB [132]	2016	USA	Randomized double-blind crossover study	ambient coarse particulate matter (PM) versus filtered air	immediately, and 2 hours after exposures.	Heart rate variability, endothelial function, and arterial compliance were not significantly affected.
Cai Y [117]	2016	Multiple	Systematic review and meta-analysis	17 studies	Systematic review and meta-analysis. A pooled odds ratio (OR) for hypertension in association with each 10 µg/m(3) increase in air pollutant was calculated by a random-effects model	Short-term exposure to SO_2 (OR=1.046), PM2.5 (OR=1.069) and PM10 (OR=1.024) and long-term exposure to NO_2 (OR=1.034) and PM10 (OR=1.054) had significant associations with hypertension.
Bao W-W [102]	2016	Multiple	Systematic review	5 studies	Systematic review of pooled data	Ambient PM was positively associated with hypertension (OR = 1.03; 95% CI: 0.99-1.06), but this was not statistically significant.
Lee WH [113]	2016	South Korea	Cross-sectional study	Community Health Survey conducted in 108 communities in 2008-2010	Data on pollutants were collected from the National Institute of Environmental Research. Distributed lag model with generalized estimating equations were used.	An association between the long-term exposure (5 years) to air pollutants (PM10, NO_2, and CO) and the regional prevalence of chronic cardiovascular disease (hypertension, stroke, myocardial infarction, and angina) was noted.

(Table 3) cont.....

Author	Year	Country/Place	Study Type	Study Population	Methods	Main Findings
Sohn J [107]	2016	Seoul, Korea	Retrospective time-series study	All emergency department visits from 2005 to 2009	The medical records within the 5 years of each acute coronary event were obtained from Health Insurance Review and Assessment Service. Generalised additive model was used.	Ambient PM10 is significantly associated with emergency department visits for coronary events, especially in males with hypertension, diabetes mellitus, or who are aged ≥ 80 years.
Chen CC [105]	2018	Taiwan	Case-crossover study	-	An odds ratio (OR) for number of hospital admissions for hypertension associated with each interquartile range increase in each gaseous air pollutant was calculated	Significant correlation was observed between number of hospital admissions for hypertension and ozone (O_3) levels both on warm and cool days, with OR of 1.2 and 1.2, respectively. No significant associations were found between levels of other gaseous (except ozone) pollutants and risk of hospital admissions for hypertension.

Short-Term Effects of Air Pollution

Fine particulate matter (that is less than 2.5 mm - PM2.5) is commonly produced as a by-product of fossil fuel combustion during power generation and in factories and vehicle traffic. Air pollution due to PM2.5 is a leading risk factor for cardiovascular morbidity and mortality [36, 97]. Numerous studies and a meta-analysis have found acute short-term exposure to air pollution to raise blood pressure (usually by 1-2 mm Hg per 10 mg/m^3) over a few hours to days [36, 97 - 100].

A more abrupt blood pressure raising effect (7.3/9.5 mm Hg per 10mg/m^3) has also been noted in a meta-analysis of a smaller number of studies [100]. The risk of cardiovascular related mortality increased by around 1% for each 10 mg/m^3

increase in PM2.5 [36]. A study of 2078 heart disease patients in Michigan, found typical daily variations of ambient PM2.5 within the previous few days to be independently associated with a significant rise in blood pressure [14]. More importantly, average PM2.5 levels were within the day-to-day United States National Ambient Air Quality Standards [36]. Extreme PM2.5 elevations detected in China were associated with both short-term and long-term elevations in blood pressure [98, 99].

A meta-analysis across 28 countries including a cumulative number of 6.2 million cardiovascular events across, showed a small but yet significant relationship between hospital admissions for stroke and mortality with an increase in PM2.5 levels in the preceding week. Furthermore, a similar association was also shown for levels of other air pollutants such as sulfur dioxide (SO_2), nitrogen dioxide (NO_2) and carbon monoxide (CO) [101]. Another systematic review of five studies showed a positively associated between ambient PM and hypertension, but this was not statistically significant [102]. Several randomized, double-blind, controlled exposures to PM2.5 and particulate matter of varying sizes have shown that even acute inhalation of such particles of varying sizes and sources were all capable of elevating blood pressure (2-10 mm Hg) over a few hours [97, 103].

Several studies have found elevated concentrations of air pollutants to be associated with an increase in hospital admissions, and emergency hospital visits for hypertension-related diseases. A study from Beijing, China found that an increase of $10\mu g/m^3$ in levels of SO_2 and NO_2 was associated with a significant increase in emergency hospital visits due to hypertensive disorders [104]. Another study from Taiwan found a similar association with ozone but not with the other gasses [105]. In 6,532 patients from Alberta, Canada, recent exposure to ambient levels of air pollutants increased blood pressure by clinically relevant amounts [106]. A time-series analysis was conducted in Seoul, Korea to look for an association between ambient PM10 air pollution and emergency department visits for cardiovascular disease and found an increased risk among those with hypertension [107]. A meta-analysis by Pedersen *et al* found evidence that pregnancy-induced hypertensive disorders were significantly associated with several parameters of air pollution [108], such as $5\mu g/m^3$ increment in PM2.5, 10-$\mu g/m^3$ increment in NO_2, and 10 $\mu g/m^3$ increment in PM10 [108]. In a large study of more than 100,000 participants from Stockholm, Sweden, there was a fairly strong association between vehicle exhaust levels close to residential areas and outcomes of pregnancy-induced hypertensive disorders. This was so even after adjustment for important confounding factors [109]. However, a more recent study from New York City, USA found that although there was a positive association between air pollutants and gestational hypertension, no significant associations were found between PM2.5 or NO_2 in the first or second trimester and any related outcomes after adjustment for individual confounding factors [110].

Long-term Effects of Air Pollution

Possible associations between long-term traffic-related air pollution and elevations in blood pressure have been studied [97]. More importantly, from a global perspective, this may occur even in a relatively clean environment [103]. A study from Canada that included more than 33,000 participants followed up over a period of 14 years, found a rise of PM2.5 levels by 10 mg/m^3 was associated with a 13% higher incidence of hypertension [111]. A similar finding was found with chronic traffic-related pollution among black women living in Los Angeles [95]. Furthermore, living in regions with higher PM2.5 in the United States of America was found to increase hypertension-related mortality over the long term [112].

Among 113,926 participants in the European Study of Cohorts for Air Pollution Effects (ESCAPE) study, the traffic load on major roads (within 100m of the residence) was associated with small but statistically significant elevations in systolic and diastolic blood pressure [69]. An analysis was done among 108 communities in South Korea from 2008-2010, found an association between long-term exposure to PM10, NO_2, and CO and the regional prevalence of cardiovascular diseases such as hypertension, stroke, and ischaemic heart disease [113]. There was a trend towards an increased prevalence of hypertension with higher concentrations of PM10. A similar association was also seen in participants younger than 30 years and may point to air pollution being a significant causative agent of hypertension even in younger individuals [113]. There have been some conflicting results among the elderly. For example, a study on elderly residents from Taipei found higher diastolic blood pressure to be associated with one-year exposures to PM10, PM2.5-10, PM2.5 but no significant association with the prevalence of hypertension [114].

Although evidence points to a strong positive association between air pollution and hypertension, this may still be due to confounding factors. For example, noise pollution is an important confounding factor associated with air pollution. Thus, some recent studies have investigated the independent effect of such factors in relation to hypertension. In the KORA study done in Germany, traffic noise and PM2.5 were both found to be associated with a higher prevalence of hypertension [64]. Even after adjusting for the noise pollution, a 1μg/m^3 increase in PM2.5 caused an increase in blood pressure [64]. In a population-based cohort study from Spain (included 3,700 participants, older than 35 years), there was a positive association between long-term exposure to NO_2 and systolic blood pressure after adjustment for transportation noise [115]. In individuals who were not under medication, a $10\mu g/m^3$ increase in NO_2 levels was associated with a 1.34 mmHg rise of systolic blood pressure. The association of NO_2 with systolic and diastolic blood pressures were stronger in those with cardiovascular disease. Furthermore, the association with systolic blood pressure was stronger in individuals exposed to high traffic density and traffic noise. This suggests a possible synergistic effect of noise and air pollution [115]. Several systematic reviews and meta-analyses have found evidence for an association of air pollution with hypertension. Zhang *et al* found a positive association between PM10 and both systolic and diastolic blood pressures; PM2.5 was only associated with systolic blood pressures [116]. In another analysis, short-term exposure to SO_2, PM2.5, and PM10 and long-term exposure to NO_2 and PM10 showed significant associations with hypertension [117]. The effects of short-term PM10 exposure was considerably lower than the equivalent long-term exposure, probably because only some of the effects due to long-term exposure were highlighted [118].

Other sources of air pollution, such as exposure to second-hand smoke from cigarettes, could also elevate blood pressure. Second-hand smoke increases the risk of raised home blood pressure readings [119 - 123] and long-term exposure to second-hand smoke also promotes the development of chronic hypertension [124, 125].

Pathophysiology of Air Pollution-Related Hypertension

The acute deleterious effects of air pollution on cardiovascular health are probably due to a number of factors. Studies have consistently found a significant association between environmental air concentrations and blood pressure elevations occurring within hours or days [9, 10]. Airborne particular matter with a diameter of less than 2.5 μm (PM2.5), are found to be the principal causative agent of cardiovascular morbidity and mortality [126 - 128].

Several biological pathways have been proposed for explaining the pathophysiological mechanisms involved in air pollution-related hypertension [36, 97]. The inhaled PM2.5 interacts with several pulmonary receptors such as transient receptor potential channels and free nerve endings and in turn initiate a number of nervous system reflex arcs. Such interactions lead to dysregulation of the autonomic nervous system. Simultaneously, fine particles deposited in the airways initiate an inflammatory response releasing a host of inflammatory mediators (cytokines, chemokines, and oxidized biological molecules). These inflammatory mediators and activated immune cells move into the systemic circulation, act on vascular endothelium and cause adverse cardiovascular effects. Some pro-oxidative inhaled particles such as nanoparticles, metals and organic compounds may also translocate directly into the systemic circulation and cause direct toxic effects. Arterial vasoconstriction and endothelial dysfunction caused by such processes may lead to an increase in blood pressure [36, 103].

Several experimental studies have found acute elevations in blood pressure and arterial stiffness following exposure to increased concentrations of PM2.5 [129 - 131]. In healthy adults, increased arterial blood pressure was noted following acute exposure to PM2.5 and PM10 [132]. Brachial ultrasound scan studies found chronic PM2.5 exposure to be significantly associated with decreased endothelial function [133]. Chronic exposure to out-door air pollutants may result in endothelial dysfunction and arterial stiffness. Endothelial dysfunction and arterial stiffness indicates early vascular aging and are closely linked with the pathogenesis of hypertension [134, 135]. Outdoor ozone concentrations were found to be positively associated with aortic stiffness in hypertensive women and may point towards increased susceptibility to air pollutants in hypertensive patients [136]. Moreover, long-term exposure to NO_2 and SO_2 were significantly linked to an increase in arterial stiffness [134].

Thus, endothelial dysfunction caused by direct and indirect effects (through oxidative stress, autonomic nervous system imbalance, activation of the hypothalamo-pituitary-adrenal axis, increase in pro-inflammatory mediators and prothrombotic pathways) may have a synergistic role in causing arterial stiffness and narrowing of major blood vessels. Increased peripheral vascular resistance could then lead to hypertension and other cardiovascular disorders [90, 137, 138].

Clinical Relevance of Air Pollution-Related Hypertension

Exposure to air pollutants may give rise to clinically relevant increases in blood pressure. Visits to the Emergency Department for hypertension and hypertension-related emergencies are found to be high on the days that follow high air-pollution [97, 106]. Increased mortality rates due to hypertension-related disorders are associated with chronic PM2.5 exposure [112]. Presently, the regulatory authorities in developed countries are able to implement effective strategies for reducing levels of air pollution, but this is not the case in low-income countries [93]. Some personal-level interventions may be helpful including wearing facemasks while out-doors or closing outside windows when residing in polluted cities or using in-home filtration systems [139]. Within a few months of implementing public smoking ordinances, decreased inhalation of second-hand smoke reduced the incidence of cardiovascular events by 10-20% [140].

High Altitude Related Hypertension

Higher altitudes are well-known to increase blood pressure. Short-term ascent to above 2500 m generally elicits a pressor response, but studies also suggest lower altitudes (1200 m) may cause a similar effect [141 - 143]. The rise in blood pressure may occur within a few days and is independent of the often simultaneous exposure to cold [141 - 146]. The extent of the associated hemodynamic changes may differ between different individuals and races [141, 143]. The rapidity of ascent has a positive association with elevated blood pressure and those who acclimatize gradually usually show smaller elevations in blood pressure [143]. When remaining at higher altitudes, the vascular pressor response may persist for weeks to months [142, 147, 148].

Some studies have assessed possible medical interventions for controlling blood pressure elevations at high altitude [149, 150]. Among 45 individuals climbing to a base camp in Mt. Everest, a gradual increase in systolic blood pressure (10-15 mm Hg) and plasma norepinephrine levels was seen whilst ascending from 3400 to 5400 m [149]. These hemodynamic responses were triggered acutely and continued throughout the study period. Treatment with angiotensin receptor blockade (ARB) was tried and only a mild blood pressure response that was not clinically relevant was seen. At 3400m, a decrease in blood pressure of 4 mm Hg was noted when compared with placebo, but no significant difference was seen at higher altitudes (5400 m) [149]. In another study that included 89 individuals with mild hypertension climbing 3260m in the Andes, a combination of an ARB and calcium channel blocker was not effective in reducing the high altitude related pressor response [150]. However, at all altitudes, those using combination-therapy, had significantly lower absolute blood pressures compared to placebo.

Although an acute rise in blood pressure is well reported, evidence on chronic hypertension due to high altitude is conflicting [145 - 147, 151] (Table **4**). This is likely due to the presence of several confounding factors such as concurrent exposure to cold, geographical variations and genetic, and lifestyle-related factors of the studied populations [151]. A meta-analysis of eight studies done in Tibetian individuals (n=516,913) living at 3000 to 4300 m above sea level, found a 100 m increase in altitude to be independently associated with a 2% increase in the prevalence of hypertension [148].

Table 4. Summary of studies in the effects of high altitude on blood pressure.

Author	Year	Country/Place	Study Type	Study Population	Methods	Main Findings
Hasler E [141]	1997	Kilimanjaro	Prospective study	Five white and four black people	Serial blood pressure measurements	Changes in systolic blood pressure and body weight during exposure to high

(Table 4) cont.....

Author	Year	Country/Place	Study Type	Study Population	Methods	Main Findings
						altitudes varied between whites and blacks. Diastolic blood pressure and heart rate remained constant. Fluid balance, acclimatisation, physical fitness or genetics could explain these findings.
Sizlan A [142]	2008	Turkey	Prospective cohort study	15 healthy, young, Turkish male subjects	Subjects were transported to a mountain hotel (altitude 1,860 m), where the measurements were repeated once every 15 days during a 10-month period.	Compared with control measurements, high altitude increased systolic blood pressure (SBP) in all subjects, but in Month 4 and Month 6, SBP returned to control values, and remained elevated thereafter
Faeh D [145]	2009	Switzerland	Prospective, census-based record linkage study	1.64 million German Swiss residents born in Switzerland	Mortality data from 1990 to 2000, sociodemographic information, (men and women between 40 and 84 years of age living at altitudes of 259 to 1960 m) were obtained and analysed	The protective effect of living at higher altitude on coronary heart disease and stroke mortality was consistent and became stronger after adjustment for potential confounders. This could be explained by factors related to climate.
[149]Parati G [149]	2014	Himalayas	Randomised Controlled clinical trial	47 healthy, normotensive lowlanders were randomized to	Conventional and Ambulatory blood pressures were measured at baseline and on treatment:	Ambulatory blood pressure increases progressively with increasing altitude, remaining elevated after 3 weeks.

(Table 4) cont.....

Author	Year	Country/Place	Study Type	Study Population	Methods	Main Findings
				placebo versus treatment group	after 8 weeks at sea level, and under acute exposure to 3400 and 5400 m altitude, the latter upon arrival and after 12 days.	An angiotensin receptor blockade maintains a mild blood pressure-lowering efficacy at 3400 m but not at 5400 m.
[150]Bilo G [150]	2015	Andes	Randomised Controlled clinical trial	89 subjects randomised to placebo versus drug treatment	Twenty-four-hour ambulatory blood pressure monitoring was performed off-treatment, after 6 weeks of treatment at sea level, on treatment during acute exposure to high altitude (3260 m) and immediately after return to sea level	24-hour blood pressure increases significantly during acute high-altitude exposure in both groups especially in hypertensive subjects. Treatment with angiotensin receptor blocker-calcium channel blocker combination is effective and safe in this condition.
Minji C [148]	2015	Tibet	Systematic review	22 eligible articles of which eight cross-sectional studies with a total of 16 913 participants	Systematic review and analysis of pooled data	A scatter plot of altitude against overall prevalence revealed a statistically significant correlation. Meta-regression analysis revealed a 2% increase in the prevalence of hypertension with every 100 m increase in altitude. The locations and socioeconomic status of subjects affected the awareness and subsequent treatment and control of hypertension.

Pathophysiology of High Altitude Related Hypertension

The most important biological pathway is likely to be hypoxia-induced (because of the lower partial pressure of oxygen at higher altitudes) activation of the chemoreflex at the level of the carotid body. This, in turn, would lead to augmentation of sympathetic outflow [143, 146, 147, 149, 150]. Other possible pathways include increased arterial stiffness, endothelin release, and heightened overall blood viscosity [143, 144].

Clinical Implications of High Altitude Related Hypertension

The current recommendations are based on expert opinion and include proper acclimatization and careful monitoring of BP during times spent at higher altitude [146, 152]. Individuals should be asked to monitor their BP during travel or seasonal relocation to higher altitudes (perhaps even at altitudes of 1200 m above sea level in at-risk patients) [149, 150]. Beta blockers and ARBs do not seem to prevent the BP-raising response. However, ARB plus calcium channel blocker therapy may provide some partial protection by lowering the absolute BP [149, 150]. The optimal medication regime and other management strategies to control high altitude-related BP elevations remain to be defined [143].

Other Environmental Factors-Related Hypertension

Several other environmental factors have been found to be associated with higher blood pressure levels. These include persistent exposure to organic pollutants, strong odors (*e.g.*, nearby hog farms), heavy metals (*i.e.*, lead, cadmium, arsenic), and chemicals used in plastics (*e.g.*, bisphenol A) and food wraps (*e.g.*, phthalates) [2, 153 - 167]. Residing at more extreme Northern or Southern latitudes and earthquake prone areas were also found to be associated with higher blood pressures [153, 154, 168] (Table 5).

Table 5. Summary of studies on the effects of other environmental factors on blood pressure.

Author	Year	Country/Place	Study Type	Study Population	Risk Factor Assessed	Methods	Main Findings
Sergeev AV [164]	2005	USA	Cross-sectional study	About 2.5 million hospital discharge records annually from 1993-2000	Persistent organic pollutants	Hospital discharge data were compared with areas with high exposure to persistent organic pollutants	In a subset of persistent organic pollutants-exposed areas the rate of hospitalization for coronary heart disease was 35.8% greater and for myocardial infarction 39.1% greater than in clean sites.

(Table 5) cont.....

Author	Year	Country/ Place	Study Type	Study Population	Risk Factor Assessed	Methods	Main Findings
Kang HK [165]	2006	Vietnam	Case control study	1,499 Vietnam veterans and a group of 1,428 non-Vietnam veterans	Dioxin (herbicide toxin)	Computer-assisted telephone interview system. Exposure to herbicides was assessed by analysing serum specimens from a sample of 897 veterans for dioxin. Logistic regression analyses.	Hypertension, OR=1.32 (1.08-1.61) significantly elevated among those Vietnam veterans who sprayed herbicides.
Wang SL [166]	2008	Taiwan	Retrospective analysis	1,054 Yucheng ("oil disease") victims	Persistent organic pollutants	examination of victims against neighbourhood reference subjects using a protocol blinded for persistent organic pollutants exposure	Yucheng women diagnosed with chloracne had adjusted ORs of 3.5 (1.7-7.2) for hypertension compared with those who were chloracne free.
Gallagher CM [160]	2010	Multiple	Systematic review and meta-analysis	12 studies	Blood and urine cadmium	Systematic review and calculation of pooled data.	A positive association between blood cadmium and blood pressure was noted among women. Associations between urine cadmium and hypertension suggest inverse relationships.
Abhyankar LN [159]	2012	Multiple countries	Systematic review	11 cross-sectional studies	Arsenic	Systematic review and calculation of pooled odds ratio	The pooled odds ratio for hypertension comparing the highest and lowest arsenic exposure categories was 1.27, p=0.001. An association between arsenic and the prevalence of hypertension was noted.

(Table 5) cont.....

Author	Year	Country/ Place	Study Type	Study Population	Risk Factor Assessed	Methods	Main Findings
Mozaffarian D [167]	2012	USA	Nested case-control studies in two separate prospective cohorts	6,045 US men and women free of hypertension	Blood mercury levels	Review of medical records and direct blood pressure measurement, and blood mercury levels	No clinically apparent adverse effects of methylmercury exposure on risk of hypertension in men or women were detected.
Wing S [158]	2013	North Carolina, USA	Prospective study	101 non-smoking adult volunteers	Hog odour	Baseline blood pressure measurement, reported levels of hog odour on a 9-point scale and measurement of blood pressure twice using an automated oscillometric device for 2 weeks	Reported stress was strongly associated with acute blood pressure increases and malodour was weekly associated. Adjustment for stress reduced the odour-blood pressure association
[163]Park SK [163]	2013	USA	Cross-sectional study	6607 adults aged 20 years or older	Blood and urine mercury	Medical examination and blood and urine mercury levels were measured	No association of hypertension with blood mercury was noted but a suggestive inverse association with urinary mercury was seen.
[155]Ranciere F [155]	2015	Multiple	Systematic review	Thirty-three studies with sample size ranging from 239 to 4811	Bisphenol A	Systematic review and meta-analysis	Evidence for a positive association between Bisphenol A concentrations and cardiovascular disease and hypertension was found in 4/5 and 2/3 of the cross-sectional studies, respectively. With a pooled odds ratio 1.41 (95% CI: 1.12-1.79) for hypertension.

(Table 5) cont.....

Author	Year	Country/ Place	Study Type	Study Population	Risk Factor Assessed	Methods	Main Findings
[156]Trasande L [156]	2015	USA	Cross-sectional study	1619 participants aged 6-19 years	Phthalate	Dietary quantification, and measurement of phthalate in urine sample, anthropometry and blood pressure measurements.	Phthalate were associated with higher age-, sex- and height-standardized blood pressure in univariate analysis. For each log unit increase in metabolites, a 0.105 standard deviation unit increase in systolic blood pressure z score was identified (P=0.004). However, multivariate analysis showed no significance.
[162]Lu Y [162]	2015	China	Cross-sectional study	1447 adults older than 20 years of ag	Blood lead levels	Participants underwent physical examinations in hospitals within a lead-polluted area of China from January to December 2013	Changes in both systolic and diastolic blood Pressure were associated with changes in blood lead level (P=.012, P=.001),This relationship was strongest among people 20-45 years of age. Young women's blood pressures were more affected.
[168]Ohira T [168]	2017	Japan	Prospective study	31 252 Japanese participants aged 40 to 74 years	Earth quake	Examined data collected from general health check-ups conducted in 13 communities following a major earth quake	Mean blood pressure significantly increased in both evacuees and non-evacuees after the disaster, with greater changes in blood pressure among the former.

(Table 5) cont.....

Author	Year	Country/ Place	Study Type	Study Population	Risk Factor Assessed	Methods	Main Findings
							For men, after adjustment for confounding variables, the hazard ratio slightly decreased to 1.20, but the association was essentially unchanged.

OVERALL CLINICAL IMPLICATIONS AND PREVENTIVE MEASURES

It is clear that several environmental factors have been found to affect blood pressure and other cardiovascular disorders. As some of these effects are clinically relevant, clinicians, patients with hypertension or cardiovascular disease and individuals at high risk for cardiovascular disease would need to be aware of these. Healthcare providers should advise their patients about the associated risks of different environmental exposures and how to mitigate their effects. In several instances, complete avoidance of such environmental factors may not be practical, but steps could be taken to reduce exposure or prevent prolonged exposure. Close attention to monitoring blood pressure during such exposures is necessary and in individuals with hypertension, treatment schedules may need adjustment to ensure more optimal blood pressure control.

CONSENT FOR PUBLICATION

Not applicable.

CONFLICT OF INTEREST

The authors declare no conflict of interest, financial or otherwise.

ACKNOWLEDGEMENT

Declare none.

REFERENCES

[1]   Foëx P, Sear J. Hypertension: pathophysiology and treatment. Contin Educ Anaesth Crit Care Pain 2004; 4: 71-5.
       [http://dx.doi.org/10.1093/bjaceaccp/mkh020]

[2]   Brook RD, Weder AB, Rajagopalan S. "Environmental hypertensionology" the effects of environmental factors on blood pressure in clinical practice and research. J Clin Hypertens

(Greenwich) 2011; 13(11): 836-42.
[http://dx.doi.org/10.1111/j.1751-7176.2011.00543.x] [PMID: 22051429]

[3]   Hänninen O, Knol AB, Jantunen M, *et al.* Environmental burden of disease in Europe: assessing nine risk factors in six countries. Environ Health Perspect 2014; 122(5): 439-46.
[http://dx.doi.org/10.1289/ehp.1206154] [PMID: 24584099]

[4]   Forouzanfar MH, Alexander L, Anderson HR, *et al.* Global, regional, and national comparative risk assessment of 79 behavioural, environmental and occupational, and metabolic risks or clusters of risks in 188 countries, 1990-2013: a systematic analysis for the Global Burden of Disease Study 2013. Lancet 2015; 386(10010): 2287-323.
[http://dx.doi.org/10.1016/S0140-6736(15)00128-2] [PMID: 26364544]

[5]   Analitis A, Katsouyanni K, Biggeri A, *et al.* Effects of cold weather on mortality: results from 15 European cities within the PHEWE project. Am J Epidemiol 2008; 168(12): 1397-408.
[http://dx.doi.org/10.1093/aje/kwn266] [PMID: 18952849]

[6]   Marti-Soler H, Gonseth S, Gubelmann C, *et al.* Seasonal variation of overall and cardiovascular mortality: a study in 19 countries from different geographic locations. PLoS One 2014; 9(11)e113500
[http://dx.doi.org/10.1371/journal.pone.0113500] [PMID: 25419711]

[7]   Danet S, Richard F, Montaye M, *et al.* Unhealthy effects of atmospheric temperature and pressure on the occurrence of myocardial infarction and coronary deaths. A 10-year survey: the Lille-World Health Organization MONICA project (Monitoring trends and determinants in cardiovascular disease). Circulation 1999; 100(1): E1-7.
[http://dx.doi.org/10.1161/01.CIR.100.1.e1] [PMID: 10393689]

[8]   Mercer JB. Cold-an underrated risk factor for health. Environ Res 2003; 92(1): 8-13.
[http://dx.doi.org/10.1016/S0013-9351(02)00009-9] [PMID: 12706750]

[9]   Yang L, Li L, Lewington S, *et al.* Outdoor temperature, blood pressure, and cardiovascular disease mortality among 23 000 individuals with diagnosed cardiovascular diseases from China. Eur Heart J 2015; 36(19): 1178-85.
[http://dx.doi.org/10.1093/eurheartj/ehv023] [PMID: 25690792]

[10]   Chen Q, Wang J, Tian J, *et al.* Association between ambient temperature and blood pressure and blood pressure regulators: 1831 hypertensive patients followed up for three years. PLoS One 2013; 8(12)e84522
[http://dx.doi.org/10.1371/journal.pone.0084522] [PMID: 24391962]

[11]   Konecny T, Kara T, Somers VK. Obstructive sleep apnea and hypertension: an update. Hypertension 2014; 63(2): 203-9.
[http://dx.doi.org/10.1161/HYPERTENSIONAHA.113.00613] [PMID: 24379177]

[12]   Fedecostante M, Barbatelli P, Guerra F, Espinosa E, Dessì-Fulgheri P, Sarzani R. Summer does not always mean lower: seasonality of 24 h, daytime, and night-time blood pressure. J Hypertens 2012; 30(7): 1392-8.
[http://dx.doi.org/10.1097/HJH.0b013e328354668a] [PMID: 22595956]

[13]   Modesti PA, Morabito M, Massetti L, *et al.* Seasonal blood pressure changes novelty and significance: An independent relationship with temperature and daylight hours. Hypertension 2013; 61: 908-14.
[http://dx.doi.org/10.1161/HYPERTENSIONAHA.111.00315] [PMID: 23381792]

[14]   Giorgini P, Rubenfire M, Das R, *et al* Particulate matter air pollution and ambient temperature: opposing effects on blood pressure in high-risk cardiac patients. J Hypertens 2015; 33(10): 2032-8.
[http://dx.doi.org/10.1097/HJH.0000000000000663] [PMID: 26203968]

[15]   Modesti PA, Morabito M, Bertolozzi I, *et al.* Weather-related changes in 24-hour blood pressure profile: effects of age and implications for hypertension management. Hypertension 2006; 47(2): 155-61.
[http://dx.doi.org/10.1161/01.HYP.0000199192.17126.d4] [PMID: 16380524]

[16]   Brook RD, Shin HH, Bard RL, *et al.* Can personal exposures to higher nighttime and early-morning temperatures increase blood pressure? J Clin Hypertens (Greenwich) 2011; 13(12): 881-8.
[http://dx.doi.org/10.1111/j.1751-7176.2011.00545.x] [PMID: 22142347]

[17]   Lewington S, Li L, Sherliker P, *et al.* Seasonal variation in blood pressure and its relationship with outdoor temperature in 10 diverse regions of China: the China Kadoorie Biobank. J Hypertens 2012; 30(7): 1383-91.
[http://dx.doi.org/10.1097/HJH.0b013e32835465b5] [PMID: 22688260]

[18]   Sun Z, Cade R, Morales C. Role of central angiotensin II receptors in cold-induced hypertension. Am J Hypertens 2002; 15(1 Pt 1): 85-92.
[http://dx.doi.org/10.1016/S0895-7061(01)02230-0] [PMID: 11824866]

[19]   Zeiher AM, Drexler H, Wollschlaeger H, Saurbier B, Just H. Coronary vasomotion in response to sympathetic stimulation in humans: importance of the functional integrity of the endothelium. J Am Coll Cardiol 1989; 14(5): 1181-90.
[http://dx.doi.org/10.1016/0735-1097(89)90414-2] [PMID: 2808971]

[20]   Cuspidi C, Ochoa JE, Parati G. Seasonal variations in blood pressure: a complex phenomenon. J Hypertens 2012; 30(7): 1315-20.
[http://dx.doi.org/10.1097/HJH.0b013e328355d7f9] [PMID: 22706390]

[21]   Keatinge WR, Coleshaw SR, Cotter F, Mattock M, Murphy M, Chelliah R. Increases in platelet and red cell counts, blood viscosity, and arterial pressure during mild surface cooling: factors in mortality from coronary and cerebral thrombosis in winter. Br Med J (Clin Res Ed) 1984; 289(6456): 1405-8.
[http://dx.doi.org/10.1136/bmj.289.6456.1405] [PMID: 6437575]

[22]   Backman C, Holm S, Linderholm H. Reaction to cold of patients with coronary insufficiency. Ups J Med Sci 1979; 84(2): 181-7.
[http://dx.doi.org/10.3109/03009737909179154] [PMID: 483494]

[23]   Minami J, Kawano Y, Ishimitsu T, Yoshimi H, Takishita S. Seasonal variations in office, home and 24 h ambulatory blood pressure in patients with essential hypertension. J Hypertens 1996; 14(12): 1421-5.
[http://dx.doi.org/10.1097/00004872-199612000-00006] [PMID: 8986924]

[24]   Woodhouse PR, Khaw K-T, Plummer M. Seasonal variation of blood pressure and its relationship to ambient temperature in an elderly population. J Hypertens 1993; 11(11): 1267-74.
[http://dx.doi.org/10.1097/00004872-199311000-00015] [PMID: 8301109]

[25]   Alpérovitch A, Lacombe J-M, Hanon O, *et al.* Relationship between blood pressure and outdoor temperature in a large sample of elderly individuals: the Three-City study. Arch Intern Med 2009; 169(1): 75-80.
[http://dx.doi.org/10.1001/archinternmed.2008.512] [PMID: 19139327]

[26]   Seals DR, Esler MD. Human ageing and the sympathoadrenal system. J Physiol 2000; 528(Pt 3): 407-17.
[http://dx.doi.org/10.1111/j.1469-7793.2000.00407.x] [PMID: 11060120]

[27]   Lindgren K, Hagelin E, Hansén N, Lind L. Baroreceptor sensitivity is impaired in elderly subjects with metabolic syndrome and insulin resistance. J Hypertens 2006; 24(1): 143-50.
[http://dx.doi.org/10.1097/01.hjh.0000198024.91976.c2] [PMID: 16331112]

[28]   Lindqvist PG, Epstein E, Nielsen K, Landin-Olsson M, Ingvar C, Olsson H. Avoidance of sun exposure as a risk factor for major causes of death: a competing risk analysis of the Melanoma in Southern Sweden cohort. J Intern Med 2016; 280(4): 375-87.
[http://dx.doi.org/10.1111/joim.12496] [PMID: 26992108]

[29]   Gavhed D, Mäkinen T, Holmér I, Rintamäki H. Face temperature and cardiorespiratory responses to wind in thermoneutral and cool subjects exposed to -10 degrees C. Eur J Appl Physiol 2000; 83(4 -5): 449-56.
[http://dx.doi.org/10.1007/s004210000262] [PMID: 11138588]

[30]   Bruno R, Taddei S. Tis bitter cold and I am sick at heart : A establishing the relationship between outdoor temperature, blood pressure, and cardiovascular mortality. Oxford University Press 2015.

[31]   Cassol CM, Martinez D, da Silva FABS, Fischer MK, Lenz MDCS, Bós ÂJG. Is sleep apnea a winter disease?: Meteorologic and sleep laboratory evidence collected over 1 decade. Chest 2012; 142(6): 1499-507.
[http://dx.doi.org/10.1378/chest.11-0493] [PMID: 22700779]

[32]   Ke L, Ho J, Feng J, *et al.* Modifiable risk factors including sunlight exposure and fish consumption are associated with risk of hypertension in a large representative population from Macau. J Steroid Biochem Mol, Bio 2014; 144 Pt A: 152-5.
[http://dx.doi.org/10.1016/j.jsbmb.2013.10.019]

[33]   Rostand Md SG, McClure LA, Kent ST, Judd SE, Gutiérrez Md OM. Associations of blood pressure, sunlight, and vitamin D in community-dwelling adults: The reasons for geographic and racial differences in stroke (regards) study. J Hypertens 2016; 34: 1704-10.
[http://dx.doi.org/10.1097/HJH.0000000000001018]

[34]   Weller RB. Sunlight has cardiovascular benefits independently of vitamin D. Blood Purif 2016; 41(1-3): 130-4.
[http://dx.doi.org/10.1159/000441266] [PMID: 26766556]

[35]   Charkoudian N. Mechanisms and modifiers of reflex induced cutaneous vasodilation and vasoconstriction in humans. J Appl Physiol 2010; 109(4): 1221-8.
[http://dx.doi.org/10.1152/japplphysiol.00298.2010] [PMID: 20448028]

[36]   Brook RD, Rajagopalan S, Pope CA III, *et al.* Particulate matter air pollution and cardiovascular disease: An update to the scientific statement from the American Heart Association. Circulation 2010; 121(21): 2331-78.
[http://dx.doi.org/10.1161/CIR.0b013e3181dbece1] [PMID: 20458016]

[37]   Somers VK, White DP, Amin R, *et al.* Sleep apnea and cardiovascular disease: An american heart association/american college of cardiology foundation scientific statement from the american heart association council for high blood pressure research professional education committee, council on clinical cardiology, stroke council, and council on cardiovascular nursing in collaboration with the national heart, lung, and blood institute national center on sleep disorders research (national institutes of health). Circulation 2008; 118(10): 1080-111.
[http://dx.doi.org/10.1161/CIRCULATIONAHA.107.189420] [PMID: 18725495]

[38]   Mente A, O'Donnell M, Rangarajan S, *et al.* Associations of urinary sodium excretion with cardiovascular events in individuals with and without hypertension: a pooled analysis of data from four studies. Lancet 2016; 388(10043): 465-75.
[http://dx.doi.org/10.1016/S0140-6736(16)30467-6] [PMID: 27216139]

[39]   Hamilton SL, Clemes SA, Griffiths PL. UK adults exhibit higher step counts in summer compared to winter months. Ann Hum Biol 2008; 35(2): 154-69.
[http://dx.doi.org/10.1080/03014460801908058] [PMID: 18428010]

[40]   Su D, Du H, Zhang X, *et al.* Season and outdoor temperature in relation to detection and control of hypertension in a large rural Chinese population. Int J Epidemiol 2014; 43(6): 1835-45.
[http://dx.doi.org/10.1093/ije/dyu158] [PMID: 25135908]

[41]   Handler J. Seasonal variability of blood pressure in California. J Clin Hypertens (Greenwich) 2011; 13(11): 856-60.
[http://dx.doi.org/10.1111/j.1751-7176.2011.00537.x] [PMID: 22051432]

[42]   Charach G, Rabinovich PD, Weintraub M. Seasonal changes in blood pressure and frequency of related complications in elderly Israeli patients with essential hypertension. Gerontology 2004; 50(5): 315-21.
[http://dx.doi.org/10.1159/000079130] [PMID: 15331861]

[43]   Madsen C, Nafstad P. Associations between environmental exposure and blood pressure among participants in the Oslo Health Study (HUBRO). Eur J Epidemiol 2006; 21(7): 485-91.
[http://dx.doi.org/10.1007/s10654-006-9025-x] [PMID: 16858621]

[44]   Münzel T, Gori T, Babisch W, Basner M. Cardiovascular effects of environmental noise exposure. Eur Heart J 2014; 35(13): 829-36.
[http://dx.doi.org/10.1093/eurheartj/ehu030] [PMID: 24616334]

[45]   Chang T-Y, Lai Y-A, Hsieh H-H, Lai J-S, Liu C-S. Effects of environmental noise exposure on ambulatory blood pressure in young adults. Environ Res 2009; 109(7): 900-5.
[http://dx.doi.org/10.1016/j.envres.2009.05.008] [PMID: 19559411]

[46]   Haralabidis AS, Dimakopoulou K, Vigna-Taglianti F, *et al.* Acute effects of night-time noise exposure on blood pressure in populations living near airports. Eur Heart J 2008; 29(5): 658-64.
[http://dx.doi.org/10.1093/eurheartj/ehn013] [PMID: 18270210]

[47]   Jarup L, Babisch W, Houthuijs D, *et al.* Hypertension and exposure to noise near airports: the HYENA study. Environ Health Perspect 2008; 116(3): 329-33.
[http://dx.doi.org/10.1289/ehp.10775] [PMID: 18335099]

[48]   Barregard L, Bonde E, Ohrström E. Risk of hypertension from exposure to road traffic noise in a population-based sample. Occup Environ Med 2009; 66(6): 410-5.
[http://dx.doi.org/10.1136/oem.2008.042804] [PMID: 19188199]

[49]   Davies HW, Vlaanderen JJ, Henderson SB, Brauer M. Correlation between co-exposures to noise and air pollution from traffic sources. Occup Environ Med 2009; 66(5): 347-50.
[http://dx.doi.org/10.1136/oem.2008.041764] [PMID: 19017692]

[50]   Andrén L, Hansson L, Björkman M, Jonsson A. Noise as a contributory factor in the development of elevated arterial pressure. A study of the mechanisms by which noise may raise blood pressure in man. Acta Med Scand 1980; 207(6): 493-8.
[PMID: 7424569]

[51]   Ortiz GA, Argüelles AE, Crespin HA, Villafañe CT, Villafañe CT. Modifications of epinephrine, norepinephrine, blood lipid fractions and the cardiovascular system produced by noise in an industrial medium. Horm Res 1974; 5(1): 57-64.
[http://dx.doi.org/10.1159/000178619] [PMID: 4810407]

[52]   Kalantary S, Dehghani A, Yekaninejad MS, Omidi L, Rahimzadeh M. The effects of occupational noise on blood pressure and heart rate of workers in an automotive parts industry. ARYA Atheroscler 2015; 11(4): 215-9.
[PMID: 26478728]

[53]   Ismaila SO, Odusote A. Noise exposure as a factor in the increase of blood pressure of workers in a sack manufacturing industry. Beni-Suef University Journal of Basic and Applied Sciences 2014; 3: 116-21.
[http://dx.doi.org/10.1016/j.bjbas.2014.05.004]

[54]   Singhal S, Yadav B, Hashmi S, Muzammil M. Effects of workplace noise on blood pressure and heart rate. Biomed Res 2009; 20(2): 122-6.

[55]   Lercher P, Hörtnagl J, Kofler WW. Work noise annoyance and blood pressure: combined effects with stressful working conditions. Int Arch Occup Environ Health 1993; 65(1): 23-8.
[http://dx.doi.org/10.1007/BF00586054] [PMID: 8354571]

[56]   Green MS, Schwartz K, Harari G, Najenson T. Industrial noise exposure and ambulatory blood pressure and heart rate. J Occup Med 1991; 33: 879-3.

[57]   Tomei F, Fantini S, Tomao E, Baccolo TP, Rosati MV. Hypertension and chronic exposure to noise. Arch Environ Health 2000; 55(5): 319-25.
[http://dx.doi.org/10.1080/00039890009604023] [PMID: 11063406]

[58]   Kristal-Boneh E, Melamed S, Harari G, Green MS. Acute and chronic effects of noise exposure on blood pressure and heart rate among industrial employees: the Cordis Study. Arch Environ Health 1995; 50(4): 298-304.
[http://dx.doi.org/10.1080/00039896.1995.9935958] [PMID: 7677430]

[59]   Lang T, Fouriaud C, Jacquinet-Salord MC. Length of occupational noise exposure and blood pressure. Int Arch Occup Environ Health 1992; 63(6): 369-72.
[http://dx.doi.org/10.1007/BF00386929] [PMID: 1544682]

[60]   van Kempen E, Babisch W. The quantitative relationship between road traffic noise and hypertension: a meta-analysis. J Hypertens 2012; 30(6): 1075-86.
[http://dx.doi.org/10.1097/HJH.0b013e328352ac54] [PMID: 22473017]

[61]   Kingsley SL, Eliot MN, Whitsel EA, *et al.* Residential proximity to major roadways and incident hypertension in post-menopausal women. Environ Res 2015; 142: 522-8.
[http://dx.doi.org/10.1016/j.envres.2015.08.002] [PMID: 26282224]

[62]   Foraster M, Künzli N, Aguilera I, *et al.* High blood pressure and long-term exposure to indoor noise and air pollution from road traffic. Environ Health Perspect 2014; 122(11): 1193-200.
[http://dx.doi.org/10.1289/ehp.1307156] [PMID: 25003348]

[63]   Stansfeld SA. Noise effects on health in the context of air pollution exposure. Int J Environ Res Public Health 2015; 12(10): 12735-60.
[http://dx.doi.org/10.3390/ijerph121012735] [PMID: 26473905]

[64]   Babisch W, Wolf K, Petz M, Heinrich J, Cyrys J, Peters A. Associations between traffic noise, particulate air pollution, hypertension, and isolated systolic hypertension in adults: the KORA study. Environ Health Perspect 2014; 122(5): 492-8.
[http://dx.doi.org/10.1289/ehp.1306981] [PMID: 24602804]

[65]   de Kluizenaar Y, Gansevoort RT, Miedema HM, de Jong PE. Hypertension and road traffic noise exposure. J Occup Environ Med 2007; 49(5): 484-92.
[http://dx.doi.org/10.1097/JOM.0b013e318058a9ff] [PMID: 17495691]

[66]   Sørensen M, Hvidberg M, Hoffmann B, *et al.* Exposure to road traffic and railway noise and associations with blood pressure and self-reported hypertension: a cohort study. Environ Health 2011; 10: 92.
[http://dx.doi.org/10.1186/1476-069X-10-92] [PMID: 22034939]

[67]   Pedersen M, Halldorsson TI, Olsen SF, *et al.* Impact of road traffic pollution on pre-eclampsia and pregnancy-induced hypertensive disorders. Epidemiology 2017; 28(1): 99-106.
[http://dx.doi.org/10.1097/EDE.0000000000000555] [PMID: 27648591]

[68]   Bendokiene I, Grazuleviciene R, Dedele A. Risk of hypertension related to road traffic noise among reproductive-age women. Noise Health 2011; 13(55): 371-7.
[http://dx.doi.org/10.4103/1463-1741.90288] [PMID: 22122952]

[69]   Fuks KB, Weinmayr G, Foraster M, *et al.* Arterial blood pressure and long-term exposure to traffic-related air pollution: an analysis in the European Study of Cohorts for Air Pollution Effects (ESCAPE). Environ Health Perspect 2014; 122(9): 896-905.
[http://dx.doi.org/10.1289/ehp.1307725] [PMID: 24835507]

[70]   Aydin Y, Kaltenbach M. Noise perception, heart rate and blood pressure in relation to aircraft noise in the vicinity of the Frankfurt airport. Clin Res Cardiol 2007; 96(6): 347-58.
[http://dx.doi.org/10.1007/s00392-007-0507-y] [PMID: 17393058]

[71]   van Kempen E, van Kamp I, Fischer P, *et al.* Noise exposure and children's blood pressure and heart rate: the RANCH project. Occup Environ Med 2006; 63(9): 632-9.
[http://dx.doi.org/10.1136/oem.2006.026831] [PMID: 16728500]

[72]   Babisch W, Kamp Iv. Exposure-response relationship of the association between aircraft noise and the risk of hypertension. Noise Health 2009; 11(44): 161-8.

[http://dx.doi.org/10.4103/1463-1741.53363] [PMID: 19602770]

[73]   Evrard A-S, Lefèvre M, Champelovier P, Lambert J, Laumon B. Does aircraft noise exposure increase the risk of hypertension in the population living near airports in France? Occupational & Environmental Medicine 2016. oemed-2016-103648.

[74]   Eriksson C, Bluhm G, Hilding A, Östenson C-G, Pershagen G. Aircraft noise and incidence of hypertension--gender specific effects. Environ Res 2010; 110(8): 764-72.
[http://dx.doi.org/10.1016/j.envres.2010.09.001] [PMID: 20880521]

[75]   Head GA, Burke SL. Sympathetic responses to stress and rilmenidine in 2K1C rabbits: evidence of enhanced nonvascular effector mechanism. Hypertension 2004; 43(3): 636-42.
[http://dx.doi.org/10.1161/01.HYP.0000116301.02975.aa] [PMID: 14744928]

[76]   Tucker DC, Hunt RA. Effects of long-term air jet noise and dietary sodium chloride in borderline hypertensive rats. Hypertension 1993; 22(4): 527-34.
[http://dx.doi.org/10.1161/01.HYP.22.4.527] [PMID: 8104890]

[77]   Brotman DJ, Golden SH, Wittstein IS. The cardiovascular toll of stress. Lancet 2007; 370(9592): 1089-100.
[http://dx.doi.org/10.1016/S0140-6736(07)61305-1] [PMID: 17822755]

[78]   McEwen BS. Physiology and neurobiology of stress and adaptation: central role of the brain. Physiol Rev 2007; 87(3): 873-904.
[http://dx.doi.org/10.1152/physrev.00041.2006] [PMID: 17615391]

[79]   Bruno RM, Ghiadoni L, Seravalle G, Dell'oro R, Taddei S, Grassi G. Sympathetic regulation of vascular function in health and disease. Front Physiol 2012; 3: 284.
[http://dx.doi.org/10.3389/fphys.2012.00284] [PMID: 22934037]

[80]   Selander J, Bluhm G, Theorell T, *et al.* Saliva cortisol and exposure to aircraft noise in six European countries. Environ Health Perspect 2009; 117(11): 1713-7.
[http://dx.doi.org/10.1289/ehp.0900933] [PMID: 20049122]

[81]   Lundberg U. Coping with stress: neuroendocrine reactions and implications for health. Noise Health 1999; 1(4): 67-74.
[PMID: 12689491]

[82]   Schmidt F, Kolle K, Kreuder K, *et al.* Nighttime aircraft noise impairs endothelial function and increases blood pressure in patients with or at high risk for coronary artery disease. Clin Res Cardiol 2015; 104(1): 23-30.
[http://dx.doi.org/10.1007/s00392-014-0751-x] [PMID: 25145323]

[83]   Schmidt FP, Basner M, Kröger G, *et al.* Effect of nighttime aircraft noise exposure on endothelial function and stress hormone release in healthy adults. Eur Heart J 2013; 34(45): 3508-14a.
[http://dx.doi.org/10.1093/eurheartj/eht269] [PMID: 23821397]

[84]   Dratva J, Phuleria HC, Foraster M, *et al.* Transportation noise and blood pressure in a population-based sample of adults. Environ Health Perspect 2012; 120(1): 50-5.
[http://dx.doi.org/10.1289/ehp.1103448] [PMID: 21885382]

[85]   Lusk SL, Gillespie B, Hagerty BM, Ziemba RA. Acute effects of noise on blood pressure and heart rate. Arch Environ Health 2004; 59(8): 392-9.
[http://dx.doi.org/10.3200/AEOH.59.8.392-399] [PMID: 16268115]

[86]   Björ B, Burström L, Karlsson M, Nilsson T, Näslund U, Wiklund U. Acute effects on heart rate variability when exposed to hand transmitted vibration and noise. Int Arch Occup Environ Health 2007; 81(2): 193-9.
[http://dx.doi.org/10.1007/s00420-007-0205-0] [PMID: 17541625]

[87]   Palagini L, Bruno RM, Gemignani A, Baglioni C, Ghiadoni L, Riemann D. Sleep loss and hypertension: a systematic review. Curr Pharm Des 2013; 19(13): 2409-19.
[http://dx.doi.org/10.2174/1381612811319130009] [PMID: 23173590]

[88]   Sayk F, Becker C, Teckentrup C, *et al.* To dip or not to dip: on the physiology of blood pressure decrease during nocturnal sleep in healthy humans. Hypertension 2007; 49(5): 1070-6.
[http://dx.doi.org/10.1161/HYPERTENSIONAHA.106.084343] [PMID: 17353512]

[89]   Akinseye OA, Williams SK, Seixas A, *et al.* Sleep as a mediator in the pathway linking environmental factors to hypertension: a review of the literature. International Journal of Hypertension 2015; 2015
[http://dx.doi.org/10.1155/2015/926414]

[90]   Münzel T, Sørensen M, Gori T, *et al.* Environmental stressors and cardio-metabolic disease: part II-mechanistic insights. Eur Heart J 2017; 38(8): 557-64.
[PMID: 27460891]

[91]   Hammer MS, Swinburn TK, Neitzel RL. Environmental noise pollution in the United States: developing an effective public health response. Environ Health Perspect 2014; 122(2): 115-9.
[http://dx.doi.org/10.1289/ehp.1307272] [PMID: 24311120]

[92]   Babisch W, Swart W, Houthuijs D, *et al.* Exposure modifiers of the relationships of transportation noise with high blood pressure and noise annoyance. J Acoust Soc Am 2012; 132(6): 3788-808.
[http://dx.doi.org/10.1121/1.4764881] [PMID: 23231109]

[93]   Global, regional, and national comparative risk assessment of 79 behavioural, environmental and occupational, and metabolic risks or clusters of risks, 1990-2015: a systematic analysis for the Global Burden of Disease Study 2015. Lancet 2016; 388(10053): 1659-724.
[http://dx.doi.org/10.1016/S0140-6736(16)31679-8] [PMID: 27733284]

[94]   Münzel T, Sørensen M, Gori T, *et al.* Environmental stressors and cardio-metabolic disease: part I-epidemiologic evidence supporting a role for noise and air pollution and effects of mitigation strategies. Eur Heart J 2017; 38(8): 550-6.
[PMID: 27460892]

[95]   Coogan PF, White LF, Jerrett M, *et al.* Air pollution and incidence of hypertension and diabetes mellitus in black women living in Los Angeles. Circulation 2012; 125(6): 767-72.
[http://dx.doi.org/10.1161/CIRCULATIONAHA.111.052753] [PMID: 22219348]

[96]   Fuks K, Moebus S, Hertel S, *et al.* Long-term urban particulate air pollution, traffic noise, and arterial blood pressure. Environ Health Perspect 2011; 119(12): 1706-11.
[http://dx.doi.org/10.1289/ehp.1103564] [PMID: 21827977]

[97]   Giorgini P, Di Giosia P, Grassi D, Rubenfire M, Brook RD, Ferri C. Air pollution exposure and blood pressure: an updated review of the literature. Curr Pharm Des 2016; 22(1): 28-51.
[http://dx.doi.org/10.2174/1381612822666151109111712] [PMID: 26548310]

[98]   Brook RD, Sun Z, Brook JR, *et al.* Extreme air pollution conditions adversely affect blood pressure and insulin resistance: the air pollution and cardiometabolic disease study. Hypertension 2015. HYPERTENSIONAHA. 115.06237.

[99]   Rich DQ, Kipen HM, Huang W, *et al.* Association between changes in air pollution levels during the Beijing Olympics and biomarkers of inflammation and thrombosis in healthy young adults. JAMA 2012; 307(19): 2068-78.
[http://dx.doi.org/10.1001/jama.2012.3488] [PMID: 22665106]

[100] Liang R, Zhang B, Zhao X, Ruan Y, Lian H, Fan Z. Effect of exposure to PM2.5 on blood pressure: a systematic review and meta-analysis. J Hypertens 2014; 32(11): 2130-40.
[http://dx.doi.org/10.1097/HJH.0000000000000342] [PMID: 25250520]

[101] Yang W-S, Wang X, Deng Q, Fan W-Y, Wang W-Y. An evidence-based appraisal of global association between air pollution and risk of stroke. Int J Cardiol 2014; 175(2): 307-13.
[http://dx.doi.org/10.1016/j.ijcard.2014.05.044] [PMID: 24866079]

[102] Bao W-W, Dong G-H. Ambient particulate matter air pollution exposure and hypertension.Update on Essential Hypertension. Rijeka: InTech 2016; pp. 103-11.
[http://dx.doi.org/10.5772/63923]

[103] Brook RD. The environment and blood pressure. Cardiol Clin 2017; 35(2): 213-21.
[http://dx.doi.org/10.1016/j.ccl.2016.12.003] [PMID: 28411895]

[104] Guo Y, Tong S, Li S, *et al.* Gaseous air pollution and emergency hospital visits for hypertension in Beijing, China: a time-stratified case-crossover study. Environ Health 2010; 9: 57.
[http://dx.doi.org/10.1186/1476-069X-9-57] [PMID: 20920362]

[105] Chen C-C, Yang C-Y. Association between gaseous air pollution and hospital admissions for hypertension in Taipei, Taiwan. J Toxicol Environ Health A 2018; 81(4): 53-9.
[http://dx.doi.org/10.1080/15287394.2017.1395573] [PMID: 29271700]

[106] Brook RD, Kousha T. Air pollution and emergency department visits for hypertension in Edmonton and Calgary, Canada: a case-crossover study. Am J Hypertens 2015; 28(9): 1121-6.
[http://dx.doi.org/10.1093/ajh/hpu302] [PMID: 25663064]

[107] Sohn J, You SC, Cho J, Choi YJ, Joung B, Kim C. Susceptibility to ambient particulate matter on emergency care utilization for ischemic heart disease in Seoul, Korea. Environ Sci Pollut Res Int 2016; 23(19): 19432-9.
[http://dx.doi.org/10.1007/s11356-016-7144-9] [PMID: 27380182]

[108] Pedersen M, Stayner L, Slama R, *et al.* Ambient air pollution and pregnancy-induced hypertensive disorders: a systematic review and meta-analysis. Hypertension 2014.
[http://dx.doi.org/10.1161/HYPERTENSIONAHA.114.03545]

[109] Olsson D, Mogren I, Eneroth K, Forsberg B. Traffic pollution at the home address and pregnancy outcomes in Stockholm, Sweden. BMJ Open 2015; 5(8)e007034
[http://dx.doi.org/10.1136/bmjopen-2014-007034] [PMID: 26275899]

[110] Savitz DA, Elston B, Bobb JF, *et al.* Ambient fine particulate matter, nitrogen dioxide, and hypertensive disorders of pregnancy in New York City. Epidemiology 2015; 26(5): 748-57.
[http://dx.doi.org/10.1097/EDE.0000000000000349] [PMID: 26237745]

[111] Chen H, Burnett RT, Kwong JC, *et al.* Spatial association between ambient fine particulate matter and incident hypertension. Circulation 2013. CIRCULATIONAHA. 113.003532.

[112] Pope CA, Turner MC, Burnett R, *et al.* Relationships between fine particulate air pollution, cardiometabolic disorders and cardiovascular mortality. Circulation research 2014. CIRCRESAHA. 114.305060.

[113] Lee WH, Choo J-Y, Son J-Y, Kim H. Association between long-term exposure to air pollutants and prevalence of cardiovascular disease in 108 South Korean communities in 2008-2010: A cross-sectional study. Sci Total Environ 2016; 565: 271-8.
[http://dx.doi.org/10.1016/j.scitotenv.2016.03.163] [PMID: 27177133]

[114] Chen S-Y, Wu C-F, Lee J-H, *et al.* Associations between long-term air pollutant exposures and blood pressure in elderly residents of Taipei city: a cross-sectional study. Environ Health Perspect 2015; 123(8): 779-84.
[http://dx.doi.org/10.1289/ehp.1408771] [PMID: 25793646]

[115] Foraster M, Basagaña X, Aguilera I, *et al.* Association of long-term exposure to traffic-related air pollution with blood pressure and hypertension in an adult population-based cohort in Spain (the REGICOR study). Environ Health Perspect 2014; 122(4): 404-11.
[http://dx.doi.org/10.1289/ehp.1306497] [PMID: 24531056]

[116] Zhang H, Qian J, Zhao H, *et al.* A study of the association between atmospheric particulate matter and blood pressure in the population. Blood Press 2016; 25(3): 169-76.
[http://dx.doi.org/10.3109/08037051.2015.1111019] [PMID: 26634767]

[117] Cai Y, Zhang B, Ke W, *et al.* Associations of short-term and long-term exposure to ambient air pollutants with hypertension: a systematic review and meta-analysis. Science of The Total Environment 2016; 565: 271-8.
[http://dx.doi.org/10.1161/HYPERTENSIONAHA.116.07218]

[118] Pope CA III. Mortality effects of longer term exposures to fine particulate air pollution: review of recent epidemiological evidence. Inhal Toxicol 2007; 19 (Suppl. 1): 33-8.
[http://dx.doi.org/10.1080/08958370701492961] [PMID: 17886048]

[119] Makris TK, Thomopoulos C, Papadopoulos DP, *et al.* Association of passive smoking with masked hypertension in clinically normotensive nonsmokers. Am J Hypertens 2009; 22(8): 853-9.
[http://dx.doi.org/10.1038/ajh.2009.92] [PMID: 19478792]

[120] Yarlioglues M, Kaya MG, Ardic I, *et al.* Acute effects of passive smoking on blood pressure and heart rate in healthy females. Blood Press Monit 2010; 15(5): 251-6.
[http://dx.doi.org/10.1097/MBP.0b013e32833e439f] [PMID: 20729727]

[121] Seki M, Inoue R, Ohkubo T, *et al.* Association of environmental tobacco smoke exposure with elevated home blood pressure in Japanese women: the Ohasama study. J Hypertens 2010; 28(9): 1814-20.
[http://dx.doi.org/10.1097/HJH.0b013e32833a3911] [PMID: 20453668]

[122] Heiss C, Amabile N, Lee AC, *et al.* Brief secondhand smoke exposure depresses endothelial progenitor cells activity and endothelial function: sustained vascular injury and blunted nitric oxide production. J Am Coll Cardiol 2008; 51(18): 1760-71.
[http://dx.doi.org/10.1016/j.jacc.2008.01.040] [PMID: 18452782]

[123] Bard RL, Dvonch JT, Kaciroti N, Lustig SA, Brook RD. Is acute high-dose second hand smoke exposure always harmful to microvascular function in healthy adults? Prev Cardiol 2010; 13(4): 175-9.
[http://dx.doi.org/10.1111/j.1751-7141.2010.00074.x] [PMID: 20860641]

[124] Alshaarawy O, Xiao J, Shankar A. Association of serum cotinine levels and hypertension in never smokers. Hypertension 2013; 61(2): 304-8.
[http://dx.doi.org/10.1161/HYPERTENSIONAHA.112.198218] [PMID: 23184382]

[125] Li N, Li Z, Chen S, Yang N, Ren A, Ye R. Effects of passive smoking on hypertension in rural Chinese nonsmoking women. J Hypertens 2015; 33(11): 2210-4.
[http://dx.doi.org/10.1097/HJH.0000000000000694] [PMID: 26259123]

[126] Pope CA III, Burnett RT, Thun MJ, *et al.* Lung cancer, cardiopulmonary mortality, and long-term exposure to fine particulate air pollution. JAMA 2002; 287(9): 1132-41.
[http://dx.doi.org/10.1001/jama.287.9.1132] [PMID: 11879110]

[127] Beelen R, Hoek G, van den Brandt PA, *et al.* Long-term effects of traffic-related air pollution on mortality in a Dutch cohort (NLCS-AIR study). Environ Health Perspect 2008; 116(2): 196-202.
[http://dx.doi.org/10.1289/ehp.10767] [PMID: 18288318]

[128] Laden F, Schwartz J, Speizer FE, Dockery DW. Reduction in fine particulate air pollution and mortality: Extended follow-up of the Harvard Six Cities study. Am J Respir Crit Care Med 2006; 173(6): 667-72.
[http://dx.doi.org/10.1164/rccm.200503-443OC] [PMID: 16424447]

[129] Lundbäck M, Mills NL, Lucking A, *et al.* Experimental exposure to diesel exhaust increases arterial stiffness in man. Part Fibre Toxicol 2009; 6: 7.
[http://dx.doi.org/10.1186/1743-8977-6-7] [PMID: 19284640]

[130] Mehta AJ, Zanobetti A, Koutrakis P, *et al.* Associations between short-term changes in air pollution and correlates of arterial stiffness: The Veterans Affairs Normative Aging Study, 2007-2011. Am J Epidemiol 2014; 179(?): 192-9.
[http://dx.doi.org/10.1093/aje/kwt271] [PMID: 24227017]

[131] Brook RD, Brook JR, Urch B, Vincent R, Rajagopalan S, Silverman F. Inhalation of fine particulate air pollution and ozone causes acute arterial vasoconstriction in healthy adults. Circulation 2002; 105(13): 1534-6.
[http://dx.doi.org/10.1161/01.CIR.0000013838.94747.64] [PMID: 11927516]

[132] Byrd JB, Morishita M, Bard RL, *et al.* Acute increase in blood pressure during inhalation of coarse

particulate matter air pollution from an urban location. J Am Soc Hyper 2016; 10: 133-9. e4.
[http://dx.doi.org/10.1016/j.jash.2015.11.015]

[133] Krishnan RM, Adar SD, Szpiro AA, *et al.* Vascular responses to long- and short-term exposure to fine particulate matter: MESA Air (Multi-Ethnic Study of Atherosclerosis and Air Pollution). J Am Coll Cardiol 2012; 60(21): 2158-66.
[http://dx.doi.org/10.1016/j.jacc.2012.08.973] [PMID: 23103035]

[134] Lenters V, Uiterwaal CS, Beelen R, *et al.* Long-term exposure to air pollution and vascular damage in young adults. Epidemiology 2010; 21(4): 512-20.
[http://dx.doi.org/10.1097/EDE.0b013e3181dec3a7] [PMID: 20407379]

[135] Mitchell GF. Arterial stiffness and hypertension. Hypertension 2014; 64(1): 13-8.
[http://dx.doi.org/10.1161/HYPERTENSIONAHA.114.00921] [PMID: 24752432]

[136] Di Pilla M, Bruno RM, Stea F, *et al.* Impact of seasonality and air pollutants on carotid-femoral pulse wave velocity and wave reflection in hypertensive patients. PLoS One 2017; 12(2)e0172550
[http://dx.doi.org/10.1371/journal.pone.0172550] [PMID: 28231259]

[137] Bruno RM, Penno G, Daniele G, *et al.* Type 2 diabetes mellitus worsens arterial stiffness in hypertensive patients through endothelial dysfunction. Diabetologia 2012; 55(6): 1847-55.
[http://dx.doi.org/10.1007/s00125-012-2517-1] [PMID: 22411135]

[138] Bruno RM, Di Pilla M, Ancona C, *et al.* Environmental factors and hypertension. Curr Pharm Des 2017; 23(22): 3239-46.
[http://dx.doi.org/10.2174/1381612823666170321162233] [PMID: 28356035]

[139] Morishita M, Thompson KC, Brook RD. Understanding air pollution and cardiovascular diseases: is it preventable? Curr Cardiovasc Risk Rep 2015; 9(6): 30.
[http://dx.doi.org/10.1007/s12170-015-0458-1] [PMID: 26097526]

[140] Jones MR, Barnoya J, Stranges S, Losonczy L, Navas-Acien A. Cardiovascular events following smoke-free legislations: an updated systematic review and meta-analysis. Curr Environ Health Rep 2014; 1(3): 239-49.
[http://dx.doi.org/10.1007/s40572-014-0020-1] [PMID: 25328861]

[141] Häsler E, Suter PM, Vetter W. Race specific altitude effects on blood pressure. J Hum Hypertens 1997; 11(7): 435-8.
[http://dx.doi.org/10.1038/sj.jhh.1000468] [PMID: 9283060]

[142] Sizlan A, Ogur R, Ozer M, Irmak MK. Blood pressure changes in young male subjects exposed to a median altitude. Clin Auton Res 2008; 18(2): 84-9.
[http://dx.doi.org/10.1007/s10286-008-0459-y] [PMID: 18363033]

[143] Handler J. Altitude-related hypertension. J Clin Hypertens (Greenwich) 2009; 11(3): 161-5.
[http://dx.doi.org/10.1111/j.1751-7176.2009.00083.x] [PMID: 19302431]

[144] Luks AM. Should travelers with hypertension adjust their medications when traveling to high altitude? High Alt Med Biol 2009; 10(1): 11-5.
[http://dx.doi.org/10.1089/ham.2008.1076] [PMID: 19278350]

[145] Faeh D, Gutzwiller F, Bopp M. Lower mortality from coronary heart disease and stroke at higher altitudes in Switzerland. Circulation 2009; 120(6): 495-501.
[http://dx.doi.org/10.1161/CIRCULATIONAHA.108.819250] [PMID: 19635973]

[146] Rimoldi SF, Sartori C, Seiler C, *et al.* High-altitude exposure in patients with cardiovascular disease: risk assessment and practical recommendations. Prog Cardiovasc Dis 2010; 52(6): 512-24.
[http://dx.doi.org/10.1016/j.pcad.2010.03.005] [PMID: 20417345]

[147] Dhar P, Sharma VK, Hota KB, *et al.* Autonomic cardiovascular responses in acclimatized lowlanders on prolonged stay at high altitude: a longitudinal follow up study. PLoS One 2014; 9(1)e84274
[http://dx.doi.org/10.1371/journal.pone.0084274] [PMID: 24404157]

[148] Mingji C, Onakpoya IJ, Perera R, Ward AM, Heneghan CJ. Relationship between altitude and the prevalence of hypertension in Tibet: a systematic review. Heart 2015; 101(13): 1054-60.
[http://dx.doi.org/10.1136/heartjnl-2014-307158] [PMID: 25953970]

[149] Parati G, Bilo G, Faini A, *et al.* Changes in 24 h ambulatory blood pressure and effects of angiotensin II receptor blockade during acute and prolonged high-altitude exposure: a randomized clinical trial. Eur Heart J 2014; 35(44): 3113-22.
[http://dx.doi.org/10.1093/eurheartj/ehu275] [PMID: 25161182]

[150] Bilo G, Villafuerte FC, Faini A, *et al.* Effects of living at higher altitudes on mortality: a narrative review. Aging & Disease 2015; 5: 274.

[151] Burtscher M. Effects of living at higher altitudes on mortality: a narrative review. Aging Dis 2013; 5(4): 274-80.
[PMID: 25110611]

[152] Bärtsch P, Swenson ER. Clinical practice: Acute high-altitude illnesses. N Engl J Med 2013; 368(24): 2294-302.
[http://dx.doi.org/10.1056/NEJMcp1214870] [PMID: 23758234]

[153] Young JH, Chang Y-PC, Kim JD-O, *et al.* Differential susceptibility to hypertension is due to selection during the out-of-Africa expansion. PLoS Genet 2005; 1(6)e82
[http://dx.doi.org/10.1371/journal.pgen.0010082] [PMID: 16429165]

[154] Rostand SG. Ultraviolet light may contribute to geographic and racial blood pressure differences. Hypertension 1997; 30(2 Pt 1): 150-6.
[http://dx.doi.org/10.1161/01.HYP.30.2.150] [PMID: 9260973]

[155] Rancière F, Lyons JG, Loh VH, *et al.* Bisphenol A and the risk of cardiometabolic disorders: a systematic review with meta-analysis of the epidemiological evidence. Environ Health 2015; 14: 46.
[http://dx.doi.org/10.1186/s12940-015-0036-5] [PMID: 26026606]

[156] Trasande L, Attina TM. Association of exposure to di-2-ethylhexylphthalate replacements with increased blood pressure in children and adolescents. Hypertension 2015; 66(2): 301-8.
[http://dx.doi.org/10.1161/HYPERTENSIONAHA.115.05603] [PMID: 26156503]

[157] Lind L, Lind PM. Can persistent organic pollutants and plastic-associated chemicals cause cardiovascular disease? J Intern Med 2012; 271(6): 537-53.
[http://dx.doi.org/10.1111/j.1365-2796.2012.02536.x] [PMID: 22372998]

[158] Wing S, Horton RA, Rose KM. Air pollution from industrial swine operations and blood pressure of neighboring residents. Environ Health Perspect 2013; 121(1): 92-6.
[http://dx.doi.org/10.1289/ehp.1205109] [PMID: 23111006]

[159] Abhyankar LN, Jones MR, Guallar E, Navas-Acien A. Arsenic exposure and hypertension: a systematic review. Environ Health Perspect 2012; 120(4): 494-500.
[http://dx.doi.org/10.1289/ehp.1103988] [PMID: 22138666]

[160] Gallagher CM, Meliker JR. Blood and urine cadmium, blood pressure, and hypertension: a systematic review and meta-analysis. Environ Health Perspect 2010; 118(12): 1676-84.
[http://dx.doi.org/10.1289/ehp.1002077] [PMID: 20716508]

[161] Solenkova NV, Newman JD, Berger JS, Thurston G, Hochman JS, Lamas GA. Metal pollutants and cardiovascular disease: mechanisms and consequences of exposure. Am Heart J 2014; 168(6): 812-22.
[http://dx.doi.org/10.1016/j.ahj.2014.07.007] [PMID: 25458643]

[162] Lu Y, Liu X, Deng Q, *et al.* Continuous lead exposure increases blood pressure but does not alter kidney function in adults 20-44 years of age in a lead-polluted region of China. Kidney Blood Press Res 2015; 40(3): 207-14.
[http://dx.doi.org/10.1159/000368496] [PMID: 25896505]

[163] Park SK, Lee S, Basu N, Franzblau A. Associations of blood and urinary mercury with hypertension in

U.S. adults: the NHANES 2003-2006. Environ Res 2013; 123: 25-32.
[http://dx.doi.org/10.1016/j.envres.2013.02.003] [PMID: 23472608]

[164] Sergeev AV, Carpenter DO. Hospitalization rates for coronary heart disease in relation to residence near areas contaminated with persistent organic pollutants and other pollutants. Environ Health Perspect 2005; 113(6): 756-61.
[http://dx.doi.org/10.1289/ehp.7595] [PMID: 15929900]

[165] Kang HK, Dalager NA, Needham LL, *et al.* Health status of Army Chemical Corps Vietnam veterans who sprayed defoliant in Vietnam. Am J Ind Med 2006; 49(11): 875-84.
[http://dx.doi.org/10.1002/ajim.20385] [PMID: 17006952]

[166] Wang SL, Tsai PC, Yang CY, Guo YL. Increased risk of diabetes and polychlorinated biphenyls and dioxins: a 24-year follow-up study of the Yucheng cohort. Diabetes Care 2008; 31(8): 1574-9.
[http://dx.doi.org/10.2337/dc07-2449] [PMID: 18487481]

[167] Mozaffarian D, Shi P, Morris JS, *et al.* Mercury exposure and risk of hypertension in US men and women in 2 prospective cohorts. Hypertension 2012; 60(3): 645-52.
[http://dx.doi.org/10.1161/HYPERTENSIONAHA.112.196154] [PMID: 22868395]

[168] Ohira T, Hosoya M, Yasumura S, *et al.* Evacuation and risk of hypertension after the great east Japan earthquake: The fukushima health management survey. Hypertension 2016; 68(3): 558-64.
[http://dx.doi.org/10.1161/HYPERTENSIONAHA.116.07499] [PMID: 27480836]

CHAPTER 2

Occupational Aspects of Hypertension

Umesh Jayarajah[1,3] and **Suranjith L. Seneviratne**[2,3,*]

[1] *Professorial Medical Unit, National Hospital of Sri Lanka, Colombo, Sri Lanka*

[2] *Institute of Immunity and Transplantation, Royal Free Hospital and University College London, London, UK*

[3] *Department of Surgery, Faculty of Medicine, University of Colombo, Sri Lanka*

Abstract: Occupational stress resulting from a combination of high work demands and low job decision latitude is linked with causation of hypertension in the modern society. Psychological and social factors related to occupation are known to interact with physical and genetic factors in disease pathogenesis and its manifestations. In this chapter, the possible association between job strain and blood pressure levels in various types of occupation and its importance in clinical practice have been critically analyzed. Several authors have attempted to arrive at some consensus on the relationship between occupational stress and hypertension and thus formulate potential therapeutic and preventive measures. Furthermore, this chapter summarises the current evidence-based knowledge on occupational aspects of hypertension according to different occupations. The psychosocial effects on hypertension and measures to reduce occupational stress have also been outlined.

Keywords: Blood pressure, Cardiovascular diseases, Decision latitude, Diastolic hypertension, Environmental factors, Healthcare workers, Heart disease, Hypertension, Job satisfaction, Job strain, Lifestyle, Occupational stress, Pathophysiology, Risk factors, Systolic hypertension, Teachers, Vehicle drivers, White-collar workers, Work demands, Work environment.

INTRODUCTION

There are many etiological factors for hypertension. Among them, psychological strain or stress is believed to be an important factor. Psychological and social factors are known to interact with physical and genetic factors in disease causation and its manifestations. Understanding such factors would help with the implementation of better treatment options. Psychological or social stress results from the interaction between environmental demands and controls. Stresses

* **Corresponding author Suranjith L. Seneviratne:** Institute of Immunity and Transplantation, Royal Free Hospital and University College London, London, UK; Tel: 00442078302141; E-mail: s.seneviratne@ucl.ac.uk

Hafize Uzun & Pınar Atukeren (Eds.)
All rights reserved-© 2019 Bentham Science Publishers

related to the daily routines of some occupations in the modern world continue to increase and are linked to the physical, mental, emotional, and social demands of the modern era. Certain occupations have a higher amount of the known environmental stressors [1 - 3]. Several studies have attempted to analyze the effects of occupation-related mental and physical strain on hypertension.

Evidence points to an association between occupational stain or stress and hypertension or other cardiovascular diseases. A combination of high work demands and low job decision latitude in the workplace has been linked with causation of hypertension. Job decision latitude refers to the extent to which a person is able to make decisions and exercise control over his work. The demands of the workplace are multifactorial and may be job or human-related factors. Job-related factors include work schedules (such as shift work or irregular hours, day or night shift work, rotating schedules etc.), time pressures, monotonous activities, the type of work (machine operation alone or involving human interaction), environmental conditions such as levels of lighting, heating and noise, sedentary or active tasks. Job-related factors may also include hierarchical status, decision-making authority and the degree of responsibility which in turn affects job satisfaction. Negative relationships with co-workers or superiors, including internal conflicts, unequal treatment, contradictory work demands, work overload or under stimulation may lead to occupation-related stress [3].

Job satisfaction is an important human-related factor influencing occupational stress. Other factors may include the organization of work routines, job security, levels of recognition and reward and pathways for promotion and career advancement. Personal factors such as self-esteem and the ability to cope positively with stressful situations may also play a role. Studies have found that an individual's perception that they lack control over the work that is done or that the work is stressful is a significant predictor of high blood pressure [1, 3, 4].

Variations of blood pressure in daily life may be influenced by factors referred to as cognitive processes [5]. Some of them are non-modifiable individual factors: gender, race, or ethnic group whilst others are modifiable and related to social or psychological characteristics such as job status, job security, marital status, coping mechanisms, anger expression and management, personality, lifestyle, socioeconomic factors, education level, and social support [3, 6 - 10]. The latter factors may also change with time.

Niedhammer *et al.*, suggested direct and indirect mechanisms for explaining the relationship between job strain and cardiovascular disease. The direct mechanisms, act through physiological variables such as increased blood pressure, raised serum cholesterol etc. and the indirect mechanisms through behavioral factors such as smoking and alcohol intake which in turn are sometimes influenced by the person's occupation [11].

Although most studies show some relationship between these factors with hypertension, a few did not [12 - 14]. This may partly be accounted for the different methodologies used. For example, different methods have been used for blood pressure measurement *e.g.* ambulatory, 24 hours, episodic or regular serial or during work time measurements. As blood pressure is a dynamic parameter, the method that is used would influence the findings. Job characteristics, another dynamic parameter is typically assessed only once. Furthermore, various types of questionnaires which differ in terms of complexity, content, length, applied or self-administered, different scales for measuring job stress, cross-country comparisons, cross-occupational differences, and choice of the study population have resulted in conflicting conclusions. Thus such, ambiguities may add to the complexity of the magnitude of the problem.

OBJECTIVES

Several authors have attempted to arrive at some form of consensus on the relationship between occupational stress and hypertension and thus formulate potential therapeutic and preventive measures. This chapter summarises the current evidence-based knowledge on occupational aspects of hypertension according to different occupations. The psychosocial effects on hypertension and measures to reduce occupational stress have also been outlined.

EFFECT OF JOB STRAIN ON HYPERTENSION AND ITS ASSOCIATED FACTORS

Occupational stress or job strain has complex interactions with hypertension and cardiovascular disease. Outside the home, the occupational setting is thought to be one of the most important environmental stressors in modern society [3]. Siegrist postulated that the effect of psychosocial stressors on cardiovascular disease was likely to parallel or even outweigh the contributions of more traditional occupational stressors such as physical or chemical hazards [15]. Although there is ample evidence for such interactions, any results should be interpreted with caution because of possible confounding by social factors, changes in gender roles and ethnic/cultural perspectives.

The effect that chronic stressors have depends on an individual's decision making and coping strategies. Primary environmental stressors interact with a person's psychological makeup to produce a perception of the levels of stress [1]. The magnitude of an individual's response is determined by the complex interaction of many factors including: the degree of arousal in the central nervous system, the ability to cope with the stressor, and the physiological susceptibility of the individual. These have been dubbed 'the three Ss': stressors (stimulus), stress (subjective element), and sickness (the physiological response) [16]. A similar relationship between job strain and blood pressure has been postulated via interactions between environmental stressors, psychological (personality/ susceptibility/previous experience) factors and physiological/biological factors [10]. Furthermore, interactions between environmental psychosocial stress, individual coping mechanisms and lifestyle-related factors such as obesity, alcohol consumption, and sodium and potassium intake and blood pressure levels have been described [9]. However, a meta-analysis of five US databases assessing the relationship between coronary heart disease risk factors and psychosocial dimensions of work did not show a strong association as was expected. This may be due to the use of casual rather than ambulatory blood pressure measurements in these studies [17]. Although the degree of job decision latitude was somewhat related to risk factors, the results were not consistent.

Siegrist's model described the importance of balancing effort versus reward. A lack of a balance between effort at work and rewards such as money, job promotion prospects, job security, and self-esteem may evoke negative stressful responses. Psychosocial experiences outside the work environment are also important. An individual's cumulative experiences at home and in the community during their lifespan could be described as part of the psychosocial analytical framework [15].

A link between job strain and hypertension has been reported in both women and men [18]. However, some authors such as Curtis *et al.*, found that job strain although more prevalent among women, was not predictive of high blood pressure. This may be because of confounding factors such as the use of casual rather than ambulatory BP monitoring [19]. Brisson *et al.*, found that among a group of white collar women with a university degree, family responsibilities combined with high job strain had a greater effect on blood pressure than either of these factors alone [20]. Goldstein studied ambulatory blood pressure, heart rate, and neuroendocrine responses in women nurses during work and off-work days and found increased activity of the cardiovascular and sympatho-adrenomedullary system in stressful work environments [21]. A woman's domestic role, length of employment and job demands were some of the modifiable contributory factors [21]. Radi *et al.,* found an association between job constraints and hypertension in both genders, although this was more significant among women [22]

Although female participation in the labour force has increased, a women's traditional responsibility in the home and the family has not changed accordingly [23]. Working mothers may have increased self-esteem compared to full-time homemakers, as they are not wholly dependent on their male partner. However, employment outside the home may impose several challenges and demands, causing role strain and fatigue. Adverse effects on blood pressure and other clinical parameters may result from conflicting responsibilities in relation to occupational prestige and personal income [13]. Analysis of the potential sources of domestic stress related to blood pressure found that married women had higher systolic blood pressure, whereas married women with children had higher systolic and diastolic blood pressures both at home and work [1]. Marital cohesion may interact with job strain in determining blood pressure. Even in subjects with job strain, greater marital cohesion was associated with lower systolic pressures [7].

Depression or exhaustion may be manifestations of occupational stress [13, 23]. Eaker *et al.,* found high demands to be potentially associated with high levels of stress irrespective of the level of control the person had [13]. Hierarchical status of the employee probably affects both the perception of stress and their ability to cope. Job strain may be influenced by lack of mutual support between co-workers, conflict with colleagues at a lower or higher hierarchical level and the degree of responsibility [24]. Furthermore, unfair treatment or insufficient reward may evoke stress among workers at lower hierarchical levels [25]. Middle managers with high effort and low rewards (active coping), were at a higher risk of developing hypertension compared to those with low rewards alone (passive coping) [26]. Occupations related to lower socioeconomic status are associated with an increased risk of hypertension [27].

HYPERTENSION AMONG DIFFERENT OCCUPATIONS

The nature and demands of occupations vary widely. Many studies have attempted to identify the relationship between occupation and hypertension. Some studies have analyzed specific occupation groups such as health care workers, white collar workers, transport vehicle drivers, teachers, blue collar workers, whilst others have taken a more global outlook. Studies analyzing the association of hypertension by occupation grouping are summarised in Table **1** [6, 11 - 13, 17, 19, 22, 25, 28 - 70]. Most have shown a significant association of job stain with hypertension and some of the linked risk factors include male gender, psychological stress, administrative type jobs, low decision latitude, sleep disturbance, job insecurity, and family background.

Hypertension in Healthcare Workers

Several studies (summarised in Table **2** [5, 14, 21, 71 - 75]) have found health care workers to have high levels of stress especially during the early stages of their careers. A cross-sectional study from Nigeria found a significant number of health workers to have work-related stress and perceived work stress was found to be significantly associated with a higher prevalence of hypertension [73]. Some of the main reasons for job strain in this group of workers include heavy workloads, demanding patient work, time pressures, and difficulties in balancing the work-home interface. The relative influence of these factors may vary depending on the healthcare workers gender, type of specialty and stage of career [71]. Rovik *et al.,* studied the level of stress related to work-home interference during the first nine years of a physicians' career. A lack of reduction in working hours and having several children predicted an increase in stress related to work-home interference. Neuroticism, conscientiousness, and lack of support from one's partner and colleagues appeared to be predictive of this stress [71]. A study among health care workers in the emergency room showed that both average blood pressure values and blood pressure load were significantly higher when the participants were on-call. Familial history of hypertension and professional status were the most important determinants of this response [72]. Several risk factors for hypertension have been identified among health care workers including male gender, older age, skin colour, family income, waist circumference, and body mass index [74, 75]. Medical residents working in stressful sub-specialties such as emergency medicine may lead to abnormal blood pressure behavior both during sleep and work [76]. On the other hand, a prospective study among female nurses showed no effect on the ambulatory blood pressure levels, heart rate, or heart rate variability with job strain or social support [14].

Hypertension in School Teachers and University Staff

Several studies have looked at aspects of hypertension and cardiovascular disease among school teachers and university staff (Table **3**) [77 - 82]. A case-control study on teachers from technical schools found an increase in mean systolic blood pressure in teachers older than 45 years. There was a significant difference in systolic blood pressure between the first and second halves of the fourth decade and a strong positive correlation between teachers' length of service and the level of blood pressure. Although this may be due to an increase in age, the increase of diastolic blood pressure with age was more pronounced among teachers than controls [78]. A prospective study among teachers found high job demand to be associated with higher systolic and diastolic blood pressures during the working day, after adjustment for confounding factors [79]. An association has been noted between arterial hypertension and overall health perception, service time and absenteeism [80]. Among a group of public university academics, working conditions influenced the development of illnesses including psychosomatic diseases and hypertension [81].

Table 1. Studies on job strain and hypertension related to different occupations.

Author	Year	Country/Place	Study Type	Study Population	Type of Occupation	Methods	Main Findings
Frommer MS [12]	1986	Australia	Prospective cohort study	4607 employees	Government employees	Age, occupation, body mass index, and level of perceived stress arising from financial problems were significantly associated with systolic blood pressure level.	However, The differences in systolic blood pressure among men from different occupational categories could not be explained by variation in the level of occupational stress.
						perceptions of work stress as ascertained in a questionnaire survey	
Mathews KA [34]	1987	Metropolitan Pittsburgh, USA	Prospective cohort study	241 male, ages 40–63 years, employed for a minimum of 10 years at	hourly workers	Questionnaire, Blood pressure was assessed by the random zero muddler method	Stressful work conditions as well as overall job dissatisfaction were significant predictors of diastolic blood pressure. Men with elevated diastolic blood pressure reported having little opportunity for promotion and for participating in decisions at work, an uncertain job future, unsupportive coworkers and foreman, difficulties communicating with others, and overall dissatisfaction with the job.

(Table 1) cont.....

Author	Year	Country/Place	Study Type	Study Population	Type of Occupation	Methods	Main Findings
Theorell T [42]	1988	Sweden	Prospective study	73 men and women ages 22–63 years	six different occupations (air traffic controllers, waiters, physicians, symphony orchestra musicians, baggage handlers, and airplane mechanics)	Blood pressure using sphygmomanometer, and questionnaire four times over 1 year.	Systolic blood pressure during work hours, as well as self-reported sleep disturbance, increased when demands increased in relation to decision latitude. Among subjects with a positive family history of hypertension the increase in systolic blood pressure at work was particularly pronounced, and among the men in this group a lower than expected level of morning cortisol was found measured during the period with the highest level of strain
Pieper C [17]	1989	USA	Meta-analysis of 5 data bases (NHANES I, II; National Health Examination Survey, Western Collaborative Group Study, and Exercise Heart Study) conducted during the period 1959–1980	12,555 men in five investigations	Wide range, non-specific	Casual blood pressure measurement. Using an imputation strategy, the authors attached measures of the two job characteristics above to persons in each data base by occupation while controlling for age, race, education, body mass index, and Type-A behaviour.	The main effects of job decision latitude were related to at least two risk factors; smoking and systolic blood pressure. Aspects of work, particularly decision latitude, were related to cardiovascular risk factors.

(Table 1) cont.....

Author	Year	Country/Place	Study Type	Study Population	Type of Occupation	Methods	Main Findings
Gold MR [69]	1989	New York, USA	Cross-sectional	633 people aged 16 years and older	Wide range, non-specific	Sociodemographic data, information about utilization of and barriers to health care and preventive services, cardiovascular risk factors, and blood pressure measurements	Compared to other workers, after adjustment for other independent variables, farmers had significantly lower mean blood pressure.
Chapman A [30]	1990	Sydney, Australia	Prospective study	2634 employees over five years (2100 men and 534 women)	government employees, administrators, professionals, technicians, clerks, skilled tradesmen, blue collar workers, tax investigators, tax future control, work and tax assessors	Perceived stress evaluated by questionnaire, and a principal component analysis produced six components: qualitative demands, quantitative demands, job control, future control, work support, and outside stress. Blood pressure measurement.	Only some components were associated with blood pressure change. Sex and age differences were observed. The observed interactions between job demands and control provided equivocal support for the Karasek job-strain model. The women responded to work-based support, but not necessarily as predicted.

(Table 1) cont......

Author	Year	Country/Place	Study Type	Study Population	Type of Occupation	Methods	Main Findings
Schlussel YR [41]	1990	New yolk, USA	Cross-sectional study	2616 men and 1648 women from seven worksites.	Employees of a newspaper typography department, a federal health agency, a stock brokerage, a liquor marketer, a private hospital, a sanitation collection and repair facility, and a department store warehouse (n= 259).	Descriptive study. Blood pressure using sphygmomanometer	Higher pressures were associated with worksite differences, male gender, lacking a high school education, having a clerical occupation, and being unmarried. Similar results for diastolic pressure suggest that researchers should consider worksite and job characteristics as important predictors of blood pressure differences in working populations
Schnall PL [51]	1990	New York, USA	Case control study	215 employed men ages 30–60 years (87 cases of hypertension and a random sample of 128 controls)	Employees at urban work sites	Ambulatory blood pressure at work site, ECG for left ventricular mass index, Karasek Job content questionnaire	Job strain was significantly related to hypertension. Job strain may be a risk factor for both hypertension and structural changes of the heart, as indicated by ventricular mass index, in working men.

(Table 1) cont.....

Author	Year	Country/Place	Study Type	Study Population	Type of Occupation	Methods	Main Findings
Landsbergis PA [47]	1994	USA	Cross-sectional study	Full-time male employees (n=262) at eight worksites	Not specified	Casual blood pressure screening, medical examinations, and questionnaires and an ambulatory blood pressure monitoring for 24 h on a workday.	All formulations of job strain exhibited significant associations with systolic pressure at work and home, but not with diastolic pressure. Adding organizational influence to the task-level decision latitude variable produced a stronger association for hypertension with job strain.
Carroll D [29]	1995	London, England	Prospective study	1003 male civil servants aged between 35 and 55 years	civil service departments	Blood pressure was recorded at a medical screening examination after which pressor reactions to a psychological stress task were determined. Follow up measurement of blood pressure: on average, 4.9 years later.	Reactions of systolic blood pressure to stress correlated positively with systolic blood pressure at follow up screening. Pressor reactions to psychological stress provide minimal independent prediction of blood pressure at follow up.
Light KC [49]	1995	USA	Prospective study	Study group included 72 men (40 white, 32 blacks) and 71 women (35 white, 326 blacks).	Working full time outside the home (not specified)	Ambulatory blood pressure monitoring followed by laboratory monitoring of blood pressure during resting baseline and reinstrumented with five behavioural stressors. Job status was assessed using standard classification	Women who were high-effort copers and had high status jobs had higher diastolic pressures at work and in the lab than other women. In men, low decision latitude was associated with hypertension. In women, low decision latitude was related to hyperlipidaemia

(Table 1) cont.....

Author	Year	Country/Place	Study Type	Study Population	Type of Occupation	Methods	Main Findings
Dryson EW [31]	1996	New Zealand	Cross-sectional study	A workforce of 5,467 European, Maori, Pacific Islander, and Asian employees age 40 years or older, working for 41 companies	Labourers, administrators, non-specific	A survey questionnaire giving details of total stressors and subcategories of stressors. Relative risks were calculated. Stress questionnaire and BP measurement.	Significant associations between increased stressors and male gender, young age, administrative group; and a negative association with Pacific Islander ethnicity were detected. These findings indicate areas in a workforce to which stress-reduction interventions can be directed.
Cesana G [45]	1996	Northern Italy	Cross-sectional study	635 employed normotensive or mild hypertensive subjects	Wide range, non-specific	Clinic details and 24 hour ambulatory blood pressure monitoring, Italian Mopsy questionnaire, a version of the Karasek scale	Among normotensive working men the highest mean for systolic blood pressure was found in the high-strain group in both the clinical and ambulatory measurements. Among the mild hypertensive subjects, lower mean values for ambulatory systolic and diastolic blood pressure were found in the passive and high job-strain categories.
Curtis AB [19]	1997	North Carolina, USA	Prospective cohort study	Community-based sample of 726 African-American adults. Ages 25–50.	Wide range, non-specific	Blood pressure measurement. Anthropometric, behavioural, demographic, and psychosocial data. Interview, Karasek questionnaire.	Job strain was not associated with blood pressure among men or women in this study. Job strain was more prevalent among women. The only significant outcome association for a group of men was relationship between decision latitude and hypertension prevalence.

(Table 1) cont......

Author	Year	Country/Place	Study Type	Study Population	Type of Occupation	Methods	Main Findings
Niedhammer I [11]	1998	France	Cross-sectional study	13,226 volunteers in a larger cohort who were currently working were analysed.	Employees from a company. Not specified	A questionnaire on psychosocial work factors in 1995. Cardiovascular risk factor assessment.	The potential effects of psychosocial work characteristics on cardiovascular risk factors were highlighted. The relationship is confirmed by direct mechanisms (through physiological variables) and indirect mechanisms (through behavioural risk factors) potentially involved in the relation between psychosocial work characteristics and cardiovascular disease
Peter R [38]	1998	Stockholm, Sweden	Cross sectional first screening of a prospective cohort study	4958 healthy employed men and women aged 19-70 years	Wide range, non-specific cardiovascular risk factors	Association between work stress and effort-reward imbalance and cardiovascular risk factors	Men with increased cardiovascular risk factors are more likely to suffer from high extrinsic effort and low status control. Women with increased cardiovascular risk factors were more likely to experience insufficient esteem by superiors and lack of reciprocal support.
Schnall PL [50]	1998	USA	Prospective study	Participants were 195 men, four groups: those not having job strain at either assessment (n=138), those having job strain at both times (n=15), and two crossover groups	Wide range, non-specific	Ambulatory blood pressures on two occasions 3 years apart. Job strain status, evaluated at each assessment.	The group repeatedly exposed to job strain had higher levels of blood pressure at the follow up assessment than either crossover group. Furthermore, change in job strain status partially predicted change in ambulatory blood pressure.

(Table 1) cont.....

Author	Year	Country/Place	Study Type	Study Population	Type of Occupation	Methods	Main Findings
Murata K [35]	1999	Japan	Prospective study	237 shift and 115 day workers without any obvious disorders	shift and day workers, not specified	Blood pressure, ECG, blood biochemistry. Shift/day work was compared to the corrected QT interval	Blood pressure, work duration, and biochemical data were comparable between the two working groups. The increased risk for cardiovascular mortality in shift workers may be attributable to prolongation of the corrected QT interval.
Peter R [39]	1999	Germany	Cross-sectional study	2288 male participants aged 30-55 years in the baseline screening of the Swedish WOLF study	Wide range, non-specific	Clinical examination and standardized questionnaire measuring shift work schedules, effort-reward imbalance at work, and health-adverse behaviour.	Stressful psychosocial work environment acts as a mediator of health-adverse effects of shift work on hypertension and, partly, atherogenic lipids.
Heath RL [68]	1999	Kentucky, USA	Cross-sectional study	998 males, aged 55 years and older	Farmers	self-reported hypertension and risk factors assessment though a telephone interview	Hypertension prevalence was 38%. Hypertensive older farmers were at increased risk for diabetes, stroke, arteriosclerosis, and heart attack. Logistic regression analysis identified increasing body mass index as a risk factor.
Theorell T [25]	2000	Sweden	Cross-sectional study	5720 working men and women ages 15–64. Participation rate 76%	Wide range, non-specific	The coping pattern was studied by means of a Swedish version of a self-administered questionnaire that was originally introduced by Harburg et al.	High scores for covert coping (highest quartile) were associated with an elevated prevalence ratio of hypertension among men. In women, there tended to be a relationship between low scores for open coping and hypertension.

(Table 1) cont.....

Author	Year	Country/Place	Study Type	Study Population	Type of Occupation	Methods	Main Findings
Tsutsumi A [43]	2001	Japan	Cross-sectional study	3187 men and 3400 women under 65 years of age	Wide range, non-specific	The association between job characteristics measured with Karasek questionnaire and the prevalence of hypertension were examined.	The findings provided limited proof that job strain is related to hypertension in Japanese working men. Older men in a lower social class may be more vulnerable to the hypertensive effects of job strain
Alfredsson L [28]	2002	Stockholm, Västernorrland, and Jämtland, Sweden	Prospective analytical	10,382 employed persons between ages 15 and 64	Wide range, non-specific	Medical examination. BP sphygmomanometer and questionnaire	The females, but not the males, with job strain had an increased prevalence of hypertension when compared with the subjects with relaxed psychosocial work characteristics. Occupational stress in the form of low decision latitude or job strain may have an adverse impact on HDL cholesterol in both males and females and on hypertension at least in females.
Landsbergis PA [48]	2002	New York, USA	Retrospective and prospective	1640 participants	Not specified	Retrospective compared with prospective. Psychosocial factors, ambulatory blood pressure monitoring and Job content Questionnaire	The work history questionnaire exhibited moderate validity for assessing past job characteristics, and the tool had a weak association with systolic pressures, and expected patterns of change over time.

(Table 1) cont.....

Author	Year	Country/Place	Study Type	Study Population	Type of Occupation	Methods	Main Findings
Landsbergis PA [66]	2003	New York, USA	Cross-sectional study	283 men (30-60 years)	work site employees	Job strain and ambulatory blood pressure, by level of education, occupational status, and income, and the interaction between job strain and these parameters were assessed.	Significant association between job strain and work ambulatory blood pressure was found among men with lower socioeconomic status. In the groups with high socioeconomic status, the association between job strain and ambulatory blood pressure at work was much smaller.
Eaker ED [13]	2004	Framingham USA	Prospective cohort study	Women (n= 1328) and men (n= 1711) who responded that they had been employed outside the home most of their adult years (18 years of age or older).	Wide range, non-specific	Psychosocial assessment forms. Questionnaire variables: job strain and job characteristics. Karasek questionnaire was used. The two outcomes of interest included 10- year total mortality and incident cardiovascular disease.	Findings did not support high job strain as a significant risk factor for heart disease or death in men or women over the follow up period.
Markovitz JH [33]	2004	Birmingham, Alabama; Chicago, Illinois; Minneapolis, Minnesota; and Oakland, California-USA	Prospective cohort study	A total of 3200 employed, initially normotensive participants, ages 20–32 in 1987–1988 were followed for 8 years	Wide range, non-specific	the Job Content Questionnaire was completed twice: initially and 8 years later; BP measurement	Job strain was associated with hypertension incidence for the entire cohort and among White women and men. The ratio of increasing demands relative to decreasing decision latitude was also associated with greater incidence of hypertension in the entire cohort in the multivariate model

(Table 1) cont.....

Author	Year	Country/Place	Study Type	Study Population	Type of Occupation	Methods	Main Findings
Steptoe A [52]	2004	UK	Prospective study	197 working men and women ages 45–59 years, recruited from the Whitehall II epidemiological cohort	Not specified	Ambulatory blood pressure monitoring. Effort-reward imbalance and over-commitment to work were assessed with standard questionnaires.	Over-commitment predicted systolic pressures over the day in men. Chronic neuroendocrine and cardiovascular activation may mediate in part the impact of over-commitment to work on cardiovascular disease risk in men.
Nomura K [36]	2005	Japan	Cross-sectional study	396 Japanese male workers, ages 24-39 years	Employees from an information service company	Cross-sectional Job content questionnaire. The job strain index was defined as the ratio of job demand to job control scores. Psychological responses were assessed by tension anxiety and anger-hostility scales in the Profile of Mood States.	The association between job stress and brachial pulse wave velocity was found to be inconsistent with the results of previous Western studies

(Table 1) cont.....

Author	Year	Country/Place	Study Type	Study Population	Type of Occupation	Methods	Main Findings
Radi S [22]	2005	France	A nested case control study was designed within the IHPAF cohort study.	203 subjects (142 men and 61 women) and 406 controls (284 men and 122 women) were included in the study. Mean age men: 41.8, women: 43.5.	Wide range, non-specific	Social Support Questionnaire for Transactions validated in French. Cardiovascular risk factors were also collected. The self-administrated questionnaire of Karasek was used. The cohort study was designed to assess the 1-year incidence of hypertension in a working population	Blood pressure and BMI were higher in the whole sample of men than in the sample of women. In this population of working men and women, an association between job constraints and hypertension in both genders were found. Results could suggest the role of job constraints as hypertension risk factors, particularly in women
Uchiyama S [44]	2005	Japan	Prospective cohort study	3877 participants aged 40–75	Wide range, non-specific	Karasek questionnaire and blood pressure measurement.	No significance found between long working hours and cardiovascular event. Job strain was significantly associated with risk of cardiovascular event. Active jobs and high strain jobs were associated with increased risk of cardiovascular event for treated hypertensive patients.

(Table 1) cont.....

Author	Year	Country/Place	Study Type	Study Population	Type of Occupation	Methods	Main Findings
Tobe SW [6]	2005	USA	Prospective study	248 male and female volunteers who were non-medicated, employed, and living with a significant other, all for a minimum of 6 months	Wide range, non-specific	Ambulatory blood pressure monitor and participants completed a diary that recorded time during work, spousal contact, and sleep. Job strain and marital cohesion were calculated from the Job Content Questionnaire and the Dyadic Adjustment Scale	Significant associations were found between 24-h systolic blood pressure. An interaction between 24-h systolic blood pressure, job strain, and marital cohesion was found such that greater marital cohesion was associated with lower systolic pressures in subjects with job strain.
Ducher M [32]	2006	France	Two prospective cohort studies	926 (age 41–46 years) healthy normotensive or newly diagnosed hypertensive subjects	Wide range, non-specific	Validated Questionnaire. Sitting blood pressure measurements were taken by work site physician during working hours.	Some evidence to suggest that development of systolic hypertension was significantly associated with high job strain. There was no global relationship between job strain and blood pressure levels. However, significant association between job strain and work site blood pressure in a subgroup of newly diagnosed hypertensive subjects exposed to high job strain

(Table 1) cont.....

Author	Year	Country/Place	Study Type	Study Population	Type of Occupation	Methods	Main Findings
Clays E [46]	2007	Belgium	Cross-sectional study	89 middle-age male and female workers subsample of the Belgian Job Stress Project (BELSTRESS) population	Not specified	Workers perceiving high job strain (measured by Job content questionnaire, Karasek) and an equally large group of workers perceiving no high job strain wore ambulatory blood pressure monitoring	Mean ambulatory blood pressure at work, at home, and while asleep was significantly higher in workers with job strain as compared with others. The associations between job strain and ambulatory blood pressure were independent from the covariates
Otsuka T [37]	2009	Kanagawa, Japan	Cross-sectional study	808 working men (mean age; 475 years)	Employees from a company. Not specified	Radial Augmentation index was measured using automated tonometry. Self-administered Brief Job Stress Questionnaire. High job strain was defined as the combination of high job demand and low job control	High job strain was significantly associated with an elevated radial augmentation index
Leigh JP [58]	2009	USA	Cross-sectional study	data from the 2004 Health and Retirement Survey, n = 3645 men and n = 3644 women (age 65+; age 70+; age 75+)	Wide range, non-specific	Hypertension was self-reported based on physician diagnosis and associations with risk factors and occupations were made.	In women, professionals, salespeople, private household cleaning service workers, and personal service workers and in men, salespersons, personal service workers, mechanics, construction trades, precisions production workers, and operators were significantly associated with hypertension.

(Table 1) cont.....

Author	Year	Country/Place	Study Type	Study Population	Type of Occupation	Methods	Main Findings
Alves MG [63]	2009	Brazil	Cross-sectional study	1,819 women who participated in the Estudo Pró-Saúde (Pro-Health Study)	Wide range, non-specific	The Brazilian version of the short version of the Job Stress Scale	The highest prevalence of arterial hypertension was found in the group with passive work (28.3%), followed by highly demanding work (24.8%). The group with the lowest prevalence was the one with low demands (20.9%). The risk for developing hypertension was 35% higher in women in passive work, when compared to women in jobs with low-demand.
Salavecz G [40]	2010	HAPIEE study (Poland, Russia, and the Czech Republic), the Hungarian Epidemiological Panel, the Heinz Nixdorf Recall study (Germany), and the Whitehall II study (UK).	Most were prospectively collected	overall sample consisted of 18,494 male and female workers ages 35–65 years	Wide range, non-specific	Epidemiological data from several centres were pooled and analysed.	The association of effort-reward imbalance at work and of a high degree of work related over commitment with poor self-rated health was seen in all countries, but the size of the effects differed considerably. The effects in Eastern Europe do not seem to be systematically stronger than in the West
Butrón J [62]	2010	Venezuela	Case control study	Fifty working men as cases and controls	workers exposed to a noise level higher than 85 dB	information was obtained from the occupational clinical history, based on international guidelines	There was no significant result between occupational noise-induced hearing loss, its intensity and working time with the prevalence of arterial hypertension in workers of an oil company.

(Table 1) cont.....

Author	Year	Country/Place	Study Type	Study Population	Type of Occupation	Methods	Main Findings
Schumann B [53]	2011	East Germany	Cross-sectional study	967 men and 808 women aged 45-83	Wide range, non-specific	Types of occupations were classified using the German classification of occupation and the associations with blood pressure was determined.	In men, hypertension was more prevalent in metal-processing workers, carpenters/painters, and electricians, compared to office clerks. In women, highest prevalence risk ratio was found in technicians/forewomen, scrutinisers/storekeepers, and food-processing occupations. Adjustment for education, smoking, body mass index, and current work hours did not fully explain occupational differences.
Djindjic N [55]	2012	Nis, Serbia	Cross-sectional study	989 middle-aged men and women	Wide range, non-specific	associations between aspects of the occupational stress index and arterial hypertension, diabetes mellitus (DM) type 2, and lipid disorders were analysed	High Demand, Conflict/Uncertainty, and Extrinsic Time Pressure were associated significantly with arterial hypertension in male workers. Noxious Exposures associated positively with DM and arterial hypertension in women.
Davila EP [56]	2012	Atlanta	Cross-sectional study	1999–2004 National Health and Nutrition Examination Survey data of 6928 workers aged 20 years or older	Wide range, non-specific	Types of occupations were compared with prevalence of hypertension awareness, treatment and control	Protective service workers ranked among the lowest in awareness, treatment, and control and had lower odds of hypertension control and treatment compared with executive/administrative/managerial workers; adjusting for sociodemographic, body-weight, smoking, and alcohol

(Table 1) cont.....

Author	Year	Country/Place	Study Type	Study Population	Type of Occupation	Methods	Main Findings
Miklos WE [54]	2013	Washington, USA	Cross-sectional study	Behavioral Risk Factors Surveillance System (BRFSS) survey data for 2003, 2005, 2007, and 2009	Wide range, non-specific	Types of occupations were compared with prevalence of hypertension awareness	Occupation has important associations with hypertension awareness.
Maksimov SA [57]	2013	Siberia	Cross-sectional study	3664 employees	employees in industrial enterprises and office workers	Occupations were classified into groups, blood pressure measurements takes and Quetlet index, risk factors assessed.	Quetlet index, age and occupation are highly significant for hypertension prediction in working age population. Occupation is very significant for hypertension prediction in middle-aged patients.
Wiernik E [59]	2013	Paris, France	Cross-sectional study	122 816 adults (84 994 men), aged ≥ 30 years	Wide range, non-specific	Blood pressure measurement, 4-item perceived stress scale and other confounding factors were documented.	After adjustment for all variables except occupational status, perceived stress was associated with high blood pressure. This association was no longer significant after additional adjustment for occupational status. The association between current perceived stress and blood pressure depends on occupational status.

(Table 1) cont.....

Author	Year	Country/Place	Study Type	Study Population	Type of Occupation	Methods	Main Findings
Kaur H [64]	2013	Cincinnati, USA	Cross-sectional study	17,494 adults	Wide range, non-specific	Data from the 2010 National Health Interview Survey, which included an occupational health supplement, were used to examine relationships between the prevalence of self-reported hypertension and job strain	Job insecurity and hostile work environment were found to be significantly associated with hypertension. Employees in Healthcare support occupations, Public administration industries, and Healthcare and social assistance industries were more associated with hypertension
Landsbergis PA [61]	2015	USA	Prospective study	2,517 Multi-Ethnic Study of Atherosclerosis (MESA) participants	working 20+ hours per week, non-specific	Associations were determined while eliminating the confounding factors	Lower job decision latitude is associated with hypertension prevalence in many occupations. However, associations differed by occupation: decision latitude was associated with a higher prevalence of hypertension in healthcare support occupations
Bosu WK [67]	2016	West Africa	A review article	55 articles involving 34,919 different cadres of workers from six countries	Wide range, non-specific	Review	The major determinants of mean BP and hypertension were similar and included male sex, older age group, higher socioeconomic status, obesity, alcohol consumption, plasma glucose, and sodium excretion. Ethnicity and educational level were inconsistently associated with hypertension.

(Table 1) cont.....

Author	Year	Country/Place	Study Type	Study Population	Type of Occupation	Methods	Main Findings
Lim MS [60]	2017	Korea	Cross-sectional study	240,086 participants assessed in 2011 and 2013 from the Korean Community Health Survey	Wide range, categorised	The association between leisure sedentary time on weekdays and hypertension/diabetes mellitus/hyperlipidaemia for different occupations was analysed using simple and multiple logistic regression analyses with complex sampling	The unemployed are more susceptible than other occupation groups to cardio-metabolic diseases when leisure time is sedentary
Vinholes DB [65]	2017	Brazil	multilevel analysis based on a Cross-sectional study	4818 Workers from 157 companies	Industrial workers	Blood pressure measurement, risk factor assessment, anthropometry	besides individual risk factors, being male, ageing, low schooling, alcohol abuse and higher BMI, small companies, urban setting, higher economic inequality were more associated with hypertension
Singh M [70]	2017	Southern India	Cross-sectional study	16,636 individuals (62.3% females and 37.7% males) above 15 years of age	Wide range, non-specific	door-to-door survey was conducted using modified WHO STEPS questionnaire	Farmers had significantly lower incidence of hypertension

Table 2. Hypertension and its associated factors in healthcare workers.

Author	Year	Country/Place	Study Type	Study Population	Type of Occupation	Methods	Main Findings
Del Arco-Galan C[72]	1994	USA	Cross sectional study	100	Physicians, staff, and residents working in emergency room	24 hour ambulatory blood pressure monitoring	Both average blood pressure values and blood pressure load were significantly higher when subjects were on-call. Familial history of hypertension and professional status were the most important determinants of the pressor response.
Brown DE [5]	1998	Hawaii	Cross-sectional study	Females from two ethnic groups: Filipino-Americans (n=38) and Caucasians (n= 22)	Nurses and nurse's aides	24 hour ambulatory blood pressure monitoring was performed during a typical work day, diary report	For all subjects blood pressure was higher at work. Ethnicity has an important impact on blood pressure variation. The extent of blood pressure variation in daily life
							may depend upon cognitive processes which are influenced by the cultural background and emotional state of the individual.
Goldstein IB [21]	1999	USA	Prospective study	138, ages 25–50	Registered nurses	Ambulatory blood pressure and heart rate were recorded over 24-hour periods on 2 work and 2 off days (during the luteal and follicular phases of menstrual cycle, evaluation of cortisol and catecholamines). Questionnaires.	The work environment leads to increased activity of the cardiovascular and sympathoadrenal medullary system in healthy women. However, the effects are modified by the woman's domestic role, by the length of employment, and by the demands of the job

(Table 2) cont.....

Author	Year	Country/Place	Study Type	Study Population	Type of Occupation	Methods	Main Findings
Mion D [74]	2004	Brazil	Cross-sectional study	864 individuals	Hospital employees	Blood pressure measurement, risk factor assessment, anthropometry	Hypertension prevalence was 26%. The multivariate logistic regression model revealed a statistically significant association of hypertension with gender, age, skin colour, family income, and body mass index.
Riese H [14]	2004	Nertherlands	prospective study	159 participants	Female nurses	Ambulatory blood pressure. Job demands, decision latitude, and social support were measured with the Karasek job content questionnaire, which was administered twice with an average interval of 12.2 months	No effect on the ambulatory levels of blood pressure, heart rate, or heart rate variability was found for job strain by itself or in interaction with social support.
							High job strain among young female nurses is not associated with an unfavourable ambulatory cardiovascular profile.
Fialho G [76]	2006	Brazil	Cross-sectional study	61 residents	Medical residents working in the emergency room	Ambulatory blood pressure monitoring during a 24-h shift work in the emergency room (ER) and comparison with a common working day	Working in the ER on a 24-h shift leads to abnormal blood pressure behaviour in medical residents both during sleep and work, thus suggesting that this type of work may be a risk factor for cardiovascular disease.

(Table 2) cont.....

Author	Year	Country/Place	Study Type	Study Population	Type of Occupation	Methods	Main Findings
Rovik JO [71]	2007	Norway	Prospective cohort study	Physicians graduating from all four Norwegian universities n= 63 responded at various time points with a mean observation period of 9.2 years.	Physicians	Established job stress questionnaire (Cooper/Tyssen), with emphasis on dimensions of the work-home interference	Stress related to the work-home interference increases through the first 9 years of physicians' careers, in contrast to decreasing specific patient-work stressors. Lack of reduction in working hours and having many children predicted an increase in stress related to the work home interference. Neuroticism, conscientiousness, and lack of support from one's partner and colleagues, appeared to be predictive of this stress.
Owolabi AO [73]	2012	Nigeria	Cross-sectional study	324	Health workers	Blood pressure using sphygmomanometer, anthropometry, standard questionnaire	A significant number of health workers in this study was afflicted by work-related stress and perceived work stress was found to be significantly associated with higher hypertension prevalence
Egbi OG [75]	2015	Nigeria	Cross-sectional study	231 participants	Employees at the Federal Medical Centre	Blood pressure measurement, risk factor assessment, anthropometry	Prevalence of hypertension was 23.8%. In multivariate regression analysis, only older age and abnormal waist circumference predicted hypertension.

Table 3. Hypertension and its associated factors in school teachers and university staff.

Author	Year	Country/Place	Study Type	Study Population	Type of Occupation	Methods	Main Findings
Brodsky CM [77]	1977	NA	Qualitative	31 teachers and 21 prison guards who complained of occupational pressure.	Teachers, Prison guards	Psychiatric evaluation, case report	The pressure-prone job is one in which the goals or objectives are contradictory, lines of support are ill defined, and there is role ambiguity, with no hope for improvement. A triggering event makes the worker aware of his vulnerability and at the same time feel isolated. Internal and external forces make it impossible for the worker to resign. Physical and psychological symptoms have a insidious onset and progress in severity.
Deyanov C [78]	1994	Sofia, Bulgaria	Case control study	168 females between 25 and 55 years of age	School teachers from comprehensive and technical schools	103 female employees (designers, researchers) served as controls. BP using sphygmomanometer, questionnaires	An abrupt elevation of systolic blood pressure was observed in teachers>45 years old and a significant difference during the first and second half of the fourth decade was found.

(Table 3) cont.....

Author	Year	Country/Place	Study Type	Study Population	Type of Occupation	Methods	Main Findings
							A strong positive correlation between teachers' length of service and blood pressure was revealed. The elevation of the diastolic blood pressure with age was more pronounced among the teachers than among the controls.
Steptoe A [79]	2000	UK	Prospective study	81 (26 men, 55 women), 36 of whom experienced persistent high job demands over 1 year, while 45 reported lower job demands.	School teachers	Assessment of cardiovascular responses to standardized behavioural tasks, job demands, and ambulatory blood pressure over a working day and evening after 12 months	Systolic and diastolic pressure during the working day were greater in high job demand participants who were stress reactive than in other groups, after adjustment for confounding factors
Cisneros-Blas Y [81]	2009	Mexico	Cross-sectional and retrospective	120	Academic workers at a Public University in Mexico City	Blood pressure measurement, standardised questionnaire	The working conditions influence on the development of illness, with evidence for psychosomatic diseases and increased blood pressure

(Table 3) cont.....

Author	Year	Country/Place	Study Type	Study Population	Type of Occupation	Methods	Main Findings
Pimenta AM [82]	2012	Brazil	Cross-sectional study	211 workers of both genders, aged between 30 and 64 years,	Workers of health campus of a public university	Standardised questionnaire	The prevalence of systemic hypertension and cardiovascular risk was higher among night workers. Nocturnal labour, highly demanding shift scale and work control, and time at work were positively associated with high cardiovascular risk.
Santos MN [80]	2013	Brazil	Cross-sectional study	414; females (96.1%)	Teachers	Blood pressure measurement, standardised questionnaire	There was an association between arterial hypertension and stress index with the overall health perception, as well as time working as a teacher, and absenteeism.

Hypertension in White Collar Workers

White-collar workers are those that carry out managerial or administrative work. In this group, a sedentary lifestyle with high levels of job strain may lead to metabolic disorders. The important studies related to this occupational group has been summarised in Table **4** [20, 26, 83 - 99]. A prospective study among white-collar workers (including senior management staff, professionals, technical and office staff) found job strain to have a significant effect on systolic blood pressure. Lower levels of social support was an important risk factor for the rise in blood pressure [89]. A prospective study in white collar workers found overtime work to be associated with hypertension [83]. In a cross-sectional study of female white collar workers, high family responsibilities were associated with significant increases in diurnal systolic and diastolic blood pressures. High family responsibilities and job strain when combined had a greater effect on blood pressure [20]. Studies have found 12.4% to 69% of bank employees to have hypertension. However, as most of these studies were cross-sectional, this may be an over-estimate [90, 93, 95, 96, 98, 99]. Socio-demographic factors like increased age, male gender, family history of hypertension, mode of travel, physical activity, overweight, years of service, intake of coffee and smoking were significantly associated with hypertension [99].

Table 4. Hypertension and its associated factors in white collar workers.

Author	Year	Country/Place	Study Type	Study Population	Type of Occupation	Methods	Main Findings
Hayashi T [83]	1996	Japan	Prospective study	NA	Workers, white collar employees	Comparison between four groups using ambulatory blood pressure monitoring, fatigue—Japanese questionnaire by Japan society for occupational health.	For those with normal blood pressure and those with mild hypertension, the ambulatory pressures of the overtime groups was higher than that of the control groups. These results indicate that the burden on the cardiovascular system of white collar workers increases with overtime work
Lindquist TL [84]	1997	Australia	Cross-sectional study	Men (n = 337) and women (n = 317)	Government tax office workers	Questionnaires for assessment of work-related stress, coping strategies, and lifestyle. Seven resting blood pressure measurements were recorded serially on each of two occasions a week apart.	There were no direct associations between measures of work stress and blood pressure. Body mass index and lifestyle factors in the form of alcohol consumption, exercise, and diet were related to blood pressure in men and women.
Peter R [26]	1997	Germany	Cross-sectional study	189 male middle-aged (40-55 years)	Middle managers in a car-producing company	Staff records were obtained. Blood pressure measured by sphygmomanometer. Structural review and questionnaires (Siegrist).	Concurrent high effort and low reward (active coping) were at substantially elevated risk of exhibiting manifest hypertension. Those characterized by passive coping (low occupational rewards only)

(Table 4) cont.....

Author	Year	Country/Place	Study Type	Study Population	Type of Occupation	Methods	Main Findings
							were more likely to experience sickness absence. Both findings are in accordance with stress-theoretical considerations on different health outcomes of active vs. passive coping
Prunier-Poulmaire [85]	1998	France	cross-sectional survey	Employees from forty-four national units	French customs service workers	A questionnaire designed for the evaluation of specific job. The three variables were included in a series of logistic regression analyses on the health aspects of the customs officers.	The results point to a need for a multifaceted approach to research and intervention regarding the difficulties encountered by shift workers, from both the occupational medicine and the work design point of view.
Chor D [86]	1998	Rio de Janeiro, Brazil	Cross-sectional study	1183 employees	Government owned bank employees	Blood pressure measurement, risk factor assessment, anthropometry	There were no important differences among hypertensives and non-hypertensives with respect to the prevalence of smoking, alcohol and physical activities.
Brisson C [20]	1999	Quebec, Canada	Cross-sectional study	199 white collar women with and without children employed in eight organizations (selected from a population of 3183 women of all ages)	White collar workers	24 hour Ambulatory blood pressure monitoring on working day. Job content questionnaire, Karasek	Large family responsibilities were associated with significant increases in diurnal systolic and diastolic blood pressure among women holding a university degree. In these women, the combined exposure of large family responsibilities and high job strain tended to have a greater effect on BP than the exposure to only one of these factors

(Table 4) cont.....

Author	Year	Country/Place	Study Type	Study Population	Type of Occupation	Methods	Main Findings
Vrijkotte TG [87]	2000	Netherlands	Cross-sectional study	109 males	white collar workers	Ambulatory blood pressure monitoring, diary, chronic stress Siegrist's model	The detrimental effects of work stress are partly mediated by increased heart rate reactivity to a stressful workday, an increase in systolic blood pressure level, and lower vagal tone
Nakanishi N [88]	2001	Japan	Prospective cohort study	941 hypertension free aged 35–54 years	Male white collar workers	Prospectively followed up for five years. Risk factor assessment	88 men developed hypertension during 4531 person years. From the multiple regression analyses, working hours per day remained as an independent negative factor for the slopes of systolic and diastolic blood pressure.
Guimont C [89]	2006	Quebec Canada	Prospective study	8395 white-collar workers	Senior management, professional, technical, and office workers.	A demographic questionnaire, BP at clinic, Karasek's Job-Strain Model	Exposure to cumulative job strain had a modest but significant effect on SBP among men. Men and women with low levels of social support at work appeared to be at higher risk for increases in blood pressure.
Maroof KA [90]	2007	Meerut, India	Cross-sectional study	176 males (88.0%) and 24 females (12.0%)	Bank employees	Blood pressure measurement, risk factor assessment, anthropometry	Prevalence of hypertension was found to be 69.5%. Hypertension was significantly associated with age 45 years, alcohol intake, waist circumference, body mass index and diabetes

(Table 4) cont.....

Author	Year	Country/Place	Study Type	Study Population	Type of Occupation	Methods	Main Findings
Maina G [91]	2008	Italy	Cross-sectional study	104 volunteers male and female	Call centre operators	Daily cortisol profiles consisting of seven time points were measured across 2 work days and 1 leisure day to determine the cortisol awakening response and the cortisol output in the day. Karasek, Siegrist and demographic questionnaires	The two work stress models differentially affect salivary cortisol output. This finding suggests that combining the information from two complementary job stress models results in improved knowledge on the psychobiological correlates of the psychosocial work environment.
Trudel X [92]	2010	Canada	Cross-sectional study	2357 workers (80% participation, 61% women; mean age, 44 years)	White collar workers recruited from public organizations	Blood pressure using sphygmomanometer and ambulatory monitoring, and job content questionnaire.	Mild hypertension is associated with job strain in men. Workers in "active" job situations may be more likely to have the condition. No significant association with a higher prevalence of MH was observed in women.
Momin MH [93]	2012	Surat, India	Cross-sectional study	1493 employees	Bank employees	Blood pressure measurement, risk factor assessment, anthropometry	Prevalence of hypertension was 30.4% and prehypertension was 34.5%. Prevalence was high among persons with age 50 years and above, among males, small family size, among separated/divorced, and higher socioeconomic group.

(Table 4) cont.....

Author	Year	Country/Place	Study Type	Study Population	Type of Occupation	Methods	Main Findings
Salaroli LB [94]	2013	Vitória, Brazil	Cross-sectional study	521 working men and women >20 years of age	Bank employees	Sociodemographic, lifestyle, anthropometric, biochemical, and hemodynamic characteristics were collected. A logistic regression model was used for analysis	Occupation can be correlated with the development of metabolic syndrome (presence of dyslipidaemia, glucose intolerance, hypertension, overweight, abdominal obesity, type 2 diabetes mellitus and cardiovascular disease).
Ismail IM [95]	2013	Sullia, India	Cross-sectional study	117 employees	Bank employees	Blood pressure measurement, risk factor assessment, anthropometry	The prevalence of hypertension was 39.3%. Increasing age, family history of hypertension, body mass index $\geq$ 25 kg/m 2 and abnormal waist-hip ratio were significantly more frequent among the hypertensive than normotensive population.
Ganesh Kumar S [96]	2014	Puducherry, India	Cross-sectional study	192 (128 male and 64 female)	Bank employees	Blood pressure measurement, risk factor assessment, standard questionnaires	The prevalence of hypertension and pre-hypertension was 44.3% and 41.1% respectively. Consumption of extra salt, and physical activity $\geq$2 hours per day were associated with hypertension.
Diwe KC [97]	2015	Nigeria	Cross-sectional study	194 employees	Bank employees	Blood pressure measurement, risk factor assessment, anthropometry	The prevalence of hypertension was 12.4%. Alcohol consumption and obesity in bankers were the commonest cardiovascular risk factors
Fikadu G [98]	2016	Ethiopia	Cross-sectional study	1866 participants	Bank employees (30%) and teachers (70%)	Blood pressure measurement, risk factor assessment, anthropometry	Prevalence of hypertension was 21%. Associations were males, age, middle and higher income.

(Table 4) cont.....

Author	Year	Country/Place	Study Type	Study Population	Type of Occupation	Methods	Main Findings
Brahmankar TR [99]	2017	Maharashtra, India	Cross-sectional study	340 employees	Bank employees	Blood pressure measurement, risk factor assessment, anthropometry	Overall prevalence of hypertension was 39.7% and that of pre-hypertension was 41.8% among the study population. Socio-demographic factors like age, male gender, family history of hypertension, mode of travel, physical activity, overweight, years of service, intake of coffee and smoking were significantly associated with hypertension

Hypertension in Blue Collar Workers

Blue collar workers refer to non-agricultural manual workers. Studies done on such workers are summarised in Table **5** [8, 34, 100, 101]. An increase in job strain due to overwork and lack of job decision latitude has been described in these studies. A case-control study among manual workers found that hypertension was strongly associated with an uncertain job future, dissatisfaction with co-workers and a lack of promotion. In addition, psychosocial interactions between suppressed anger and job stress had significant predictive value for hypertension. Thus, psychological factors such as poor coping characteristics may be an important modifier in the relationship between job strain and hypertension [8]. A cross-sectional study among manual workers found job decision latitude and work demand to be associated with important cardiovascular risk factors such as hypertension, dyslipidemia, and homocysteinemia [100]. A prospective cohort study of a group of blue collar workers in Japan found that job stress due to complicated machine operation, was a significant predictor of diastolic hypertension. In contrast, job overload, physical discomfort, human relations, and job dissatisfaction did not have a significant influence on hypertension [101]. Another prospective study among hourly workers found stressful work conditions and overall job dissatisfaction to be significantly associated with diastolic blood pressure. Furthermore, hypertension was also associated with a lack of promotion and decision-making capacity, job uncertainty, unsupportive co-workers and lack of communication [34].

Hypertension in Heavy Vehicle Drivers

Studies on hypertension among heavy vehicle drivers are summarised in Table **6** [102 - 110]. In a review of 34 studies, professional drivers, specifically urban transport operators were reported to have an increased risk of hypertension and cardiovascular disease [111]. Several cross-sectional studies have identified a high prevalence of hypertension among bus drivers and commercial truck drivers. Several associated risk factors such as overweight, supporting a large family, dietary habits, family history of cardiovascular diseases, trip duration, trip distance, and sedentary behavior have been identified [103, 104, 108 - 110]. However, some studies did not find a significant association of job demands with hypertension, after correction for possible confounding factors [105, 106]. Heavy vehicle drivers are a unique occupational group, that need to perform complex tasks requiring rapid responses to unexpected hazards whilst following a rigid time schedule. Frequent shift work, a high level of responsibility for passengers and equipment, and low levels of job decision latitude are some important stressors in the job [112]. Due to the wide range of psychological and physical stressors, heavy vehicle drivers are prone to higher levels of hypertension than other manual workers [113]. Gobel performed a detailed assessment of job strain in different types of bus drivers and found short-haul bus drivers to be exposed to high-density traffic and frequent stops, often involving multiple simultaneous executions of tasks, performed with compulsory monotonous body posture and under exposure to vibration and noise [114]. Furthermore, there is contradictory demands made on bus drivers such as safety while adhering to timetables, repetitive and sedentary work balanced against vigilance and the processing of a multitude of signals, with little or no control over the pace of work and schedules [115].

Hypertension in Fire Fighters, Police Officers, Prison Guards, and Other Emergency Responders

Firefighters, police officers, prison guards, and other emergency responders comprise a unique group of occupations [116], comprising strenuous duties and high risk situations. These may interact with their personal risk profiles to adversely affect blood pressure (Table **7** [72, 76, 77, 116 - 118]). These occupations may comprise of long periods of relative inactivity punctuated by unpredictable, potentially life-threatening and stressful bursts of high intensity work activity. Furthermore, fatigue and sleep disruption due to the irregular working hours may have a negative impact on their health and lead to an increased risk of chronic disease and mortality [119].

Table 5. Hypertension and its associated factors among blue collar workers.

Author	Year	Country/Place	Study Type	Study Population	Type of Occupation	Methods	Main Findings
Cottington EM [8]	1986	Metropolitan Pittsburgh, PA, area USA	Controlled study	The study population consisted of a random sample of 366 male hourly workers, aged 40-63 years, employed at one of two plants	Manual workers	A psychosocial questionnaire measuring job stress, coronary-prone behaviour, trait anxiety, anger, life stress, and specific coping behaviours associated with occupational noise exposure. Resting BP and reaction of BP to acute stress or test was measured.	Hypertension was more strongly associated with dissatisfaction with co-workers, uncertain job future and promotions among men who suppress their anger. Interactions between suppressed anger and job stress significantly predicted hypertension status. These findings suggest that a coping-related characteristic such as anger expression may be an important modifier of the relationship between job stress and hypertension
Matthews KA [34]	1987	Metropolitan Pittsburgh, USA	Prospective cohort study	241 male, ages 40–63 years, employed for a minimum of 10 years at	Hourly workers	Questionnaire, Blood pressure was assessed by the random zero muddler method	Stressful work conditions as well as overall job dissatisfaction were significant predictors of diastolic blood pressure.

(Table 5) cont.....

Author	Year	Country/Place	Study Type	Study Population	Type of Occupation	Methods	Main Findings
							Men with elevated diastolic blood pressure reported having little opportunity for promotion and for participating in decisions at work, an uncertain job future, unsupportive co-workers and foreman, difficulties communicating with others, and overall dissatisfaction with the job.
Kawakami N [101]	1989	Japan	Prospective cohort study	373 males without hypertension were followed for one year.	blue collar worker	Five kinds of perceived job-stress were a+H7ssessed by means of mailed questionnaires	Job stress from complicated machine operation was found to be a significant predictor of DBP increase. Job overload, physical discomfort, human relations, and job dissatisfaction, on the other hand, bore no significant relation to systolic and DBP increases. The use of production machines involving complicated

(Table 5) cont.....

Author	Year	Country/Place	Study Type	Study Population	Type of Occupation	Methods	Main Findings
							operations and newly developed technology might be a risk factor for high DBP.
Kang MG [100]	2005	South Korea	Cross-sectional study	152 eligible participants were analysed from a sample of 1,071 workers in 20 companies	Manual workers	Karasek's Job Strain Model, BP measurement	Decision latitude was associated with cholesterol, triglyceride, and homocysteine and that work demand was related to smoking and systolic blood pressure. Job was significantly related to higher levels of homocysteine. Job stress is associated with cardiovascular risk factors and might contribute to the development of CV disease

Three-quarters of emergency responders have pre-hypertension or hypertension. The elevated blood pressure levels are also inadequately controlled and thus strongly linked to cardiovascular disease morbidity and mortality [116]. However, Sega *et al* found that blood pressure was not increased in a group of air traffic controllers. This may be because they are a highly selected group having a good health profile and suitable training to adequately cope with stress [39, 118]. Studies have found that irregular bursts of physical exertion and sedentary behavior in-between, unhealthy diet and shift work, increased noise exposure (for example due to sirens, machine engines, mechanical rescue equipment), post-traumatic stress disorder, high job demand, and low job decision latitudes may have a negative impact on health and lead to an increased risk of hypertension and cardiovascular disease [116, 120, 121].

Table 6. Hypertension and its associated factors in heavy vehicle drivers.

Author	Year	Coutry/Place	Study Type	Study Population	Type of Occupation	Methods	Main Findings
Ragland DR [112]	1987	USA	Cross-sectional study	1500 black and white male bus drivers from a large urban transit system	Bus drivers: 80% operate diesel and electronic buses, 20% operate light rail vehicles and cable cars	Drivers were compared to three groups: individuals from both a national (HANES II) and local health survey and individuals undergoing baseline health examinations before employment as bus drivers. Blood pressure using sphygmomanometer.	Hypertension rates for bus drivers were significantly greater than rates for each of the three comparison groups. These findings may support exposure to the occupation of driving a bus may carry increased health risk
Albright CL [105]	1992	USA	Prospective study	1396 biracial drivers	Urban bus drivers	Standard questionnaire, anthropometric measurements	Although univariate analysis showed a significant association with job demands and job strain, the multivariate analysis following
							elimination of possible confounding factors did not reveal any significant association with hypertension.
Stoohs RA [109]	1993	USA	Case control study	193 subjects	Commercial truck drivers	Blood pressure measuremt, risk factor assessment and validated questionnaires for obstructive sleep apnea	Significant association between hypertension and obstructive sleep apnea and body mass index was noted.

(Table 6) cont.....

Author	Year	Coutry/Place	Study Type	Study Population	Type of Occupation	Methods	Main Findings
Lakshman A [104]	2014	Kerala, India	Cross-sectional study	179 (aged 21-60)	Male bus drivers of Corporation Bus	Blood pressure, height, and weight of subjects were measured, and relevance was obtained using a structured questionnaire.	Prevalence of hypertension was high among bus drivers (41.9% had prehypertension, and 41.3% had hypertension) Age > 35 years, elevated BMI, supporting a large family, and dietary habits associated with the job showed significant association with hypertension
Sangaleti CT [110]	2014	Southern Brazil	Cross-sectional study	250 males (18-60 years)	Long-distance truck drivers	Assessment of social habits and demographic data and an evaluation of risk factors for cardiovascular disease	Hypertension was confirmed in 45.2%. Odds of hypertension increased with abdominal obesity, age and the family history of premature cardiovascular disease.
Taklikar S [107]	2015	Kolkata, India	Cross-sectional study	210	Bus drivers	Occupational stress was assessed by using Stress- related health complaints questionnaire.	Hypertension was seen among 24%. Occupational stress is associated with hypertension,
							gastrointestinal and musculoskeletal problems among bus drivers.

(Table 6) cont.....

Author	Year	Coutry/Place	Study Type	Study Population	Type of Occupation	Methods	Main Findings
Biglari H [106]	2016	Iran	Cross-sectional study	220	Intercity drivers	Stardard questionnaires. After a 10-h fasting period, systolic and diastolic blood pressure was recorded. Intravenous blood samples were taken to determine cholesterol, triglyceride and blood glucose levels.	There was no significant relationship between occupational stress and diastolic blood pressure among the drivers
Jayarajah U [103]	2017	Colombo, Sri Lanka	Cross-sectional study	120	Male bus drivers of Corporation Bus	Serial blood pressure measurement and pretested questionnaire	Prevalence of hypertension was significantly associated with obesity, average trip duration and distance/ sedentary behaviour.
Chankaramangalam MA [108]	2017	South India	Cross-sectional study	175	Truck drivers	Standard questionnaire, anthropometric measurements	The prevalence of overweight was 50% and the prevalence of hypertension was 40%. In multivariate data analysis, history of chronic disease was the only significant associated with hypertension.

Hypertension Among other Occupational Categories

Among pilots, chronic noise exposure was found to be an important occupational-related environmental risk factor for hypertension [122]. Studies done in farmers have shown conflicting results. A cross-sectional survey of farmers in Kentucky, the USA using a self-reported questionnaire and telephone interview found the prevalence of hypertension to be 38%. This may be an under-estimate as an onsite medical evaluation was not done. Hypertensive older farmers were at increased risk for diabetes, stroke, arteriosclerosis, and cardiovascular diseases. Further-more, logistic regression analysis also found high body mass index to be a risk factor [68]. Similarly, a case-control study from Italy found farmers to have a higher prevalence of systolic and diastolic hypertension and electrocardiogram

(ECG) abnormalities compared with controls [123]. In contrast, a few community surveys have found farmers to be at a significantly lower risk of developing hypertension compared to other occupations. Increased physical activity compared to other occupations was postulated as a possible reason [69, 70].

Table 7. Hypertension in fire fighters, police officers, prison guards and other emergency responders.

Author	Year	Country/Place	Study Type	Study Population	Type of Occupation	Methods	Main Findings
Brodsky CM [77]	1977	NA	Qualitative	31 teachers and 21 prison guards who	Teachers, Prison guards	Psychiatric evaluation, case report	The pressure-prone job is one in which the goals
Brodsky CM[77]				complained of occupational pressure.			or objectives are contradictory, lines of support are ill defined, and there is role ambiguity, with no hope for improvement. A triggering event makes the worker aware of his vulnerability and at the same time feel isolated. Internal and external forces make it impossible for the worker to resign. Physical and psychological symptoms have a insidious onset and progress in severity.

(Table 7) cont.....

Author	Year	Country/Place	Study Type	Study Population	Type of Occupation	Methods	Main Findings
Del Arco-Galan C [72]	1994	USA	Cross sectional study	100	Physicians, staff, and residents working in emergency room	24 hour ambulatory blood pressure monitoring	Both average blood pressure values and blood pressure load were significantly higher when subjects were on-call. Familial history of hypertension and professional status were the most important determinants of the pressor response.
Goldberg P [117]	1996	Prison in France	Cross-sectional study	Men and women aged 20–64	All kinds of prison personnel (prison guards, administrative staff, socio-educational workers, technicians, health care workers, and managers.	Postal self-administered questionnaire was used to assess sociodemographic factors, work conditions, and physical and mental disorders. Multiple logistic regression analyses were conducted to determine the effects of work conditions and social relationships on the mental health of prison staff.	The factors concerning the subjective evaluation of work conditions and social support were more closely related to mental disorders than work conditions. In addition, seniority was associated with depressive symptoms and anxiety among the men.

(Table 7) cont.....

Author	Year	Country/Place	Study Type	Study Population	Type of Occupation	Methods	Main Findings
Sega R [118]	1998	Italy	Cross-sectional study	80	Air traffic controllers	The 24 h blood pressure monitoring was obtained during two working shifts separated by one night of rest. Data were compared with those of an age matched male sample.	Conventional diastolic pressures and heart rate were similar in cases and controls, whereas conventional systolic pressures was significantly greater in the former than in the latter group. Daily life blood pressure was not increased in the sample.
Fialho G [76]	2006	Brazil	Cross-sectional study	61 residents	Medical residents in working in emergency room	Ambulatory blood pressure monitoring during a 24-h shift work in the emergency room and comparison with a common working day	Working in the ER on a 24-h shift leads to abnormal blood pressure behaviour in medical residents both during sleep and work,
							thus suggesting that this type of work may be a risk factor for cardiovascular disease. thus suggesting that this type of work may be a risk factor for cardiovascular disease.

(Table 7) cont.....

Author	Year	Country/Place	Study Type	Study Population	Type of Occupation	Methods	Main Findings
Kales SN [116]	2009	USA and other countries	Review	NA	Fire-fighters, Police Officers, and Other Emergency Responders	Review	Approximately three-quarters of emergency responders have prehypertension or hypertension, a proportion which is expected to increase, based on the obesity epidemic. Elevated blood pressure is also inadequately controlled in these professionals and strongly linked to cardiovascular disease morbidity and mortality.

PREVENTIVE STRATEGIES AND IMPLICATIONS IN MANAGEMENT

In view of the effect of occupation on hypertension, suitable preventive strategies and interventions have been suggested [3]. When managing hypertension in patients with high occupational stress, suitable steps to minimize job strain are needed. When formulating workplace health promotion programs, individual coping strategies and lifestyle modifications should be targeted as much as the work environment. Some of these strategies include population-based wellness strategies such as encouraging aerobic exercise, maintaining a healthy weight, sleep hygiene, stress management; screening and counseling for individuals at higher risk of occupational stress and the early identification and treatment of hypertension. Time-limited work clearance should be considered so that persons with hypertension do not continue to work for long hours with uncontrolled blood pressure [116].

The role of psychosocial work characteristics (job control and psychological demands) on leisure time physical activity has been studied. Workers in low-strain jobs were found to have increased leisure time physical activity [124]. High-strain jobs may discourage workers from engaging in leisure time physical activity and thus negatively impact their health. Thus steps to increase leisure time physical activity in such groups would be important. However, longer working hours and lower annual incomes in those from poorer socioeconomic groups may lead to practical difficulties in performing such leisure time activities. Specific employment groups at increased risk of stress should be identified and preventive measures implemented [15]. As proposed by Siegrist et al such interventions could be implemented within single companies/organizations at the individual level (reduction of commitment), the interpersonal level (improvement of leadership, providing esteem rewards), and the organizational level (compensatory wage systems, gain-sharing, non-monetary gratifications) [15]. The introduction of anti-stress programs in the workplace was shown to reverse autonomic symptoms [125]. It is important that managers provide proper training for workers and define clear goals and lines of authority.

CONSENT FOR PUBLICATION

Not applicable.

CONFLICT OF INTEREST

The authors declare no conflict of interest, financial or otherwise.

ACKNOWLEDGEMENT

Declare none.

REFERENCES

[1]   Pickering TG, Devereux RB, James GD, *et al.* Environmental influences on blood pressure and the role of job strain. J Hypertens Suppl 1996; 14(5): S179-85.
        [PMID: 9120676]

[2]   Tsutsumi A, Kawakami N. A review of empirical studies on the model of effort-reward imbalance at work: reducing occupational stress by implementing a new theory. Soc Sci Med 2004; 59(11): 2335-59.
        [http://dx.doi.org/10.1016/j.socscimed.2004.03.030] [PMID: 15450708]

[3]   Rosenthal T, Alter A. Occupational stress and hypertension. J Am Soc Hypertens 2012; 6(1): 2-22.
        [http://dx.doi.org/10.1016/j.jash.2011.09.002] [PMID: 22024667]

[4]   Schnall PL, Landsbergis PA, Pieper CF, *et al.* The impact of anticipation of job loss on psychological distress and worksite blood pressure. Am J Ind Med 1992; 21(3): 417-32.
        [http://dx.doi.org/10.1002/ajim.4700210314] [PMID: 1585951]

[5]   Brown DE, James GD, Nordloh L. Comparison of factors affecting daily variation of blood pressure in Filipino-American and Caucasian nurses in Hawaii. Am J Phys Anthropol 1998; 106(3): 373-83.
        [http://dx.doi.org/10.1002/(SICI)1096-8644(199807)106:3<373::AID-AJPA9>3.0.CO;2-N] [PMID: 9696152]

[6]   Tobe SW, Kiss A, Szalai JP, Perkins N, Tsigoulis M, Baker B. Impact of job and marital strain on ambulatory blood pressure results from the double exposure study. Am J Hypertens 2005; 18(8): 1046-51.
        [http://dx.doi.org/10.1016/j.amjhyper.2005.03.734] [PMID: 16109318]

[7]   Tobe SW, Kiss A, Sainsbury S, Jesin M, Geerts R, Baker B. The impact of job strain and marital cohesion on ambulatory blood pressure during 1 year: the double exposure study. Am J Hypertens 2007; 20(2): 148-53.
[http://dx.doi.org/10.1016/j.amjhyper.2006.07.011] [PMID: 17261459]

[8]   Cottington EM, Matthews KA, Talbott E, Kuller LH. Occupational stress, suppressed anger, and hypertension. Psychosom Med 1986; 48(3-4): 249-60.
[http://dx.doi.org/10.1097/00006842-198603000-00010] [PMID: 3704088]

[9]   Beilin LJ. Stress, coping, lifestyle and hypertension: a paradigm for research, prevention and non-pharmacological management of hypertension. Clin Exp Hypertens 1997; 19(5-6): 739-52.
[http://dx.doi.org/10.3109/10641969709083183] [PMID: 9247752]

[10]   Schwartz JE, Pickering TG, Landsbergis PA. Work-related stress and blood pressure: current theoretical models and considerations from a behavioral medicine perspective. J Occup Health Psychol 1996; 1(3): 287-310.
[http://dx.doi.org/10.1037/1076-8998.1.3.287] [PMID: 9547052]

[11]   Niedhammer I, Goldberg M, Leclerc A, David S, Bugel I, Landre M-F. Psychosocial work environment and cardiovascular risk factors in an occupational cohort in France. J Epidemiol Community Health 1998; 52(2): 93-100.
[http://dx.doi.org/10.1136/jech.52.2.93] [PMID: 9578855]

[12]   Frommer MS, Edye BV, Mandryk JA, Grammeno GL, Berry G, Ferguson DA. Systolic blood pressure in relation to occupation and perceived work stress. Scand J Work Environ Health 1986; 12(5): 476-85.
[http://dx.doi.org/10.5271/sjweh.2115] [PMID: 3491422]

[13]   Eaker ED, Sullivan LM, Kelly-Hayes M, D'Agostino RB Sr, Benjamin EJ. Does job strain increase the risk for coronary heart disease or death in men and women? The Framingham Offspring Study. Am J Epidemiol 2004; 159(10): 950-8.
[http://dx.doi.org/10.1093/aje/kwh127] [PMID: 15128607]

[14]   Riese H, Van Doornen LJ, Houtman IL, De Geus EJ. Job strain in relation to ambulatory blood pressure, heart rate, and heart rate variability among female nurses. Scand J Work Environ Health 2004; 30(6): 477-85.
[http://dx.doi.org/10.5271/sjweh.837] [PMID: 15635758]

[15]   Siegrist J. Effort-reward imbalance at work and cardiovascular diseases. Int J Occup Med Environ Health 2010; 23(3): 279-85.
[http://dx.doi.org/10.2478/v10001-010-0013-8] [PMID: 20934954]

[16]   Kristensen TS. Job stress and cardiovascular disease: a theoretic critical review. J Occup Health Psychol 1996; 1(3): 246-60.
[http://dx.doi.org/10.1037/1076-8998.1.3.246] [PMID: 9547050]

[17]   Pieper C, LaCroix AZ, Karasek RA. The relation of psychosocial dimensions of work with coronary heart disease risk factors: a meta-analysis of five United States data bases. Am J Epidemiol 1989; 129(3): 483-94.
[http://dx.doi.org/10.1093/oxfordjournals.aje.a115159] [PMID: 2916541]

[18]   Pickering T. The effects of occupational stress on blood pressure in men and women. Acta Physiol Scand Suppl 1997; 640: 125-8.
[PMID: 9401623]

[19]   Curtis AB, James SA, Raghunathan TE, Alcser KH. Job strain and blood pressure in African Americans: the Pitt County Study. Am J Public Health 1997; 87(8): 1297-302.
[http://dx.doi.org/10.2105/AJPH.87.8.1297] [PMID: 9279264]

[20]   Brisson C, Laflamme N, Moisan J, Milot A, Mâsse B, Vézina M. Effect of family responsibilities and job strain on ambulatory blood pressure among white-collar women. Psychosom Med 1999; 61(2):

205-13.
[http://dx.doi.org/10.1097/00006842-199903000-00013] [PMID: 10204974]

[21] Goldstein IB, Shapiro D, Chicz-DeMet A, Guthrie D. Ambulatory blood pressure, heart rate, and neuroendocrine responses in women nurses during work and off work days. Psychosom Med 1999; 61(3): 387-96.
[http://dx.doi.org/10.1097/00006842-199905000-00020] [PMID: 10367621]

[22] Radi S, Lang T, Lauwers-Cancès V, *et al.* Job constraints and arterial hypertension: different effects in men and women: the IHPAF II case control study. Occup Environ Med 2005; 62(10): 711-7.
[http://dx.doi.org/10.1136/oem.2004.012955] [PMID: 16169917]

[23] Lundberg U. Influence of paid and unpaid work on psychophysiological stress responses of men and women. J Occup Health Psychol 1996; 1(2): 117-30.
[http://dx.doi.org/10.1037/1076-8998.1.2.117] [PMID: 9547041]

[24] Schieman S, Whitestone YK, Van Gundy K. The nature of work and the stress of higher status. J Health Soc Behav 2006; 47(3): 242-57.
[http://dx.doi.org/10.1177/002214650604700304] [PMID: 17066775]

[25] Theorell T, Alfredsson L, Westerholm P, Falck B. Coping with unfair treatment at work--what is the relationship between coping and hypertension in middle-aged men and Women? An epidemiological study of working men and women in Stockholm (the WOLF study). Psychother Psychosom 2000; 69(2): 86-94.
[http://dx.doi.org/10.1159/000012371] [PMID: 10671829]

[26] Peter R, Siegrist J. Chronic work stress, sickness absence, and hypertension in middle managers: general or specific sociological explanations? Soc Sci Med 1997; 45(7): 1111-20.
[http://dx.doi.org/10.1016/S0277-9536(97)00039-7] [PMID: 9257402]

[27] Steptoe A, Marmot M. Socioeconomic status and coronary heart disease: a psychobiological perspective. Popul Dev Rev 2004; 30: 133-50.

[28] Alfredsson L, Hammar N, Fransson E, *et al.* Job strain and major risk factors for coronary heart disease among employed males and females in a Swedish study on work, lipids and fibrinogen. Scand J Work Environ Health 2002; 28(4): 238-48.
[http://dx.doi.org/10.5271/sjweh.671] [PMID: 12199425]

[29] Carroll D, Smith GD, Sheffield D, Shipley MJ, Marmot MG. Pressor reactions to psychological stress and prediction of future blood pressure: data from the Whitehall II Study. BMJ 1995; 310(6982): 771-6.
[http://dx.doi.org/10.1136/bmj.310.6982.771] [PMID: 7711581]

[30] Chapman A, Mandryk JA, Frommer MS, Edye BV, Ferguson DA. Chronic perceived work stress and blood pressure among Australian government employees. Scand J Work Environ Health 1990; 16(4): 258-69.
[http://dx.doi.org/10.5271/sjweh.1786] [PMID: 2389133]

[31] Dryson EW, Scragg RKR, Metcalf PA, Baker JR. Stress at work: an evaluation of occupational stressors as reported by a multicultural New Zealand workforce. Int J Occup Environ Health 1996; 2(1): 18-25.
[http://dx.doi.org/10.1179/oeh.1996.2.1.18] [PMID: 9933861]

[32] Ducher M, Cerutti C, Chatellier G, Fauvel JP. Is high job strain associated with hypertension genesis? Am J Hypertens 2006; 19(7): 694-700.
[http://dx.doi.org/10.1016/j.amjhyper.2005.12.016] [PMID: 16814123]

[33] Markovitz JH, Matthews KA, Whooley M, Lewis CE, Greenlund KJ. Increases in job strain are associated with incident hypertension in the CARDIA Study. Ann Behav Med 2004; 28(1): 4-9.
[http://dx.doi.org/10.1207/s15324796abm2801_2] [PMID: 15249254]

[34] Matthews KA, Cottington EM, Talbott E, Kuller LH, Siegel JM. Stressful work conditions and

diastolic blood pressure among blue collar factory workers. Am J Epidemiol 1987; 126(2): 280-91.
[http://dx.doi.org/10.1093/aje/126.2.280] [PMID: 3605056]

[35] Murata K, Yano E, Shinozaki T. Cardiovascular dysfunction due to shift work. J Occup Environ Med 1999; 41(9): 748-53.
[http://dx.doi.org/10.1097/00043764-199909000-00006] [PMID: 10491790]

[36] Nomura K, Nakao M, Karita K, Nishikitani M, Yano E. Association between work-related psychological stress and arterial stiffness measured by brachial-ankle pulse-wave velocity in young Japanese males from an information service company. Scand J Work Environ Health 2005; 31(5): 352-9.
[http://dx.doi.org/10.5271/sjweh.918] [PMID: 16273961]

[37] Otsuka T, Kawada T, Ibuki C, Kusama Y. Relationship between job strain and radial arterial wave reflection in middle-aged male workers. Prev Med 2009; 49(2-3): 260-4.
[http://dx.doi.org/10.1016/j.ypmed.2009.07.005] [PMID: 19616573]

[38] Peter R, Alfredsson L, Hammar N, Siegrist J, Theorell T, Westerholm P. High effort, low reward, and cardiovascular risk factors in employed Swedish men and women: baseline results from the WOLF Study. J Epidemiol Community Health 1998; 52(9): 540-7.
[http://dx.doi.org/10.1136/jech.52.9.540] [PMID: 10320854]

[39] Peter R, Alfredsson L, Knutsson A, Siegrist J, Westerholm P. Does a stressful psychosocial work environment mediate the effects of shift work on cardiovascular risk factors? Scand J Work Environ Health 1999; 25(4): 376-81.
[http://dx.doi.org/10.5271/sjweh.448] [PMID: 10505664]

[40] Salavecz G, Chandola T, Pikhart H, *et al.* Work stress and health in Western European and post-communist countries: an East-West comparison study. J Epidemiol Community Health 2010; 64(1): 57-62.
[http://dx.doi.org/10.1136/jech.2008.075978] [PMID: 19692735]

[41] Schlussel YR, Schnall PL, Zimbler M, Warren K, Pickering TG. The effect of work environments on blood pressure: evidence from seven New York organizations. J Hypertens 1990; 8(7): 679-85.
[http://dx.doi.org/10.1097/00004872-199007000-00012] [PMID: 2168459]

[42] Theorell T, Perski A, Åkerstedt T, *et al.* Changes in job strain in relation to changes in physiological state. A longitudinal study. Scand J Work Environ Health 1988; 14(3): 189-96.
[http://dx.doi.org/10.5271/sjweh.1932] [PMID: 3393855]

[43] Tsutsumi A, Kayaba K, Tsutsumi K, Igarashi M. Association between job strain and prevalence of hypertension: a cross sectional analysis in a Japanese working population with a wide range of occupations: the Jichi Medical School cohort study. Occup Environ Med 2001; 58(6): 367-73.
[http://dx.doi.org/10.1136/oem.58.6.367] [PMID: 11351051]

[44] Uchiyama S, Kurasawa T, Sekizawa T, Nakatsuka H. Job strain and risk of cardiovascular events in treated hypertensive Japanese workers: hypertension follow-up group study. J Occup Health 2005; 47(2): 102-11.
[http://dx.doi.org/10.1539/joh.47.102] [PMID: 15824474]

[45] Cesana G, Ferrario M, Sega R, *et al.* Job strain and ambulatory blood pressure levels in a population-based employed sample of men from northern Italy. Scand J Work Environ Health 1996; 22(4): 294-305.
[http://dx.doi.org/10.5271/sjweh.144] [PMID: 8881018]

[46] Clays E, Leynen F, De Bacquer D, *et al.* High job strain and ambulatory blood pressure in middle-aged men and women from the Belgian job stress study. J Occup Environ Med 2007; 49(4): 360-7.
[http://dx.doi.org/10.1097/JOM.0b013e31803b94e2] [PMID: 17426519]

[47] Landsbergis PA, Schnall PL, Warren K, Pickering TG, Schwartz JE. Association between ambulatory blood pressure and alternative formulations of job strain. Scand J Work Environ Health 1994; 20(5): 349-63.

[http://dx.doi.org/10.5271/sjweh.1386] [PMID: 7863299]

[48]   Landsbergis PA, Schnall PL, Pickering TG, Schwartz JE. Validity and reliability of a work history questionnaire derived from the Job Content Questionnaire. J Occup Environ Med 2002; 44(11): 1037-47.
[http://dx.doi.org/10.1097/00043764-200211000-00010] [PMID: 12448355]

[49]   Light KC, Brownley KA, Turner JR, *et al.* Job status and high-effort coping influence work blood pressure in women and blacks. Hypertension 1995; 25(4 Pt 1): 554-9.
[http://dx.doi.org/10.1161/01.HYP.25.4.554] [PMID: 7721397]

[50]   Schnall PL, Schwartz JE, Landsbergis PA, Warren K, Pickering TG. A longitudinal study of job strain and ambulatory blood pressure: results from a three-year follow-up. Psychosom Med 1998; 60(6): 697-706.
[http://dx.doi.org/10.1097/00006842-199811000-00007] [PMID: 9847028]

[51]   Schnall PL, Pieper C, Schwartz JE, *et al.* The relationship between 'job strain,' workplace diastolic blood pressure, and left ventricular mass index. Results of a case-control study. JAMA 1990; 263(14): 1929-35.
[http://dx.doi.org/10.1001/jama.1990.03440140055031] [PMID: 2138234]

[52]   Steptoe A, Siegrist J, Kirschbaum C, Marmot M. Effort-reward imbalance, overcommitment, and measures of cortisol and blood pressure over the working day. Psychosom Med 2004; 66(3): 323-9.
[PMID: 15184690]

[53]   Schumann B, Seidler A, Kluttig A, Werdan K, Haerting J, Greiser KH. Association of occupation with prevalent hypertension in an elderly East German population: an exploratory cross-sectional analysis. Int Arch Occup Environ Health 2011; 84(4): 361-9.
[http://dx.doi.org/10.1007/s00420-010-0584-5] [PMID: 20957489]

[54]   Miklos WE. Occupation and Hypertension Awareness, Washington BRFSS 2003, 2005, 2007, and 2009 2013.

[55]   Djindjic N, Jovanovic J, Djindjic B, Jovanovic M, Jovanovic JJ. Associations between the occupational stress index and hypertension, type 2 diabetes mellitus, and lipid disorders in middle-aged men and women. Ann Occup Hyg 2012; 56(9): 1051-62.
[PMID: 22986427]

[56]   Davila EP, Kuklina EV, Valderrama AL, Yoon PW, Rolle I, Nsubuga P. Prevalence, management, and control of hypertension among US workers: does occupation matter? J Occup Environ Med 2012; 54(9): 1150-6.
[http://dx.doi.org/10.1097/JOM.0b013e318256f675] [PMID: 22885710]

[57]   Maksimov SA, Artamonova GV. Modeling of arterial hypertension's risk in occupational groups. Russian Open Medical Journal 2013; 2: 0104.
[http://dx.doi.org/10.15275/rusomj.2013.0104]

[58]   Leigh JP, Du J. Hypertension and occupation among seniors. J Occup Environ Med 2009; 51(6): 661-71.
[http://dx.doi.org/10.1097/JOM.0b013e31819f1d85] [PMID: 19415032]

[59]   Wiernik E, Pannier B, Czernichow S, *et al.* Occupational status moderates the association between current perceived stress and high blood pressure: evidence from the IPC cohort study. Hypertension 2013.
[http://dx.doi.org/10.1161/HYPERTENSIONAHA.111.00302]

[60]   Lim MS, Park B, Kong IG, *et al.* Leisure sedentary time is differentially associated with hypertension, diabetes mellitus, and hyperlipidemia depending on occupation. BMC Public Health 2017; 17(1): 278.
[http://dx.doi.org/10.1186/s12889-017-4192-0] [PMID: 28335768]

[61]   Landsbergis PA, Diez-Roux AV, Fujishiro K, *et al.* Job strain, occupational category, systolic blood pressure, and hypertension prevalence: The multi-ethnic study of atherosclerosis. J Occup Environ

Med 2015; 57(11): 1178-84.
[http://dx.doi.org/10.1097/JOM.0000000000000533] [PMID: 26539765]

[62] Butrón J, Colina-Chourio J. Efecto del ruido sobre la presión arterial en trabajadores de una empresa petrolera venezolana. Invest Clin 2010; 51: 301-14.

[63] Chor D, Faerstein E, Werneck GL, Lopes CS. Estresse no trabalho e hipertensão arterial em mulheres no Estudo Pró-Saúde: Estudo Pró-Saúde (Pro-Health Study). Rev Saude Publica 2009; 43: 893-6.
[http://dx.doi.org/10.1590/S0034-89102009000500019]

[64] Kaur H, Luckhaupt SE, Li J, Alterman T, Calvert GM. Workplace psychosocial factors associated with hypertension in the U.S. workforce: a cross-sectional study based on the 2010 national health interview survey. Am J Ind Med 2014; 57(9): 1011-21.
[http://dx.doi.org/10.1002/ajim.22345] [PMID: 25137617]

[65] Vinholes DB, Bassanesi SL, Chaves Junior HC, *et al.* Association of workplace and population characteristics with prevalence of hypertension among Brazilian industry workers: a multilevel analysis. BMJ Open 2017; 7(8)e015755
[http://dx.doi.org/10.1136/bmjopen-2016-015755] [PMID: 28827245]

[66] Landsbergis PA, Schnall PL, Pickering TG, Warren K, Schwartz JE. Lower socioeconomic status among men in relation to the association between job strain and blood pressure. Scand J Work Environ Health 2003; 29(3): 206-15.
[http://dx.doi.org/10.5271/sjweh.723] [PMID: 12828390]

[67] Bosu WK. Determinants of mean blood pressure and hypertension among workers in West Africa. Int J Hypertens 2016; 20163192149
[http://dx.doi.org/10.1155/2016/3192149] [PMID: 26949543]

[68] Heath RL, Browning SR, Reed DB. Prevalence and risk factors for hypertension among older Kentucky farmers. J Agromed 1999; 6: 43-58.
[http://dx.doi.org/10.1300/J096v06n01_05]

[69] Gold MR, Franks P. Farming: Primary prevention for hypertension? Effects of employment type on blood pressure. J Rural Health 1989; 5: 257-65.
[http://dx.doi.org/10.1111/j.1748-0361.1989.tb00986.x]

[70] Singh M, Kotwal A, Mittal C, Babu SR, Bharti S, Ram CVS. Prevalence and correlates of hypertension in a semi-rural population of Southern India. J Hum Hypertens 2017; 32(1): 66-74.
[http://dx.doi.org/10.1038/s41371-017-0010-5] [PMID: 29180803]

[71] Røvik JO, Tyssen R, Hem E, *et al.* Job stress in young physicians with an emphasis on the work-home interface: a nine-year, nationwide and longitudinal study of its course and predictors. Ind Health 2007; 45(5): 662-71.
[http://dx.doi.org/10.2486/indhealth.45.662] [PMID: 18057809]

[72] del Arco-Galán C, Súarez-Fernández C, Gabriel-Sánchez R. What happens to blood pressure when on-call? Am J Hypertens 1994; 7(5): 396-401.
[http://dx.doi.org/10.1093/ajh/7.5.396] [PMID: 8060571]

[73] Owolabi AO, Owolabi MO. OlaOlorun AD, Olofin A. Work-related stress perception and hypertension amongst health workers of a mission hospital in Oyo State, south-western Nigeria. Afr J Prim Health Care Fam Med 2012; 4: 1-7.
[http://dx.doi.org/10.4102/phcfm.v4i1.307]

[74] Mion D Jr, Pierin AM, Bambirra AP, *et al.* Hypertension in employees of a University General Hospital. Rev Hosp Clin Fac Med Sao Paulo 2004; 59(6): 329-36.
[http://dx.doi.org/10.1590/S0041-87812004000600004] [PMID: 15654485]

[75] Egbi OG, Rotifa S, Jumbo J. Prevalence of hypertension and its correlates among employees of a tertiary hospital in Yenagoa, Nigeria. Ann Afr Med 2015; 14(1): 8-17.
[http://dx.doi.org/10.4103/1596-3519.148709] [PMID: 25567690]

[76]   Fialho G, Cavichio L, Povoa R, Pimenta J. Effects of 24-h shift work in the emergency room on ambulatory blood pressure monitoring values of medical residents. Am J Hypertens 2006; 19(10): 1005-9.
[http://dx.doi.org/10.1016/j.amjhyper.2006.03.007] [PMID: 17027818]

[77]   Brodsky CM. Long-term work stress in teachers and prison guards. J Occup Med 1977; 19(2): 133-8.
[http://dx.doi.org/10.1097/00043764-197702000-00007] [PMID: 839288]

[78]   Deyanov C, Hadjiolova I, Mincheva L. Prevalence of arterial hypertension among school teachers in Sofia. Rev Environ Health 1994; 10(1): 47-50.
[http://dx.doi.org/10.1515/REVEH.1994.10.1.47] [PMID: 8029526]

[79]   Steptoe A, Cropley M. Persistent high job demands and reactivity to mental stress predict future ambulatory blood pressure. J Hypertens 2000; 18(5): 581-6.
[http://dx.doi.org/10.1097/00004872-200018050-00011] [PMID: 10826561]

[80]   Marques AC. Condições de saúde, estilo de vida e características de trabalho de professores de uma cidade do sul do Brasil. Cien Saude Colet 2013; 18: 837-46.
[http://dx.doi.org/10.1590/S1413-81232013000300029]

[81]   Cisneros Blas Y, Ramírez Sandoval MdLP. Prevalencia de enfermedades en trabajadores académicos de una universidad pública según seguro de gastos médicos. Salud de los Trabajadores 2009; 17: 121-31.

[82]   Pimenta AM, Kac G, Souza RRC, Ferreira LM, Silqueira SM. Night-shift work and cardiovascular risk among employees of a public university. Rev Assoc Med Bras (1992) 2012; 58(2): 168-77.
[http://dx.doi.org/10.1016/S0104-4230(12)70177-X] [PMID: 22569611]

[83]   Hayashi T, Kobayashi Y, Yamaoka K, Yano E. Effect of overtime work on 24-hour ambulatory blood pressure. J Occup Environ Med 1996; 38(10): 1007-11.
[http://dx.doi.org/10.1097/00043764-199610000-00010] [PMID: 8899576]

[84]   Lindquist TL, Beilin LJ, Knuiman MW. Influence of lifestyle, coping, and job stress on blood pressure in men and women. Hypertension 1997; 29(1 Pt 1): 1-7.
[http://dx.doi.org/10.1161/01.HYP.29.1.1] [PMID: 9039072]

[85]   Prunier-Poulmaire S, Gadbois C, Volkoff S. Combined effects of shift systems and work requirements on customs officers. Scand J Work Environ Health 1998; 24 (Suppl. 3): 134-40.
[PMID: 9916830]

[86]   Chor D. [High blood pressure among bank employees in Rio de Janeiro. Life-style and treatment]. Arq Bras Cardiol 1998; 71(5): 653-60. [High blood pressure among bank employees in Rio de Janeiro. Life-style and treatment].
[PMID: 10347947]

[87]   Vrijkotte TG, van Doornen LJ, de Geus EJ. Effects of work stress on ambulatory blood pressure, heart rate, and heart rate variability. Hypertension 2000; 35(4): 880-6.
[http://dx.doi.org/10.1161/01.HYP.35.4.880] [PMID: 10775555]

[88]   Nakanishi N, Yoshida H, Nagano K, Kawashimo H, Nakamura K, Tatara K. Long working hours and risk for hypertension in Japanese male white collar workers. J Epidemiol Community Health 2001; 55(5): 316-22.
[http://dx.doi.org/10.1136/jech.55.5.316] [PMID: 11297649]

[89]   Guimont C, Brisson C, Dagenais GR, *et al.* Effects of job strain on blood pressure: a prospective study of male and female white-collar workers. Am J Public Health 2006; 96(8): 1436-43.
[http://dx.doi.org/10.2105/AJPH.2004.057679] [PMID: 16809603]

[90]   Maroof KA, Parashar P, Bansal R, Ahmad S. A study on hypertension among the bank employees of Meerut district of Uttar Pradesh. Indian J Public Health 2007; 51(4): 225-7.
[PMID: 18232162]

[91]   Maina G, Bovenzi M, Palmas A, Larese Filon F. Associations between two job stress models and measures of salivary cortisol. Int Arch Occup Environ Health 2009; 82(9): 1141-50.
[http://dx.doi.org/10.1007/s00420-009-0439-0] [PMID: 19554345]

[92]   Trudel X, Brisson C, Milot A. Job strain and masked hypertension. Psychosom Med 2010; 72(8): 786-93.
[http://dx.doi.org/10.1097/PSY.0b013e3181eaf327] [PMID: 20639388]

[93]   Momin MH, Desai VK, Kavishwar AB. Study of socio-demographic factors affecting prevalence of hypertension among bank employees of Surat City. Indian J Public Health 2012; 56(1): 44-8.
[http://dx.doi.org/10.4103/0019-557X.96970] [PMID: 22684172]

[94]   Salaroli LB, Saliba RAD, Zandonade E, Molina MdelC, Bissoli NS. Prevalence of metabolic syndrome and related factors in bank employees according to different defining criteria, Vitória/ES, Brazil. Clinics (São Paulo) 2013; 68(1): 69-74.
[http://dx.doi.org/10.6061/clinics/2013(01)OA11] [PMID: 23420160]

[95]   Ismail I, Kulkarni A, Kamble S, Borker S, Rekha R, Amruth M. Prevalence of hypertension and its risk factors among bank employees of Sullia Taluk, Karnataka. Sahel Medical Journal 2013; 16: 139-43.
[http://dx.doi.org/10.4103/1118-8561.125553]

[96]   Ganesh Kumar S, Deivanai Sundaram N. Prevalence and risk factors of hypertension among bank employees in urban Puducherry, India. Int J Occup Environ Med 2014; 5(2): 94-100.
[PMID: 24748000]

[97]   Diwe K, Enwere O, Uwakwe K, Duru C, Chineke H. Prevalence and awareness of hypertension and associated risk factors among bank workers in Owerri, Nigeria. Int J Med Biomed Res 2015; 4: 142-8.
[http://dx.doi.org/10.14194/ijmbr.4.3.5]

[98]   Fikadu G, Lemma S. Socioeconomic status and hypertension among teachers and bankers in addis ababa, Ethiopia. Int J Hypertens 2016; 20164143962
[http://dx.doi.org/10.1155/2016/4143962] [PMID: 27313874]

[99]   Brahmankar TR, Prabhu PM. Prevalence and risk factors of hypertension among the bank employees of Western Maharashtra–a cross sectional study. International Journal Of Community Medicine And Public Health 2017; 4: 1267-77.
[http://dx.doi.org/10.18203/2394-6040.ijcmph20171361]

[100]   Kang MG, Koh SB, Cha BS, Park JK, Baik SK, Chang SJ. Job stress and cardiovascular risk factors in male workers. Prev Med 2005; 40(5): 583-8.
[http://dx.doi.org/10.1016/j.ypmed.2004.07.018] [PMID: 15749142]

[101]   Kawakami N, Haratani T, Kaneko T, Araki S. Perceived job-stress and blood pressure increase among Japanese blue collar workers: one-year follow-up study. Ind Health 1989; 27(2): 71-81.
[http://dx.doi.org/10.2486/indhealth.27.71] [PMID: 2745163]

[102]   Ragland DR, Winkleby MA, Schwalbe J, *et al.* Prevalence of hypertension in bus drivers. Int J Epidemiol 1987; 16(2): 208-14.
[http://dx.doi.org/10.1093/ije/16.2.208] [PMID: 3497118]

[103]   Jayarajah U, Jayakody AJ, Jayaneth JM, Wijeratne S. Prevalence of hypertension and its associated factors among a group of bus drivers in Colombo, Sri Lanka. The international journal of occupational and environmental medicine 2017; 8: 986-58-9.

[104]   Lakshman A, Manikath N, Rahim A, Anilakumari V. Prevalence and risk factors of hypertension among male occupational bus drivers in North Kerala, South India: A Cross-sectional Study. ISRN preventive medicine 2014 2014.

[105]   Albright CL, Winkleby MA, Ragland DR, Fisher J, Syme SL. Job strain and prevalence of hypertension in a biracial population of urban bus drivers. Am J Public Health 1992; 82(7): 984-9.
[http://dx.doi.org/10.2105/AJPH.82.7.984] [PMID: 1609917]

[106] Biglari H, Ebrahimi MH, Salehi M, Poursadeghiyan M, Ahmadnezhad I, Abbasi M. Relationship between occupational stress and cardiovascular diseases risk factors in drivers. Int J Occup Med Environ Health 2016; 29(6): 895-901.
[http://dx.doi.org/10.13075/ijomeh.1896.00125] [PMID: 27869240]

[107] Taklikar C. Occupational stress and its associated health disorders among bus drivers. International Journal Of Community Medicine And Public Health 2017; 3: 208-11.

[108] Chankaramangalam MA, Ramamoorthy V, Muthuraja D, An P, Saravanan E. Factors associated with hypertension among truck drivers: A cross sectional study at a check post on a national highway in South India. Int J Med Res Health Sci 2017; 6: 126-9.

[109] Stoohs RA, Guilleminault C, Dement WC. Sleep apnea and hypertension in commercial truck drivers. Sleep 1993; 16(8 Suppl): S11-3.

[110] Sangaleti CT, Trincaus MR, Baratieri T, *et al.* Prevalence of cardiovascular risk factors among truck drivers in the South of Brazil. BMC Public Health 2014; 14: 1063.
[http://dx.doi.org/10.1186/1471-2458-14-1063] [PMID: 25304259]

[111] Belkić K, Schnall P, Landsbergis P, Baker D. The workplace and cardiovascular health: conclusions and thoughts for a future agenda. Occup Med 2000; 15(1): 307-321, v-vi. [v-vi.].
[PMID: 10702092]

[112] Ragland DR, Winkleby MA, Schwalbe J, *et al.* Prevalence of hypertension in bus drivers. AAOHN J 1989; 37(2): 71-8.
[http://dx.doi.org/10.1177/216507998903700204] [PMID: 2914031]

[113] Friedman R, Schwartz JE, Schnall PL, *et al.* Psychological variables in hypertension: relationship to casual or ambulatory blood pressure in men. Psychosom Med 2001; 63(1): 19-31.
[http://dx.doi.org/10.1097/00006842-200101000-00003] [PMID: 11211061]

[114] Göbel M, Springer J, Scherff J. Stress and strain of short haul bus drivers: psychophysiology as a design oriented method for analysis. Ergonomics 1998; 41(5): 563-80.
[http://dx.doi.org/10.1080/001401398186757] [PMID: 9613219]

[115] Rydstedt LW, Johansson G, Evans GW. The human side of the road: improving the working conditions of urban bus drivers. J Occup Health Psychol 1998; 3(2): 161-71.
[http://dx.doi.org/10.1037/1076-8998.3.2.161] [PMID: 9585915]

[116] Kales SN, Tsismenakis AJ, Zhang C, Soteriades ES. Blood pressure in firefighters, police officers, and other emergency responders. Am J Hypertens 2009; 22(1): 11-20.
[http://dx.doi.org/10.1038/ajh.2008.296] [PMID: 18927545]

[117] Goldberg P, David S, Landre MF, Goldberg M, Dassa S, Fuhrer R. Work conditions and mental health among prison staff in France. Scand J Work Environ Health 1996; 22(1): 45-54.
[http://dx.doi.org/10.5271/sjweh.108] [PMID: 8685673]

[118] Sega R, Cesana G, Costa G, Ferrario M, Bombelli M, Mancia G. Ambulatory blood pressure in air traffic controllers. Am J Hypertens 1998; 11(2): 208-12.
[http://dx.doi.org/10.1016/S0895-7061(97)00321-X] [PMID: 9524050]

[119] Wirth M, Burch J, Violanti J, *et al.* Shiftwork duration and the awakening cortisol response among police officers. Chronobiol Int 2011; 28(5): 446-57.
[http://dx.doi.org/10.3109/07420528.2011.573112] [PMID: 21721860]

[120] Violanti JM, Fekedulegn D, Hartley TA, *et al.* Police trauma and cardiovascular disease: association between PTSD symptoms and metabolic syndrome. Int J Emerg Ment Health 2006; 8(4): 227-37.
[PMID: 17131769]

[121] Bishop GD, Enkelmann HC, Tong EM, *et al.* Job demands, decisional control, and cardiovascular responses. J Occup Health Psychol 2003; 8(2): 146-56.
[http://dx.doi.org/10.1037/1076-8998.8.2.146] [PMID: 12703880]

[122] Tomei F, De Sio S, Tomao E, *et al.* Occupational exposure to noise and hypertension in pilots. Int J Environ Health Res 2005; 15(2): 99-106.
[http://dx.doi.org/10.1080/09603120500061534] [PMID: 16026021]

[123] Tomei G, Sancini A, Tomei F, *et al.* Prevalence of systemic arterial hypertension, electrocardiogram abnormalities, and noise-induced hearing loss in agricultural workers. Arch Environ Occup Health 2013; 68(4): 196-203.
[http://dx.doi.org/10.1080/19338244.2012.701245] [PMID: 23697692]

[124] Choi B, Schnall PL, Yang H, *et al.* Psychosocial working conditions and active leisure-time physical activity in middle-aged us workers. Int J Occup Med Environ Health 2010; 23(3): 239-53.
[http://dx.doi.org/10.2478/v10001-010-0029-0] [PMID: 20934957]

[125] Lucini D, Riva S, Pizzinelli P, Pagani M. Stress management at the worksite: reversal of symptoms profile and cardiovascular dysregulation. Hypertension 2007; 49(2): 291-7.
[http://dx.doi.org/10.1161/01.HYP.0000255034.42285.58] [PMID: 17210835]

CHAPTER 3

Antihypertensive Drug Interactions

Cigdem Usul Afsar[1] and **Sibel Ozyazgan**[2,*]

[1] *Department of Internal Medicine and Medical Oncology, Acıbadem Mehmet Ali Aydınlar University Medical Faculty, Istanbul, Turkey*

[2] *Department of Pharmacology and Clinical Pharmacology, Istanbul University, Cerrahpasa Medical Faculty, Istanbul, Turkey*

Abstract: Systemic hypertension is a chronic disease which results in complications such as heart failure, renal failure or stroke. Polypharmacy is getting more important in this population. There are many mechanisms by which drugs may interact, mostly pharmacokinetic (absorption, distribution, metabolism, and elimination) or pharmacodynamic, or additive toxicity. Absorption of drugs can be affected by foods, antacids and antidiarrhoeals.

Distribution of the drugs can be changed by the volumetric status of the body and binding of drugs to proteins such as p-glycoproteins.

The most important class of drug interactions involves the cytochrome P450 (CYP) microsomal enzyme system, which metabolizes a variety of drugs and herbal products. Cytochrome P450 enzymes metabolize approximately 60% of prescribed drugs, with CYP3A4 responsible for about half of this metabolism.

Diuretics are renally eliminated and more vulnerable to drug interactions which take place in the kidney. Probenecid, nonselective nonsteroidal antiinflammatory drugs (NSAIDs), beta-lactam antibiotics, valproic acid, methotrexate, cimetidine and antivirals decrease the tubular secretion of loop diuretics from the proximal tubulus.

Pharmacodynamic interactions between similarly acting drugs may lead to additive or even over-additive effects (potentiation). A good example for antihypertensive drugs is the combination of intravenous verapamil and a β-blocker, which may cause additive impairment and increase the risk of A-V (atrio-ventricular) block.

The interaction of antihypertensives and NSAIDs is another important type of interaction. In this chapter, we mentioned all the interactions of antihypertensive agents through kinetic and dynamic ways.

* **Corresponding author Sibel Ozyazgan:** Department of Pharmacology and Clinical Pharmacology, Istanbul University, Cerrahpasa Medical Faculty, Istanbul, Turkey; Tel: +90-212-4143000; Fax: +90-212-6320050; E-mail: ozyazgans@yahoo.com

Hafize Uzun & Pınar Atukeren (Eds.)

Keywords: Systemic hypertension, Polypharmacy, Pharmacokinetic, Absorption, Distribution, Elimination, Pharmacodynamic, Additive toxicity, Antidiarrhoeals, Pharmacokinetic interactions, Cytochrome P450, Losartan, Kinins, Eplerenone, Propranolol, Bioavailability, Antihypertensives, Diuretics, Digoxin, Renin inhibitors.

INTRODUCTION

Systemic hypertension is a chronic disease which results in complications such as heart failure, renal failure or stroke [1]. Due to these complications, hypertensive patients generally use multiple dugs. Polypharmacy is becoming more important in this population. Side effects of drugs increase and their efficacy get lower according to drug interactions. There are several factors which augment the frequency of drug interactions. Polypharmacy, older age, comorbidities, pharmacokinetic and pharmacodynamic interactions, narrow therapeutic index of some drugs are the most disputed subjects. The potential for drug-drug interactions increases with rising age, since elderly patients receive larger number of drugs, but also because the renal excretion of several therapeutic agents is impaired in the elderly, as a result of diminishing kidney function [2, 3].

There are many mechanisms by which drugs may interact, mostly pharmacokinetic (absorption, distribution, metabolism, and elimination) or pharmacodynamic, or additive toxicity [4 - 6].

Pharmacokinetic Interactions

Absorption of drugs can be affected by foods, antacids and antidiarrhoeals. Advising patients to remove the grapefruit juice and hesperidine (a flavonoid of orange juice) from their diet when treated with these drugs is very important. Peppermint oil, salty diet, vitamin C and grayonotoxin of the honey made by rhododendron genius can also influence the bioavailability of antihypertensives [7]. Vitamin C reduces the bioavailability of propranolol but the extent is too small to be of clinical significance [7]. Distribution of the drugs can be changed by the volumetric status of the body and binding of drugs to proteins such as p-glycoproteins. For example, diltiazem increases the levels of serum propranolol levels by 50% extent with binding to these proteins [4]. The most important class of drug interactions involves the cytochrome P450 (CYP) microsomal enzyme system, which metabolizes a variety of drugs and herbal products [8]. A potential for interactions with these enzymes exists with calcium channel blockers, β-adrenergic blocking agents, angiotensin-converting enzyme inhibitors, and angiotensin receptor blockers [8]. Cytochrome P450 enzymes metabolize approximately 60% of prescribed drugs, with CYP3A4 responsible for about half of this metabolism. Antihypertensive substrates of CYP3A4 are diltiazem, verapamil, nifedipine and other calcium channel blockers, losartan, some kinins (vasodilators), eplerenone (aldosterone antagonist) and propranolol (β-blocker). We summarized the inducers and inhibitos of CYP3A4 in Table **1**. Diuretics are renally eliminated and more vulnerable to drug interactions which take place in the kidney [8].

Probenecid, nonselective nonsteroidal antiinflammatory drugs (NSAIDs), beta-lactam antibiotics, valproic acid, methotrexate, cimetidine and antivirals decrease the tubular secretion of loop diuretics from the proximal tubulus [8].

Table 1. Inducers/enhancers and inhibitors of CYP3A4.

CYP 3A4 Enhancers/Inducers
Rifampicin
Alcohol
Phenobarbital
Phenytoin sodium
Carbamazepine
CYP 3A4 Inhibitors
Some antifungals (ketoconazole, itraconazole)
Protease inhibitors (ritonavir, indinavir, etc)
Grapefruit juice
Cimetidine hydrochloride
Some macrolide antibiotics (clarithromycin, erythromycin, telithromycin) and chloramphenicol
Some antidepressants (nefazodone)
Diltiazem hydrochloride
Verapamil hydrochloride
Aprepitant

In particular, CYP2D6 is responsible for the metabolism and elimination of approximately 25% of clinically used drugs. Most β-blockers (propranolol, metoprolol, timolol, carvedilol, nebivolol), debrisoquine are substrates of CYP2D6. The only strong inducer of CYP2D6 is glutethimide. Inhibitors are some SSRIs (fluoxetine, paroxetine, sertraline) and ritonavir [9].

Some therapeutic drugs are metabolized by CYP2C9, including drugs with a narrow therapeutic index such as warfarin and phenytoin and other routinely prescribed drugs such as acenocoumarol, tolbutamide, losartan, glipizide, and some nonsteroidal anti-inflammatory drugs [9]. Rifampicin and phenobarbital are inducers of 2C9 and fluconazole, some statins, cimetidine and amiodarone are examples of inhibitors [10].

Propranolol is the antihypertensive drug substrate of CYP2C19. Some inhibitors of CYP2C19 are fluconazole, chloramphenicol and fluoxetine. There is no strong inducer for CYP2C19 [11].

Certain drugs may impair the renal excretion of other agents, usually at the renal tubular level. Thiazide diuretics may decelerate the renal elimination of lithium salts and reinforce their toxicity [4 - 6].

Pharmacodynamic Interactions

This kind of interaction is more frequent but it is very difficult to measure and mechanisms are not well defined. Pharmacodynamic interactions between similarly acting drugs may lead to additive or even over-additive effects (potentiation). A good example for antihypertensive drugs is the combination of intravenous verapamil and a β-blocker, which may cause additive impairment and increase the risk of A-V block [12]. Another example of this interaction is the inhibition of the therapeutic effect of a drug by an additional agent [12]. Drugs suppressing the activity of the central nervous system increases the side effects of centrally acting antihypertensives [4 - 6].

Another topic that should be discussed is the interaction of antihypertensives and NSAIDs [13]. They can raise the blood pressure and worsen control of hypertension as a result of sodium and fluid retention as well as of decreased formation of vasodilatory prostaglandins in patients already being treated [13]. Nonselective NSAIDs should be used with caution and should be used at the lowest effective dose and for the shortest duration. If blood pressure becomes elevated while using NSAIDs, discontinuing or reducing the dose of the NSAID is generally preferred [14]. It is well-studied about acetaminophen. Aspirin, in low dose that is used as an antithrombotic agent, does not affect blood pressure or interfere with the efficacy of antihypertensive drugs [15]. It is important for patients to limit their sodium intake, monitor their blood pressure frequently and monitor their renal function after NSAIDs are initiated and when their doses are increased [16].

Drug Interactions of Antihypertensive Drugs, Classified According to Drug Class

A. Alpha Blockers (Table 2)

Table 2. The interactions of other antihypertensive drugs with alpha blockers.

Alpha Blockers and ACEI (*e.g.*; Enalapril and Bunazosin) [17]	Severe first-dose hypotension, and synergistic hypotensive effects
Alpha Blockers and Beta Blockers (*e.g.*; Prazosin) [18]	First-dose hypotension (sequential management in patients with pheochromocytoma is important)
Alpha Blockers and Calcium Channel Blockers [19]	Blood pressure may fall sharply, increase in the AUC (Area Under Curve)
Alpha Blockers and Diuretics [20]	Additive hypotensive effect, but aside from first dose hypotension (caution for congestive heart failure patients)

B. Beta Blockers (Table 3)

Table 3. The interactions of other antihypertensive drugs with beta blockers.

Beta Blockers and Calcium Channel Blockers (Dihydropyridines) [20]	Severe hypotension and heart failure
Beta Blockers and Calcium Channel Blockers (Diltiazem) [21]	Serious and potentially life-threatening bradycardia
Beta Blockers and Calcium Channel Blockers (Verapamil) [22]	Serious cardiodepression (bradycardia, asystole, sinus arrest); also with eye drops
Beta Blockers and Potassium-Depleting Diuretics [23]	Life-threatening torsade de pointes arrhythmias

C. Calcium Channel Blockers (Table 4)

Table 4. The interactions of other antihypertensive drugs with calcium channel blockers.

Calcium Channel Blockers and Calcium Channel Blockers [24]	Intestinal occlusion attributed to the concurrent use of nifedipine and diltiazem, blood pressure reduction
Calcium Channel Blockers and Clonidine [25]	Complete heart block
Calcium Channel Blockers and Diuretics [26]	Additive antihypertensive effects

D. Angiotensin Converting Enzyme İnhibitors (ACEI) and Angiotensin II (AT-II) Receptor Antagonists (Table 5)

Table 5. The interactions of other antihypertensive drugs with ACEI and AT-II antagonists.

ACEI and Angiotensin II Receptor Antagonists [27]	Increases the risk of hypotension, renal impairment and hyperkalemia in patients with heart failure
ACEI and Beta Blockers [28]	Enhanced blood pressure-lowering effects
ACEI and Calcium Channel Blockers [29]	No clinically significant pharmacokinetic interactions
ACEI and Diuretics [30-32]	First dose hypotension (dizziness, light headedness, fainting), renal impairment, n deven acute renal failure, diuretic-induced hypokalaemia
ACEI and Orlistat [33]	Hypertensive crises and intracranial haemorrhage
AT-II Antagonists and Beta Blockers [34]	Enhances the hypotensive effects
AT-II and Calcium Channel İnhibitors [35]	None
AT-II and Diuretics [36, 37]	Symptomatic hypotension, potassium levels may be either increased, decreased or not affected, bioavailability of hydrochlorothiazide may be modestly reduced

E. Diuretics

To give an example; thiazid diuretics can interact with digoxin and according to hypokalemia digoxin can become very toxic. Thiazides can impair the renal excretion of lithium ions and these ions can accumulate [12].

F. Renin Inhibitors

When administered with an ACEI, aliskiren can produce hyperkalemia, especially in diabetic patients [38].

G. Centrally Acting Antihypertensives

Fe^{+2} ions changes the enteral absorption of α-methyl-DOPA and reduces antihypertensive actions of it. Clonidine and tricyclic antidepressants affect at the same central α2-adrenoceptors [12].

CONCLUSION/FUTURE PERSPECTIVES

Polypharmacy is getting more important in hypertensive patients. Pharmacokinetic (absorption, distribution, metabolism, and elimination) and pharmacodynamic interactions are myriad frequent. As these population lives longer with new therapies, it is now more substantial to define interactions and warn the patients accurately during the use of different kinds of drugs together.

CONSENT FOR PUBLICATION

Not applicable.

CONFLICT OF INTEREST

The authors declare no conflict of interest, financial or otherwise.

ACKNOWLEDGEMENT

Declare none.

REFERENCES

[1]   Smith BE, Madigan VM. Understanding the haemodynamics of hypertension. Curr Hypertens Rep 2018; 20(4): 29.
        [http://dx.doi.org/10.1007/s11906-018-0832-8] [PMID: 29637390]

[2]   Popplewell PY, Henschke PJ. Acute admissions to a geriatric assessment unit. Med J Aust 1982; 1(8): 343-4.
        [PMID: 6806588]

[3]   Williamson J, Chopin JM. Adverse reactions to prescribed drugs in the elderly: a multicentre investigation. Age Ageing 1980; 9(2): 73-80.
        [http://dx.doi.org/10.1093/ageing/9.2.73] [PMID: 7395657]

[4]   Katzung BG. Hansten PhD. Important drug interactions.Basic and clinical pharmacology. 5th ed. Englewood Cliffs, NJ, USA: Prentice-Hall Int 1992; pp. 931-42.

[5]   Stockley IH. Drug interactions. 5th ed., London: Pharmaceutical Press 1999.

[6]   Opie LH. Cardiovascular drug interactions.Cardiovascular drug therapy. 2nd ed. Philadelphia, USA: W.B. Saunders Company 1996; pp. 347-53.

[7]   Jáuregui-Garrido B, Jáuregui-Lobera I. Interactions between antihypertensive drugs and food. Nutr Hosp 2012; 27(6): 1866-75.
        [PMID: 23588433]

[8]   Flockhart DA, Tanus-Santos JE. Implications of cytochrome P450 interactions when prescribing medication for hypertension. Arch Intern Med 2002; 162(4): 405-12.
        [http://dx.doi.org/10.1001/archinte.162.4.405] [PMID: 11863472]

[9]   Teh LK, Bertilsson L. Pharmacogenomics of CYP2D6: molecular genetics, interethnic differences and clinical importance. Drug Metab Pharmacokinet 2012; 27(1). 55-67.
        [http://dx.doi.org/10.2133/dmpk.DMPK-11-RV-121] [PMID: 22185816]

[10]   Rettie AE, Jones JP. Clinical and toxicological relevance of CYP2C9: drug-drug interactions and pharmacogenetics. Annu Rev Pharmacol Toxicol 2005; 45: 477-94.
        [http://dx.doi.org/10.1146/annurev.pharmtox.45.120403.095821] [PMID: 15822186]

[11]   Desta Z, Zhao X, Shin JG, Flockhart DA. Clinical significance of the cytochrome P450 2C19 genetic polymorphism. Clin Pharmacokinet 2002; 41(12): 913-58.

[http://dx.doi.org/10.2165/00003088-200241120-00002] [PMID: 12222994]

[12] van Zwieten PA, Farsang C. Interactions between antihypertensive agents and other drugs. Blood Press 2003; 12(5-6): 351-2.
[PMID: 14763670]

[13] Beilin LJ. Non-steroidal anti-inflammatory drugs and antihypertensive drug therapy. J Hypertens 2002; 20(5): 849-50.
[http://dx.doi.org/10.1097/00004872-200205000-00017] [PMID: 12011643]

[14] Chiam E, Weinberg L, Bailey M, McNicol L, Bellomo R. The haemodynamic effects of intravenous paracetamol (acetaminophen) in healthy volunteers: a double-blind, randomized, triple crossover trial. Br J Clin Pharmacol 2016; 81(4): 605-12.
[http://dx.doi.org/10.1111/bcp.12841] [PMID: 26606263]

[15] Chalmers JP, West MJ, Wing LM, Bune AJ, Graham JR. Effects of indomethacin, sulindac, naproxen, aspirin, and paracetamol in treated hypertensive patients. Clin Exp Hypertens A 1984; 6(6): 1077-93.
[http://dx.doi.org/10.3109/10641968409039582] [PMID: 6378437]

[16] Chan AT, Manson JE, Albert CM, *et al.* Nonsteroidal antiinflammatory drugs, acetaminophen, and the risk of cardiovascular events. Circulation 2006; 113(12): 1578-87.
[http://dx.doi.org/10.1161/CIRCULATIONAHA.105.595793] [PMID: 16534006]

[17] Baba T, Tomiyama T, Takebe K. Enhancement by an ACE inhibitor of first-dose hypotension caused by an alpha 1-blocker. N Engl J Med 1990; 322(17): 1237.
[http://dx.doi.org/10.1056/NEJM199004263221715] [PMID: 1970122]

[18] Elliott HL, McLean K, Sumner DJ, Meredith PA, Reid JL. Immediate cardiovascular responses to oral prazosin--effects of concurrent β-blockers. Clin Pharmacol Ther 1981; 29(3): 303-9.
[http://dx.doi.org/10.1038/clpt.1981.40] [PMID: 6110503]

[19] Donnelly R, Elliott HL, Meredith PA, Howie CA, Reid JL. The pharmacodynamics and pharmacokinetics of the combination of nifedipine and doxazosin. Eur J Clin Pharmacol 1993; 44(3): 279-82.
[http://dx.doi.org/10.1007/BF00271372] [PMID: 8491245]

[20] Gangji D, Juvent M, Niset G, *et al.* Study of the influence of nifedipine on the pharmacokinetics and pharmacodynamics of propranolol, metoprolol and atenolol. Br J Clin Pharmacol 1984; 17 (Suppl. 1): 29S-35S.
[http://dx.doi.org/10.1111/j.1365-2125.1984.tb02425.x] [PMID: 6146337]

[21] Sagie A, Strasberg B, Kusnieck J, Sclarovsky S. Symptomatic bradycardia induced by the combination of oral diltiazem and beta blockers. Clin Cardiol 1991; 14(4): 314-6.
[http://dx.doi.org/10.1002/clc.4960140406] [PMID: 1674455]

[22] Sakurai H, Kei M, Matsubara K, *et al.* Cardiogenic shock triggered by verapamil and atenolol: a case report of therapeutic experience with intravenous calcium. Jpn Circ J 2000; 64(11): 893-6.
[http://dx.doi.org/10.1253/jcj.64.893] [PMID: 11110438]

[23] Tan HH, Hsu LF, Kam RML, Chua T, Teo WS. A case series of sotalol-induced torsade de pointes in patients with atrial fibrillation--a tale with a twist. Ann Acad Med Singapore 2003; 32(3): 403-7.
[PMID: 12854385]

[24] Harada T, Ohtaki E, Sumiyoshi T, Hosoda S. Paralytic ileus induced by the combined use of nifedipine and diltiazem in the treatment of vasospastic angina. Cardiology 2002; 97(2): 113-4.
[http://dx.doi.org/10.1159/000057683] [PMID: 11978960]

[25] Jaffe R, Livshits T, Bursztyn M. Adverse interaction between clonidine and verapamil. Ann Pharmacother 1994; 28(7-8): 881-3.
[http://dx.doi.org/10.1177/106002809402800712] [PMID: 7949506]

[26] Weir SJ, Dimmitt DC, Lanman RC, Morrill MB, Geising DH. Steady-state pharmacokinetics of diltiazem and hydrochlorothiazide administered alone and in combination. Biopharm Drug Dispos

1998; 19(6): 365-71.
[http://dx.doi.org/10.1002/(SICI)1099-081X(199809)19:6<365::AID-BDD112>3.0.CO;2-R] [PMID: 9737817]

[27]   McMurray JJV, Östergren J, Swedberg K, *et al.* Effects of candesartan in patients with chronic heart failure and reduced left-ventricular systolic function taking angiotensin-converting-enzyme inhibitors: the CHARM-Added trial. Lancet 2003; 362(9386): 767-71.
[http://dx.doi.org/10.1016/S0140-6736(03)14283-3] [PMID: 13678869]

[28]   Wing LMH, Chalmers JP, West MJ, *et al.* Enalapril and atenolol in essential hypertension: attenuation of hypotensive effects in combination. Clin Exp Hypertens A 1988; 10(1): 119-33.
[http://dx.doi.org/10.3109/10641968809046803] [PMID: 2832102]

[29]   Sun JX, Cipriano A, Chan K, John VA. Pharmacokinetic interaction study between benazepril and amlodipine in healthy subjects. Eur J Clin Pharmacol 1994; 47(3): 285-9.
[http://dx.doi.org/10.1007/BF02570510] [PMID: 7867683]

[30]   Haïat R, Piot O, Gallois H, Hanania G. Blood pressure response to the first 36 hours of heart failure therapy with perindopril versus captopril. J Cardiovasc Pharmacol 1999; 33(6): 953-9.
[http://dx.doi.org/10.1097/00005344-199906000-00017] [PMID: 10367600]

[31]   Nilsen OG, Sellevold OFM, Romfo OS, *et al.* Pharmacokinetics and effects on renal function following cilazapril and hydrochlorothiazide alone and in combination in healthy subjects and hypertensive patients. Br J Clin Pharmacol 1989; 27 (Suppl. 2): 323S-8S.
[http://dx.doi.org/10.1111/j.1365-2125.1989.tb03499.x] [PMID: 2527546]

[32]   D'Costa DF, Basu SK, Gunasekera NPR. ACE inhibitors and diuretics causing hypokalaemia. Br J Clin Pract 1990; 44(1): 26-7.
[PMID: 2317435]

[33]   Valescia ME, Malgor LA, Farías EF, Figueras A, Laporte J-R. Interaction between orlistat and antihypertensive drugs. Ann Pharmacother 2001; 35(11): 1495-6.
[http://dx.doi.org/10.1345/aph.10346] [PMID: 11724110]

[34]   Czendlik CH, Sioufi A, Preiswerk G, Howald H. Pharmacokinetic and pharmacodynamic interaction of single doses of valsartan and atenolol. Eur J Clin Pharmacol 1997; 52(6): 451-9.
[http://dx.doi.org/10.1007/s002280050318] [PMID: 9342580]

[35]   Stangier J, Su C-APF. Pharmacokinetics of repeated oral doses of amlodipine and amlodipine plus telmisartan in healthy volunteers. J Clin Pharmacol 2000; 40(12 Pt 1): 1347-54.
[PMID: 11185633]

[36]   MacKay JH, Arcuri KE, Goldberg AI, Snapinn SM, Sweet CS. Losartan and low-dose hydrochlorothiazide in patients with essential hypertension. A double-blind, placebo-controlled trial of concomitant administration compared with individual components. Arch Intern Med 1996; 156(3): 278-85.
[http://dx.doi.org/10.1001/archinte.1996.00440030072009] [PMID: 8572837]

[37]   Wrenger E, Müller R, Moesenthin M, Welte T, Frölich JC, Neumann KH. Interaction of spironolactone with ACE inhibitors or angiotensin receptor blockers: analysis of 44 cases. BMJ 2003; 327(7407): 147-9.
[http://dx.doi.org/10.1136/bmj.327.7407.147] [PMID: 12869459]

[38]   Fu S, Wen X, Han F, Long Y, Xu G. Aliskiren therapy in hypertension and cardiovascular disease: a systematic review and a meta-analysis. Oncotarget 2017; 8(51): 89364-74.
[http://dx.doi.org/10.18632/oncotarget.19382] [PMID: 29179525]

CHAPTER 4

Pulmonary Hypertension

Pelin Uysal[1] and **Hafize Uzun**[2,*]

[1] *Department of Chest Diseases, Faculty of Medicine, Mehmet Ali Aydınlar University, Atakent Hospital, Istanbul, Turkey*

[2] *Department of Medical Biochemistry, Cerrahpaşa Faculty of Medicine, Istanbul University-Cerrahpasa, Istanbul, Turkey*

Abstract: Pulmonary hypertension (PH) is a hemodynamic and pathophysiological condition defined as right pulmonary artery pressure (PAP) determined by right heart catheterizatition (RHC) at rest, at 25 mm Hg or higher. RHC and vasoreactivity test are the gold standard methods for diagnosis, treatment and prognosis follow-up of PH. Each group has different physiopathological features. Three main features that outstand in pulmonary artery are vasoconstriction, remodeling of arterial wall and in situ thrombosis. A wide variety of biomarkers have been explored, although there is no specific marker for PH. Patients were stratified according to pathophysiological, hemodynamical features, clinical pictures and form of treatment. Differential diagnosis of PH might be difficult because of its non-specific symptoms and it might be caused by many different disorders. Exertional dyspnea disproportional with underlying cause should be warning. Findings on physical examination are related with underlying disease. Treatment of the underlying disease is important. In patients with positive vasoreactivity test might benefit from calcium channel blockers. In patients with poor prognosis, treatment with a combination protocol involves intravenous (IV) treatment. Many combination treatments are used or developing at the present time. PAH is rare and often diagnosed late. Novel circulating biomarkers could contribute to the screening of PH. Different biomarkers may lead to different relevant information in PH patients, including disease progression, response to medical and surgical therapy, and prognosis. This chapter presents an update on alterations in the diagnostic algorithm, haemodynamic definitions, biomarkers, treatment and prognose in PH. A multiparametric approach is usually preferred because PH is more of a systemic condition than an isolated cardiorespiratory illness.

Keyword: Pulmonary hypertension, Walking test, Artery pressure, Pulmonary artery, Hypoxia, Vasoconstriction, Remodeling, Arterial wall, Thrombosis, Catheterization, Diagnostic algorithm, Haemodynamic definitions, Veno-occlusive disease, Treatment, Prognose, Biomarkers, Serotonin, Endotelin-1, Thromboxane, Natriuretic peptides.

---

* **Corresponding author Hafize Uzun:** Department of Medical Biochemistry, Cerrahpaşa Faculty of Medicine, Istanbul University-Cerrahpasa Istanbul, Turkey; Tel: +902124143056; Fax: +902126332987; E-mail: huzun59@hotmail.com

INTRODUCTION

According to Pulmonary Hypertension (PH) guidelines which were jointly provided by European Society of Cardiology and European Respiratory Society (ESC/ERS) in 2015, PH is defined as a physiopathological disorder that involves more than one clinical picture and may further complicate most of cardiovascular and respiratory system diseases [1]. Normally, mean pulmonary artery pressure (PAPm) at rest is 14±3 mmHg with an upper limit of normal of approximately 20 mmHg and pulmonary vascular resistance (PVR) is 2.0 Woods units (WU). To hemodynamically state diagnose of patient as PH, PAPm which is measured at rest with RHC should be 25 mmHg or higher and PVR should be 3.0 WU or higher. While PAP is 25 mmHg and higher; if a pulmonary artery wedge pressure (PAWP) is 15 mmHg or lower diagnosis is precapillary PH, and if PAWP is higher than 15 mmHg then diagnosis is post-capillary PH (Table **1**). Exercise-induced PH was withdrawn in the latest guideline. Disproportioned PH definition used for group 2 was also withdrawn in 2015 ESC/ERS PH guideline (Table **1**). Diastolic pressure difference (DPD): (diastolic PAP – mean pulmonary capillary wedge pressure (PCWPm)) which was used for discrimination of isolated post-capillary PH and combined pre and post capillary PH, and PVR values added to this definition were simplified. Accordingly, a value of DPD below 7 mmHg and/or PVD value below 3 WU is defined as isolated post-capillary PH; while a value of DPD above 7 mmHg and a value of PVD above 3 WU are defined as combined (post-capillary and pre-capillary) PH [1].

Table 1. Haemodynamic definitions of pulmonary hypertension.

Definition	Characteristics	Clinical Group
PH	PAPm 25 mmHg	All
Pre- capillary PH	PAPm≥25 mmHg PAWP≤15 mmHg	1. Pulmonary arterial hypertension 3. PH due to lung diseases 4. Chronic thromboembolic PH 5. PH with unclear and/or multi-factorial mechanisms
Post-capillary PH Isolated post-capillary PH Combined post-capillary and pre-capillary PH	PAPm≥25 mmHg PAWP>15 mmHg DPG< mmHg and/or PVR<3 WU DPG≥7 mmHg and/or PVR> 3 WU	2.PH due to left heart disease 5.PH with unclear and/or multi-factorial mechanisms

Classification

Patients were stratified according to pathophysiological, hemodynamical features, clinical pictures and form of treatment [1 - 3]. Classification of PH was made in 1973 and since then underwent lots of changes [4]. Latest update was made in year 2015, it was again separated into 5 different groups and some arrangements were made (Table **2**) [1].

Table 2. Comprehensive clinical classification of pulmonary hypertension.

1. Pulmonary Arterial Hypertension	3. Pulmonary hypertension due to lung diseases and/or hypoxia
Idiopathic Heritable - BMPR2 mutation - Other mutation Drugs and toxins induced Associated with - Connective tissue disease - Human immunodeficiency virüs (HIV) infection - Portal hypertension - Congenital heart disease - Schistosomiasis	Chronic obstructive pulmonary disease Interstitial lung disease Other pulmonary diseases with mixed restrictive and obstructive pattern Sleep-disorders breathing Alveolar hypoventilation disorders Chronic exposure to high altitude Development lung diseases
1'. Pulmonary veno-occlusive and-or pulmonary capillary hemangiomatosis	4. Chronic thromboembolic pulmonary hypertension and other pulmonary artery obstructions
Idiopathic Heritable - EIF2AK4 mutation - Other mutation Drugs, toxins and radiation induced Associated with - Connective tissue disease - HIV infection	Chronic thromboembolic pulmonary hypertension Other pulmonary artery obstructions -Angiosarcoma -Other intravascular tumors -Arteritis -Congenital pulmonary arteries stenoses -Parasites
1". Persistent pulmonary hypertension of the newborn	
2. Pulmonary hypertension due to left heart disease	5. Pulmonary hypertension with unclear and/or multifactorial mechanisms
Left ventricular systolic dysfunction Left ventricular diastolic dysfunction Valvular disease Congenital / acquired left heart inflow / outflow tract obstruction and congenital cardiomyopathies Congenital / acquired pulmonary veins stenosis	Heamatological disorders: Chronic hemolytic anemia, myeloproliferative disorders, splenectomy Systemic disorders: Sarcoidosis, pulmonary histiocytosis, lymphangioleiomyomatosis, neurofibromatosis Metabolic disorders: Glycogen storage disease, Gaucher disease, thyroid disorders Others: Pulmonary tumoral thrombotic micro angiopathy, fibrosing mediastinitis, chronic renal failure, segmental pulmonary hypertension

Group 1 Pulmonary arterial hypertension (PAH)
Group 2 PH related to left heart diseases
Group 3 PH related to pulmonary diseases

Group 4 Chronic thromboembolic PH (CTEPH) and other pulmonary arterial (PA) occlusions
Group 5 PH with unclear or multifactorial mechanisms.

Pulmonary veno-occlusive disease (PVOD) and/or pulmonary capillary hemangiomatosis (PCH) that were included in sub-category of group 1 were extended and their forms due to and related with idiopathic, hereditary, drug, toxin and radiation were included in them. Also, persistent pulmonary hypertension of the newborn (PPHN) was arranged as a sub-category of group 1. Pediatric hearth diseases such as congenital or acquired left heart inflow/outflow tract occlusion and congenital cardiomyopathies were included in group 2. One of the most important change was that group 4 was renamed as CTEPH+PA obstructions instead of CTEPH. It was revised to include pulmonary angiosarcoma, other intravascular tumors, arthritis, congenital pulmonary artery obstruction and parasites. Precapillary PH related with chronic hemolytic anemia was removed from group 1 and evaluated in group 5 PH due to its pathological, hemodynamical differences and its response to treatment. Besides this, PH that was observed in specific areas (segmental) connected to aortopulmonary collaterals in patients with pulmonary or tricuspid atresia were added into sub-group of group 5 [1].

Epidemiology

Even though comparative epidemiologic studies are required between PH groups, prevalence of group 2 PH related with left heart diseases was the highest. In left side valvular diseases, PH prevalence increases as severity of defect and symptoms increase [5]. In group 3, in patients with chronic obstructive pulmonary disease (COPD), PH prevalence increases as severity of COPD increases. PH was identified in 20% of terminal COPD patients who were interned in the hospital [6]. In a study, group 4 chronic thromboembolic pulmonary hypertension incidence was found 3.8%, 2 years after an acute pulmonary embolus [7]. PH prevalence was reported increased with age. In a population-based study conducted in Minnesota, USA, total prevalence in general population was reported between 10% and 20% [8]. 5-year mortality ratio is around %36 in PAH. In various studies, lowest and highest PAH and IPAH prevalence in adult population were 15 and 5.9 cases in a million, respectively. Lowest PAH incidence in adults was 2.4 cases in a million per year. Idiopathic, familial or drug related PAH patients (Table **3**) [9], form half of PAH patients in general [10 - 12]. Bone morphogenetic protein receptor type 2 (BMPR2) gene is a member of transforming growth factor (TGF-B) superfamily and contribute to vascular cell proliferation. Heterozygote BMPR2 mutation has a high incidence of 75% and 25% in hereditary PAH patients and sporadic cases, respectively. Most common cause of associated pulmonary hypertension (APAH) is PAH related with connective tissue disorders (especially systemic sclerosis). Infection of human immunodeficiency virus (HIV), portal hypertension, schistosomiases is other rare causes [11, 13].

Selective serotonin-reuptake inhibitors (SSRIs) maternal use has also been linked to persistent pulmonary hypertension of the newborn. Maternal use of SSRIs in late pregnancy may be a risk factor for PPHN [14, 15].

Table 3. Drug induced pulmonary arterial hypertension [9].

Definite	Likely	Possible
Aminorex Fenfluramine Dexfenfluramine Toxic rapeseed oil Benfluorex	Amphetamine L-tryptophan Metamphetamine	Cocaine Phenylpropanolamine St John's wort Chemotherapy Selective serotonin reuptake inhibitors Pergolide

Physiopathology

Each group has different physiopathological features. Three main features that outstand in pulmonary artery are vasoconstriction, remodeling of arterial wall and in situ thrombosis. In patients with Group 1 PAH, mechanisms that increase pulmonary arterial pressure (PAP) are hemodynamically pre-capillary and might be in either or both in arterial or venous vascular bed. Based on injury of vascular wall, the balance between vasoconstrictive and proliferative mediators and vasodilatory and anti-proliferative mediators is altered. Because of the decrease in effectiveness of potassium channels in smooth muscle cells with prostacyclin and nitric oxide and increase of serotonin, endotelin-1 and thromboxane activity; PVR and PAP increase due to proliferation in intima and adventitia layers, hypertrophy in smooth muscles and plexiform structures and in situ thrombosis [3, 16]. In group 2 PH related to left heart diseases, main hemodynamic disorder that occur with reflection of increase in left ventricular diastole pressure (or left atrium) to pulmonary veins and then to pulmonary arteries. Disorders in group 2 cause post-capillary PH while disorders in other groups cause pre-capillary PH [5]. Vasoconstriction in pulmonary arteries because of pressure increase in strain receptors of left atrium and pulmonary veins and/or endothelial dysfunctions in left heart disorders, active mechanisms that cause remodeling because of genetic predisposition and high levels of endothelin might cause changes in pulmonary artery, formation of neointima and thickening of media layer and finally pulmonary hypertension. Acute vasoreactivity test is only positive if there is a vasoconstriction, however its result is negative in case of remodeling because it causes a structural change that constricts vein lumen [3, 5]. Even though there are many mechanisms responsible of PH related with pulmonary diseases, most efficient one is hypoxic vasoconstriction. Polycythemia then reduced fluidity of blood caused by erythropoiesis secondary to acidosis and hypoxia, remodeling in vein wall caused by stimulation of proinflammatory mediators secondary to carbon dioxide (CO_2) retention and chronic hypoxia and reduced area caused by pulmonary capillary bed injury are other mechanisms. Even though some recent studies do not support, it is thought that interstitial pulmonary diseases cause PH based on parenchyma injury. Also, it is thought that deep hypoxia in PH related with sleep-disordered breathing is formed with similar mechanisms [3, 6]. Group 4 chronic thromboembolic PH is late complication of acute pulmonary emboli. Chronic thrombi hold onto media layer and organized thrombi substitute normal intima and prevent blood flow by occluding partially or even totally. Also, formed web-like structures slow down blood-flow and cause remodeling of pulmonary artery bed in parallel with macrovascular obstruction [17]. Group 5 PH with unclear or multifactorial mechanisms are also pre-capillary and it is believed that many uncertain factors contribute to PH [3].

Diagnosis and Algorithm

Differential diagnosis of PH might be difficult because of its non-specific symptoms and it might be caused by many different disorders. Exertional dyspnea disproportional with underlying cause should be warning. Most important and early sign is exertional dyspnea and getting tired quickly. Chest pain or syncope with effort might be seen. Shortness of breath, fatigue, exhaustion, angina, syncope and dry cough might be present. In advanced diseases with right heart failure dyspnea, leg edema and ascites might be present even at rest.

Findings on physical examination are related with underlying disease. For example, telangiectasia ulcers at fingertips and sclerodactylia point to scleroderma while inspiratory rales should warn for interstitial pulmonary disease. Because of higher pulmonary pressures, pulmonary (P2) sound is accentuated and s4 gallop can be heard if right ventricular (RV) diastolic function disorder and pulmonary valve early systolic murmur are present. In cases with right ventricular dysfunction, findings such as jugular venous distension, hepatomegaly, peripheral edema, ascites and cold extremities, holo-systolic tricuspid insufficiency murmur might be present [1, 3].

Normal electrocardiogram (ECG) and chest x-ray do not exclude the diagnosis. However, in advanced cases ECG findings such as biphasic T wave at V1-V3, ST depression, right bundle brunch block, right axis misalignment, P pulmonale associated with right ventricular overload can be found. In late phase of PH dilatation of main pulmonary artery descending branch, disappearance of vein shadows at upper regions of lungs and increase of heart-chest ratio related with right atrium and right ventricle enlargement might be observed at chest x-ray [18, 19].

Respiratory function test and arterial blood gas (ABG) especially help with underlying and PH-causing obstructive or interstitial pulmonary disease such as COPD at group 3. Reduction of carbon monoxide diffusion capacity (DLCO) without significant volume lose should point to PAH. Reduction of DLCO is a sign of poor prognosis. In this patient, arterial oxygen level is normal or close to normal at ABG. CO_2 partial pressure might be normal or increased at COPD [20].

6-minute walking test (6MWT) is a measurement used for diagnosis and follow-up that objectively detects functional performance of the patient. Walking distance is directly proportional to functional stage of the disease and survival [3]. Biomarkers such as uric acid, brain natriuretic peptide (BNP), atrial natriuretic peptide, N-terminal pro-brain natriuretic peptide (NT-pro-BNP), troponin I and troponin T can be used for evaluation and follow-up of right ventricular failure. As shown in Fig. (1), many biomarkers have been reported in the literature showing vascular dysfunction, inflammation, myocardial stress, vascular remodelling, and organ tissue damage in PH. They are important biomarker in diagnosis and follow-up. It is important in diagnosis and follow-up. However, the most commonly used biomarker BNP / NT-proBNP level tends to be high and shows correlation with myocardial dysfunction [1] and is important in diagnosis and follow-up [21]. Serology is important for identification of diseases that cause PH. Related biomarkers should be tested for underlying diseases. For example, PAH findings can be found in %2 of patients with liver disease, so liver function tests and abdominal ultrasonography (USG) should be performed in these patients. HIV serology must be checked and again related markers should be tested at sclerosis because PAH prevalence is high and genetic tests such as BMPR-2 and activin receptor-like kinase (ALK-1) should be performed for hereditary PAH diagnosis [3, 22] (Table 4).

High-resolution computerized tomography (HRCT), contrast-enhanced computer tomography (BT) and pulmonary angiography might reveal cardiac, vascular, parenchymal and mediastinal abnormalities thus provide useful information for PH diagnosis and underlying diseases. For example, PA and RV enlargement can be identified; pulmonary artery diameter of > 29 mm and equal or higher ratio of pulmonary artery diameter/ ascending aorta diameter increase suspicion of PH. In terms of group 3 diseases, parenchymal abnormalities can be evaluated with HRCT and pulmonary BT angiography can be of use for vasculitis and pulmonary arteriovenous malformations of group 4 CTEPH and group 1 etiologies [22].

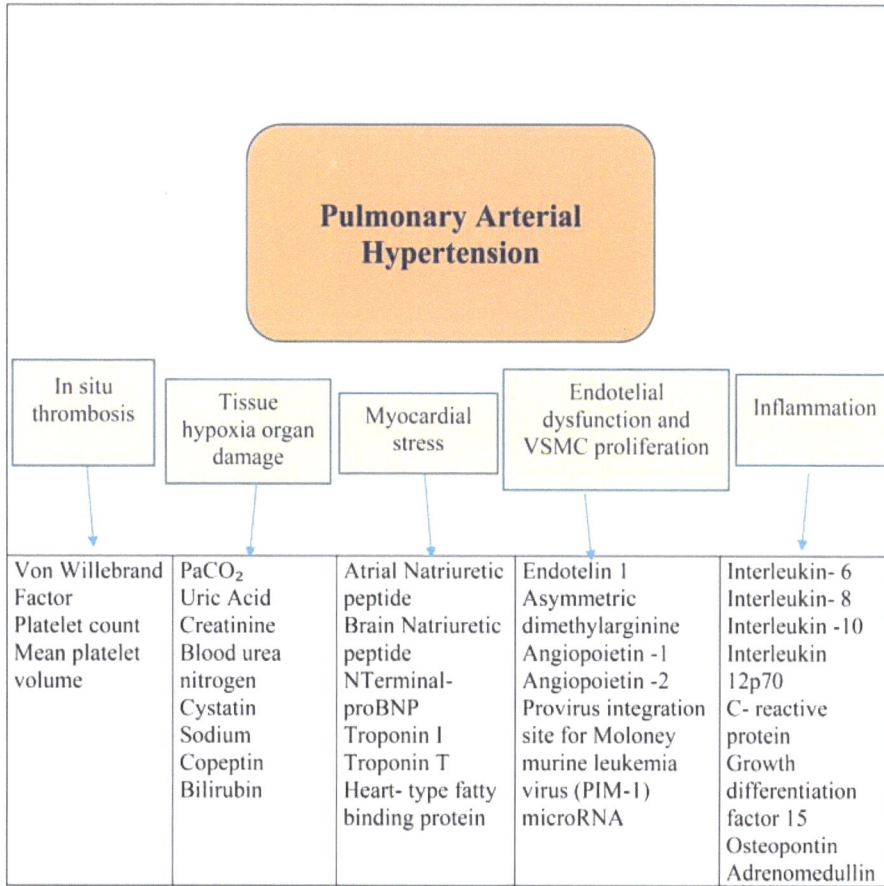

Fig. (1). Biomarkers in pulmonary arterial hypertension.

Ventilation perfusion scintigraphy is mostly used for group 4 CTEPH differential diagnosis. Its sensitivity and specificity are higher than BT angiography. CTEPH can be excluded with normal or high probability scintigraphy [23].

In suspicion of congenital cardiac diseases cardiac magnetic resonance (CMR) can be used if echocardiography (ECO) is not certain [24]. According to risk factors, symptoms, examination findings and some preliminary test results, the first and most important non-invasive diagnostic method is ECO [2, 3]. In ECO, a PAP >35-40 mmHg suggests PH. RV dilatation, "D" shaped left ventricle by flattening of interventricular septum, pericardial effusion, pulmonary arterial dilatation, increase of RV wall thickness are other ECO findings of PH [2, 3, 25]. Because ECO shows right heart functions for PH diagnosis, follow-up and survival estimation, its importance is indisputable and it can also help with diagnosis of congenital heart diseases [26]. Calculation of PAP is based on maximal tricuspid regurgitation jet velocity. A value higher than 3.4 m/sec is significant. ESC guideline classified maximal tricuspid regurgitation jet velocity based PH probability according to echocardiographic variables in PH suspected cases; and thus, cardiac catheterization requirement is considered [27, 28]. In a meta-analysis, ECO and RHC is compared for PH diagnosis, ECO sensitivity and specificity were found %83 and %72, systolic PAP correlation measured with RHC and ECO was found %70 [29]. In cases with high systolic PAP are shown in Table 1. However, in a cohort study in USA, a 10 mmHg pressure difference was shown %60 of ECO performed patients compared to catheterized patients [30].

Table 4. Diagnostic algorithm.

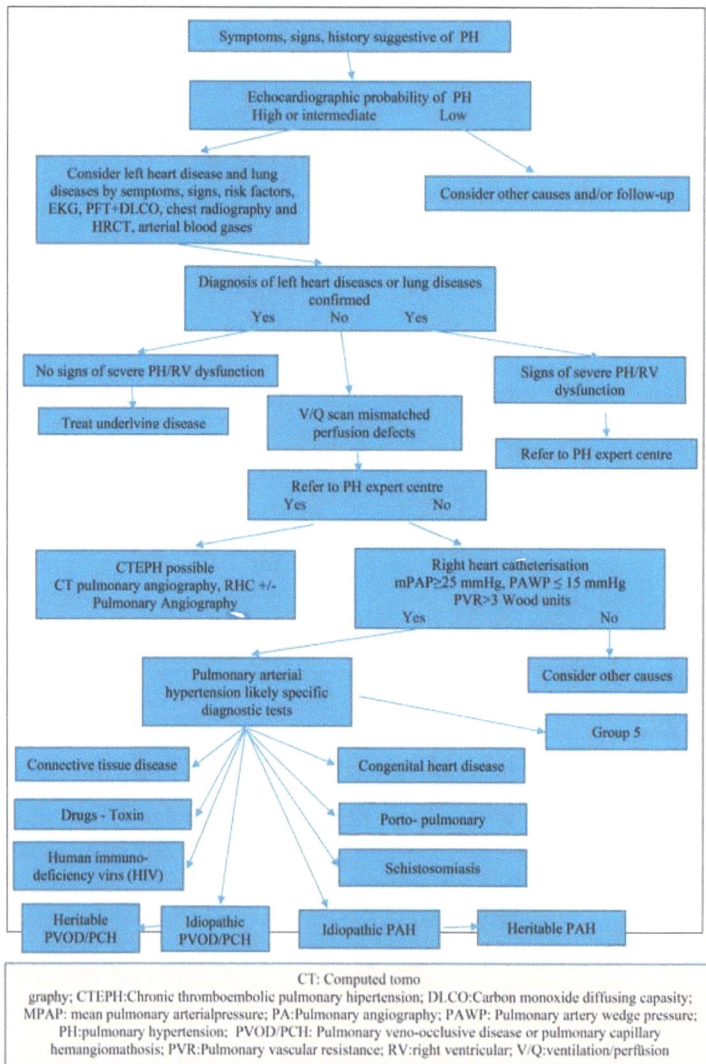

CT: Computed tomo
graphy; CTEPH:Chronic thromboembolic pulmonary hipertension; DLCO:Carbon monoxide diffusing capasity; MPAP: mean pulmonary arterialpressure; PA:Pulmonary angiography; PAWP: Pulmonary artery wedge pressure; PH:pulmonary hypertension; PVOD/PCH: Pulmonary veno-occlusive disease or pulmonary capillary hemangiomathosis; PVR:Pulmonary vascular resistance; RV:right ventricular; V/Q:ventilation/perfüsion

RHC and vasoreactivity test are the golden standard methods for diagnosis, treatment and prognosis follow-up of PH. Indicator-dilution, thermodilution and Fick method can be used for measurement of cardiac output. Cardiac index, pressures; right atrium pressure, PVR and PCWB and oxygen saturation measurements can be identified with RHC. PH diagnosis become definite when mean PAP is over 25 mmHg. If PCWB is lower than 15 mmHg it is pre-capillary PH, if it is higher than 15 mmHg it is post-capillary PH. If systemic pulmonary shunt is present, Fick method that is based on oxygen utilization rate must be used. In thermodilution method, temperature change is inversely correlated with volume of blood flow in pulmonary artery. For vasoreactivity test, 10 mmHg decrease of PAP below 40 mmHg after administering acute vasodilators such as nitric oxide (NO), adenosine or prostacyclin is considered positive. These patients might benefit from calcium channel blockers. However, clinical benefit might not be permanent and follow-up is required [1 - 3, 31, 32].

This typically includes testing to identify the clinical class and the functional capacity, which are essential to planning appropriate therapy.

Treatment and Prognosis

PH treatment varies according to etiological classification. A multidisciplinary approach is needed, treatment and monitoring should be done by expert centers. Most important change of treatment algorithm in ESC/ERS 2015 guideline was treatment redirection according to prognostic risk (Table **5**).

Table 5. PAH determinants of prognosis.

Characteristic	Good Prognosis	Poor Prognosis
Type of PAH	**Familial, connective tissue disease or liver disease related**	**Congenital heart disease**
Functional Class	3 or 4	1 or 2
Echocardiogram	Pericardial effusion	Absence of pericardial effusion
Exercise capacity	Low six minute walk distance	High six minute walk distance
Systemic blood pressure	Low	High
Right atrial pressure	Very high	Lower
Pulmonary vascular resistance	Very high	Lower
BNP levels	Significantly elevated	Minimally elevated
Kidney function	Normal	Impaired

Treatment of group 1 PAH: Currently, PAH is still incurable but a controllable disease but survival is partially extended. Target-specific treatments are developed according to PAH pathophysiology. General measurements and supportive care are important aspects of the treatment. Patients who are initiated on PAH treatment should be followed-up with 6DYT or ECO every 3 months. In patients with positive vasoreactivity test, calcium channel blockers are the first choice. In patients with poor prognosis, treatment with a combination protocol that involves IV treatment (such as IV epoprostenol) recommended. Many combination treatment is used or developing at the present time. According to 2015 guidelines, single treatment is highlighted for patients with good prognosis. Researched with significant studies after 2009 guideline and newer agents such as riociguat, selexipag and macitentan take place with agents such as ambrisentan, bosentan, sildenafil, tadalafil, iloprost and trepostinil. Ambrisentan+tadalafil combination is the first line treatment after report of ABMITION study. Double or triple treatment is recommended for patients with poor prognosis or single-treatment failure in recent studies. Sildenafil+macitentan SERAPHIN, bosentan+riociguat PATENT, endothelin receptor antagonist (ERA) selexipag with phosphodiesterase 5 inhibitor (PDE5I) GRIPHON studies can be cited as examples [1 - 3, 25, 32 - 35].

Treatment of group 2 PH related to left heart diseases: Treatment of underlying heart disease is required. Treatment might be surgical or medical [3, 5].

Treatment of group 3 PH related to pulmonary diseases: Treatment of underlying diseases is required also in this group. Most common cause of diseases in this group is COPD. Treatments such as bronchodilator treatment, oxygen and non-invasive mechanic can be administered [3, 6].

Treatment of group 4 Chronic thromboembolic PH (CTEPH) and other pulmonary arterial (PA) occlusions: Main treatment is removal of thrombus. Endarterectomy can only be performed on proximal. Pulmonary angiography is required before procedure. Experience of surgical team is crucial. If distal thrombus is present or operation is contraindicated, up-to-date medical anticoagulant treatment should be given [36].

Treatment of group 5 PH with unclear or multifactorial mechanisms: Treatment of underlying disease that causes PH is usually sufficient. Treatment of sickle cell anemia can be given as an example [37].

Also, contraception of PH patients, especially PAH patients, is important. Bosentan is reported to reduce effectivity of oral contraceptives [38]. Because it is a disorder that impairs quality of life, psychosocial support and education are important. Oxygen support should be given for high altitudes to patients with low arterial O_2 pressure and residency in areas with >2000 m altitude is not recommended [39]. Patients should be vaccinated for influenza and pneumonia because infection is a risk factor that increases mortality [2, 40, 41]. Because of higher mortality and morbidity risk for individuals that will receive a surgical operation, pre-operative and peri-operative evaluation should right ventricular functions with ECO and related specialty consultations should be done [2, 42].

CONSENT FOR PUBLICATION

Not applicable.

CONFLICT OF INTEREST

The author confirms that this chapter contents have no conflict of interest.

ACKNOWLEDGEMENTS

Declare none.

REFERENCES

[1]   Galie N, Humbert M, Vachieri JL, *et al.* 2015 ESC/ERS guidelines for the diagnosis and treatment of pulmonary hypertension: The Joint Task Force for the Diagnosis and Treatment of Pulmonary Hypertension of the European Society of Cardiology (ESC) and the European Respiratory Society (ERS). Eur Heart J 2016; 37(1): 67-119.
[http://dx.doi.org/10.1093/eurheartj/ehv317] [PMID: 26320113]

[2]   Taichman DB, Ornelas J, Chung L, *et al.* Pharmacologic therapy for pulmonary arterial hypertension in adults: CHEST guideline and expert panel report. Chest 2014; 146(2): 449-75.
[http://dx.doi.org/10.1378/chest.14-0793] [PMID: 24937180]

[3]   Mclaughlin VV, Archer SL, Badesch DB, *et al.* ACCF/AHA 2009 expert consensus document on pulmonary hypertension:a report of the American College of Cardiology Foundation Task Force on Expert Consensus Documents and the American Heart Association: developed in collaboration with, the American College of Chest Physicians, American Thoracic Society, Inc., and the Pulmonary Hypertension Association Circulation. published correction appears in Circulation 2009; 120(2): e13.

[4]   Hatano S, Strasser T. Primary pulmonary hypertension. Report on a WHO meeting. October 15-17, 1973

[5]   Guazzi M, Borlaug BA. Pulmonary hypertension due to left heart disease. Circulation 2012; 126(8): 975-90.
[http://dx.doi.org/10.1161/CIRCULATIONAHA.111.085761] [PMID: 22908015]

[6]   Seeger W, Adir Y, Barberà JA, *et al.* Pulmonary hypertension in chronic lung diseases. J Am Coll Cardiol 2013; 62(25) (Suppl.): D109-16.
[http://dx.doi.org/10.1016/j.jacc.2013.10.036] [PMID: 24355635]

[7]   Pengo V, Lensing AW, Prins MH, *et al.* Incidence of chronic thromboembolic pulmonary hypertension after pulmonary embolism. N Engl J Med 2004; 350(22): 2257-64.
[http://dx.doi.org/10.1056/NEJMoa032274] [PMID: 15163775]

[8]   Lam CS, Borlaug BA, Kane GC, Enders FT, Rodeheffer RJ, Redfield MM. Age-associated increases in pulmonary artery systolic pressure in the general population. Circulation 2009; 119(20): 2663-70.
[http://dx.doi.org/10.1161/CIRCULATIONAHA.108.838698] [PMID: 19433755]

[9]   Montani D, Seferian A, Savale L, Simonneau G, Humbert M. Drug-induced pulmonary arterial hypertension: a recent outbreak. Eur Respir Rev 2013; 22(129): 244-50.

[http://dx.doi.org/10.1183/09059180.00003313] [PMID: 23997051]

[10]   McGoon MD, Benza RL, Escribano-Subias P, *et al.* Pulmonary arterial hypertension: epidemiology and registries. J Am Coll Cardiol 2013; 62(25) (Suppl.): D51-9.
[http://dx.doi.org/10.1016/j.jacc.2013.10.023] [PMID: 24355642]

[11]   Humbert M, Sitbon O, Chaouat A, *et al.* Pulmonary arterial hypertension in France: results from a national registry. Am J Respir Crit Care Med 2006; 173(9): 1023-30.
[http://dx.doi.org/10.1164/rccm.200510-1668OC] [PMID: 16456139]

[12]   Thenappan T, Shah SJ, Rich S, Tian L, Archer SL, Gomberg-Maitland M. Survival in pulmonary arterial hypertension: a reappraisal of the NIH risk stratification equation. Eur Respir J 2010; 35(5): 1079-87.
[http://dx.doi.org/10.1183/09031936.00072709] [PMID: 20032020]

[13]   Soubrier F, Chung WK, Machado R, *et al.* Genetics and genomics of pulmonary arterial hypertension. J Am Coll Cardiol 2013; 62(25) (Suppl.): D13-21.
[http://dx.doi.org/10.1016/j.jacc.2013.10.035] [PMID: 24355637]

[14]   Tuder RM, Archer SL, Dorfmüller P, *et al.* Relevant issues in the pathology and pathobiology of pulmonary hypertension. J Am Coll Cardiol 2013; 62(25) (Suppl.): D4-D12.
[http://dx.doi.org/10.1016/j.jacc.2013.10.025] [PMID: 24355640]

[15]   Chambers CD, Johnson KA, Dick LM, Felix RJ, Jones KL. Birth outcomes in pregnant women taking fluoxetine. N Engl J Med 1996; 335(14): 1010-5.
[http://dx.doi.org/10.1056/NEJM199610033351402] [PMID: 8793924]

[16]   Chambers CD, Hernandez-Diaz S, Van Marter LJ, *et al.* Selective serotonin-reuptake inhibitors and risk of persistent pulmonary hypertension of the newborn. N Engl J Med 2006; 354(6): 579-87.
[http://dx.doi.org/10.1056/NEJMoa052744] [PMID: 16467545]

[17]   Humbert M. Pulmonary arterial hypertension and chronic thromboembolic pulmonary hypertension: pathophysiology. Eur Respir Rev 2010; 19(115): 59-63.
[http://dx.doi.org/10.1183/09059180.00007309] [PMID: 20956167]

[18]   Olsson KM, Nickel NP, Tongers J, Hoeper MM. Atrial flutter and fibrillation in patients with pulmonary hypertension. Int J Cardiol 2013; 167(5): 2300-5.
[http://dx.doi.org/10.1016/j.ijcard.2012.06.024] [PMID: 22727973]

[19]   Milne EN. Forgotten gold in diagnosing pulmonary hypertension: the plain chest radiograph. Radiographics 2012; 32(4): 1085-7.
[http://dx.doi.org/10.1148/rg.324125021] [PMID: 22786995]

[20]   Sun XG, Hansen JE, Oudiz RJ, Wasserman K. Pulmonary function in primary pulmonary hypertension. J Am Coll Cardiol 2003; 41(6): 1028-35.
[http://dx.doi.org/10.1016/S0735-1097(02)02964-9] [PMID: 12651053]

[21]   Coghlan JG, Denton CP, Grünig E, *et al.* Evidence-based detection of pulmonary arterial hypertension in systemic sclerosis: the DETECT study. Ann Rheum Dis 2014; 73(7): 1340-9.
[http://dx.doi.org/10.1136/annrheumdis-2013-203301] [PMID: 23687283]

[22]   Rajaram S, Swift AJ, Condliffe R, *et al.* CT features of pulmonary arterial hypertension and its major subtypes: a systematic CT evaluation of 292 patients from the ASPIRE Registry. Thorax 2015; 70(4): 382-7.
[http://dx.doi.org/10.1136/thoraxjnl-2014-206088] [PMID: 25523307]

[23]   Tunariu N, Gibbs SJR, Win Z, *et al.* Ventilation-perfusion scintigraphy is more sensitive than multidetector CTPA in detecting chronic thromboembolic pulmonary disease as a treatable cause of pulmonary hypertension. J Nucl Med 2007; 48(5): 680-4.
[http://dx.doi.org/10.2967/jnumed.106.039438] [PMID: 17475953]

[24]   Peacock AJ, Vonk Noordegraaf A. Cardiac magnetic resonance imaging in pulmonary arterial hypertension. Eur Respir Rev 2013; 22(130): 526-34.

[http://dx.doi.org/10.1183/09059180.00006313] [PMID: 24293468]

[25] Agency for Healthcare Research and Quality. Pulmonary arterial hypertension: Screening, management and treatment: executive summary April 25, 2013 August 18, 2015.

[26] Vonk Noordegraaf A, Galiè N. The role of the right ventricle in pulmonary arterial hypertension. Eur Respir Rev 2011; 20(122): 243-53.
[http://dx.doi.org/10.1183/09059180.00006511] [PMID: 22130817]

[27] Rudski LG, Lai WW, Afilalo J, *et al.* Guidelines for the echocardiographic assessment of the right heart in adults: a report from the American Society of Echocardiography endorsed by the European Association of Echocardiography, a registered branch of the European Society of Cardiology, and the Canadian Society of Echocardiography. J Am Soc Echocardiogr 2010; 23(7): 685-713.
[http://dx.doi.org/10.1016/j.echo.2010.05.010] [PMID: 20620859]

[28] Lang RM, Badano LP, Mor-Avi V, *et al.* Recommendations for cardiac chamber quantification by echocardiography in adults: an update from the American Society of Echocardiography and the European Association of Cardiovascular Imaging. Eur Heart J Cardiovasc Imaging 2015; 16(3): 233-70.
[http://dx.doi.org/10.1093/ehjci/jev014] [PMID: 25712077]

[29] Janda S, Shahidi N, Gin K, Swiston J. Diagnostic accuracy of echocardiography for pulmonary hypertension: a systematic review and metaanalysis (published correction appears in Heart. 2011; 97(13):1112). Heart 2011; 97(8): 612-22.
[http://dx.doi.org/10.1136/hrt.2010.212084] [PMID: 21357375]

[30] Farber HW, Foreman AJ, Miller DP, McGoon MD. REVEAL Registry: correlation of right heart catheterization and echocardiography in patients with pulmonary arterial hypertension. Congest Heart Fail 2011; 17(2): 56-64.
[http://dx.doi.org/10.1111/j.1751-7133.2010.00202.x] [PMID: 21449993]

[31] Hoeper MM, Lee SH, Voswinckel R, *et al.* Complications of right heart catheterization procedures in experienced centers. J Am Coll Cardiol 2006; 48: 2546-52.
[http://dx.doi.org/10.1016/j.jacc.2006.07.061] [PMID: 17174196]

[32] Sitbon O, Humbert M, Jaïs X, *et al.* Long-term response to calcium channel blockers in idiopathic pulmonary arterial hypertension. Circulation 2005; 111(23): 3105-11.
[http://dx.doi.org/10.1161/CIRCULATIONAHA.104.488486] [PMID: 15939821]

[33] Galiè N, Barberà JA, Frost AE, *et al.* Initial use of ambrisentan plus tadalafil in pulmonary arterial hypertension. N Engl J Med 2015; 373(9): 834-44.
[http://dx.doi.org/10.1056/NEJMoa1413687] [PMID: 26308684]

[34] Ghofrani HA, Galiè N, Grimminger F, *et al.* Riociguat for the treatment of pulmonary arterial hypertension. N Engl J Med 2013; 369(4): 330-40.
[http://dx.doi.org/10.1056/NEJMoa1209655] [PMID: 23883378]

[35] Sitbon O, Channick R, Chin KM, *et al.* Selexipag for the treatment of pulmonary arterial hypertension. N Engl J Med 2015; 373(26): 2522-33.
[http://dx.doi.org/10.1056/NEJMoa1503184] [PMID: 26699168]

[36] Kim NH, Delcroix M, Jenkins DP, *et al.* Chronic thromboembolic pulmonary hypertension. J Am Coll Cardiol 2013; 62(25) (Suppl.): D92-9.
[http://dx.doi.org/10.1016/j.jacc.2013.10.024] [PMID: 24355646]

[37] Klings ES, Machado RF, Barst RJ, *et al.* An official American Thoracic Society clinical practice guideline: diagnosis, risk stratification, and management of pulmonary hypertension of sickle cell disease. Am J Respir Crit Care Med 2014; 189(6): 727-40.
[http://dx.doi.org/10.1164/rccm.201401-0065ST] [PMID: 24628312]

[38] Olsson KM, Jais X. Birth control and pregnancy management in pulmonary hypertension. Semin Respir Crit Care Med 2013; 34(5): 681-8.

[http://dx.doi.org/10.1055/s-0033-1355438] [PMID: 24037634]

[39] Kingman M, Hinzmann B, Sweet O, Vachiéry JL. Living with pulmonary hypertension: unique insights from an international ethnographic study. BMJ Open 2014; 4(5)e004735
[http://dx.doi.org/10.1136/bmjopen-2013-004735] [PMID: 24838724]

[40] Kim DK, Bridges CB, Harriman KH. Advisory Committee on Immunization Practices recommended immunization schedule for adults aged 19 years or older United States, 2016. MMWR Morb Mortal Wkly Rep 2016; 65(4): 88-90.
[http://dx.doi.org/10.15585/mmwr.mm6504a5] [PMID: 26845417]

[41] Tomczyk S, Bennett NM, Stoecker C, *et al.* Use of 13-valent pneumococcal conjugate vaccine and 23-valent pneumococcal polysaccharide vaccine among adults aged ≥65 years: recommendations of the Advisory Committee on Immunization Practices (ACIP). MMWR Morb Mortal Wkly Rep 2014; 63(37): 822-5.
[PMID: 25233284]

[42] Kinger JR, Frantz RP, Eds. Diagnosis and Management of Pulmonary Hypertension. New York, NY: Humana Press 2015; pp. 437-64.
[http://dx.doi.org/10.1007/978-1-4939-2636-7]

CHAPTER 5

Hypertension in Thyroid Disorders

Lebriz Uslu-Beşli[1] and **Pınar Atukeren**[2,*]

[1] *Department of Nuclear Medicine, Cerrahpaşa Faculty of Medicine, Istanbul University-Cerrahpasa, Istanbul, Turkey*

[2] *Department of Medical Biochemistry, Cerrahpaşa Faculty of Medicine, Istanbul University-Cerrahpasa, Istanbul, Turkey*

Abstract: Although prevalence of hypertension is high in the population, underlying pathology can be determined only in the 10% of the cases and called secondary hypertension. Endocrine disorders are the second most common cause of secondary hypertension after renal diseases. Thyroid diseases are relatively rare causes of secondary hypertension; however, thyroid dysfunction is common in the population. Thyroid hormones affect all physiological systems, including cardiovascular system and blood pressure regulation. Both hypothyroidism and hyperthyroidism can cause hypertension using different mechanisms of action. Hyperthyroidism generally results in increased cardiac output and systolic hypertension, whereas hypothyroidism is associated with increased peripheral vascular resistance, causing diastolic hypertension. As hypertension due to an underlying thyroid disease is reversible if early and adequate therapy is given, thyroid disease related hypertension has to be excluded in hypertensive patients.

This chapter summarizes the present knowledge on the pathogenesis of thyroid disease related hypertension, as well as common thyroid diseases related with hypertension, their diagnosis and treatment alternatives.

Keywords: Blood pressure, Cardiac output, Diastolic hypertension, Graves' disease, Hashimoto's thyroiditis, Hypertension, Hyperthyroidism, Hypothyroidism, Systolic hypertension, Thyroid, Thyrotoxicosis, Thyroid cancer, T3, T4, TSH, TRH, TPO, MIT, DIT, D2 enzyme.

THYROID HORMONE SYNTHESIS AND FUNCTIONS

Thyroid gland function, hormone synthesis and secretion are stimulated by thyroid stimulating hormone (TSH), which is secreted by pituitary gland. TSH secretion is regulated by hypothalamic thyrotropin-releasing hormone (TRH)

---

[*] **Corresponding author Pinar Atukeren:** Department of Medical Biochemistry, Cerrahpaşa Faculty of Medicine, Istanbul University-Cerrahpasa, Istanbul, Turkey; Tel: +902124143056; Fax: +902126332987; E-mail: p_atukeren@yahoo.com

(Fig. **1**). Thyroid hormone synthesis begins with iodide (I⁻) uptake, which is actively transported into thyroid follicular cells (thyrocytes) by sodium-iodide symporter (NIS) at the basal cell membrane (Fig. **2**). At the apical cell membrane, thyroid peroxidase (TPO) oxidizes iodide and catalyzes iodination of tyrosyl residues in the thyroglobulin within the follicular lumen, resulting in formation of monoiodotyrosines (MIT) and diiodotyrosines (DIT). TPO also catalyzes the coupling of MIT and DIT to form thyroxine (T_4) and triiodothyronine (T_3). The resulting iodinated thyroglobulin is stored as colloid in follicular lumen until thyroid cells are stimulated for thyroid hormone secretion.

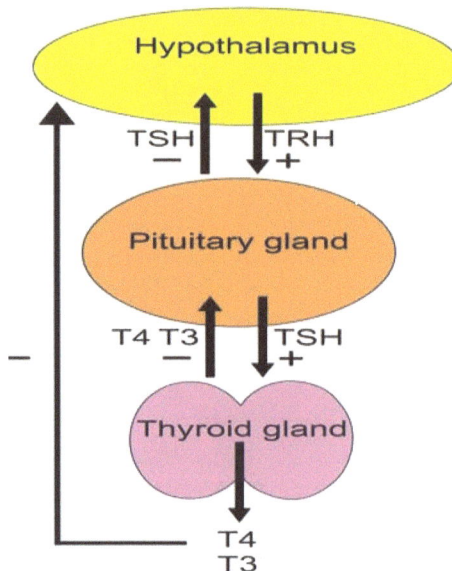

Fig. (1). Hypothalamic-pituitary-thyroid gland axis.

Upon stimulation of thyrocytes by TSH, iodinated thyroglobulin enters thyrocytes and is hydrolyzed within lysosomes to form T_4, T_3, MIT and DIT again. T_4 and T_3 are released into blood, whereas MIT and DIT are deiodinated within thyrocytes and released iodide is recycled for another thyroid hormone synthesis. The majority of secreted thyroid hormones are in the form of T_4 (80%). On contrary, the majority of T_3 is derived from conversion of T_4 to T_3 in the peripheral tissues mainly via type-2 5'-deiodinase 2 (D2) enzyme but also via type-1 5'-deiodinase (D1) enzyme, both of which catalyze deiodination in the outer ring of T_4 [1 - 4]. T_3 is the most active form of thyroid hormones with a short half-life and contributes in the regulation of cells via thyroid hormone receptors, which are ligand-dependent transcription factors on cellular membrane. Type-3 5'-deiodinase (D3) catalyzes deiodination in the inner ring of T_4, resulting in production of reverse T_3 (rT_3), which is an inactive form of T_3. D3 can also deiodinize and therefore deactivate T_3 [1]. D1-D3 enzymes contain selenocysteine and selenium deficiency may contribute to impaired conversion of T_4 to T_3 [5, 6].

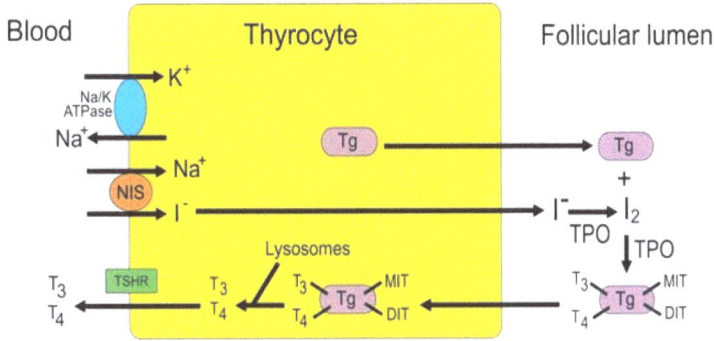

Fig. (2). Thyroid hormone synthesis pathway. NIS: Na^+/I^- symporter; TSHR: Thyroid stimulating hormone receptor; Tg: Thyroglobulin; TPO: Thyroid peroxidase; MIT: Monoiodotyrosine; DIT: Diiodotyrosine.

Several regulatory mechanisms control thyroid hormone synthesis, secretion and peripheral conversion. Decreased serum levels of T_4 increase D2 activity, which in turn increases the amount of serum T_3 [4, 7]. Decreased circulating T_4 and T_3 levels also activate synthesis of TRH and TSH secretion, which in turn upregulates thyrocytes for thyroid hormone synthesis and secretion [8, 9]. On contrary, increased levels of T_4 and T_3 act as a feedback inhibitor downregulating both TRH and TSH secretion [1, 8]. Age, diet, exercise, environmental temperature, altitude, hypoxia, microgravity, circadian rhythms, drugs and several other factors act on the rate and amount of thyroid hormone synthesis [10]. Liver synthesizes several plasma proteins, which are thyroxine-binding globulin, prealbumin and albumin that bind more than 99% of the plasma thyroid hormones and limit plasma free T_4 and free T_3 concentration [11]. Thyroid hormones are deiodinated and conjugated mainly in liver and secreted into bile, then reabsorbed from the gut and finally excreted via kidneys [12, 13].

Thyroid hormones enter target cells most likely *via* plasma membrane transporters or via passive diffusion and T_4 can be converted to more active T_3 intracellularly by deiodinases [14]. Thyroid hormones bind to special nuclear receptors, called thyroid hormone receptors (TR), which act as hormone-activated transcription factors and modulate gene expression [15, 16]. TR binding affinity of T_3 is 10-15 times higher than T_4 [17]. Binding of thyroid hormone to TR leads to conformational change on TR resulting in induction of target gene expression and thereby increasing messenger RNA (mRNA) and protein expression [14]. The most profound effects of thyroid hormones are on metabolic rate and cardiovascular function, but effects of thyroid hormones can be seen on all body systems, including brain functions, gut motility, bone formation, bone marrow function, liver metabolism, kidney function and pulmonary system [11, 18 - 24]. Thyroid hormones also exhibit non-genomic effects on plasma membrane and cytoplasmic proteins [25, 26]

Deiodinase activity can be altered in various clinical settings, such as critical illnesses, drug use and pregnancy [27]. In the presence of a critical illness plasma D3 increases and T_3 level decreases within a few hours after the onset of disease and the severity of these changes is directly related with the severity of the disease [28]. Amiodarone and anti-arrhythmic drugs inhibit D3 activity, thus serum T_4 level is increased and T_3 level is decreased [29]. Vascular tumors with high D3 activity can create hypothyroidism by deactivating T_3 [30]. During pregnancy fetoplacental and uterine D3 activity are increased, which may increase thyroid hormone requirement in pregnant women [31 - 33].

THYROID DISEASES RELATED WITH HYPERTENSION

Hyperthyroidism

Hyperthyroidism is defined as overactive thyroid gland, resulting in excess serum thyroid hormone levels and increased metabolic rate. Thyrotoxicosis is defined as excessive serum thyroid hormone levels, which can be either due to hyperfunctioning thyroid gland or destruction of thyroid cells and release of excessive amount of thyroid hormones stored in thyroid follicles. The symptoms related with thyrotoxicosis are tachycardia, palpitations, exercise intolerance, fatigue, heat intolerance, widened pulse pressure, dyspnea on exertion, weight loss, sweating, nervousness, irritability, tremor, skin and hair thinning, irregularity in menstrual cycle, difficulty in concentration and sleeping disorders [34, 35]. Long-term uncontrolled hypertension can also result in atrial fibrillation and heart failure [36]. Hyperthyroidism is generally associated with decreased vascular resistance and increased systolic hypertension.

Causes of Hyperthyroidism

The most common cause of hyperthyroidism is *Graves' disease*, which is an autoimmune disorder with a classical triad of hyperthyroidism, exophthalmos and pretibial myxedema.

TSH receptor antibodies (TRAB) play the main role in the pathogenesis of the disease. TRAB binds to and activates TSH receptors leading to diffuse hyperplasia of thyroid gland and overproduction of the thyroid hormones. Several immune system elements play role in the pathogenesis of exophthalmos, including T and B-lymphocyte-based immune reaction against TSH receptors in orbita, as well as many genetic and environmental factors contributing to the disease development [37].

Toxic adenoma (Plummer's disease) and *toxic multinodular goiter* are defined as presence of hyperfunctioning one or multiple thyroid nodules, which have gained autonomy and produced thyroid hormones independent from TSH stimulation. Both are more common in iodine-deficient areas.

Thyrotropin-induced thyrotoxicosis is a rare disorder, which is originated from TSH-secreting tumors, particularly pituitary adenomas. Excessive TSH production stimulates thyroid gland TSH receptors, resulting in overproduction of thyroid hormones. *Trophoblastic tumors*, including hydatidiform moles and choriocarcinomas can also produce hyperthyroidism by secretion of human chorionic gonadotropin (hCG), which is similar to TSH in structure and therefore can bind to TSH receptors and stimulate thyroid gland. Some *teratomas* can harbor embryogenic thyroid tissue, which can rarely create hyperthyroidism.

Some *drugs*, including potassium iodine, amiodarone, intravenous contrast agents with iodine or excessive level of thyroid hormone supplements (factitial thyrotoxicosis) can also produce thyrotoxicosis.

Thyroditis can produce elevated serum thyroid hormone levels due to thyroid follicle destruction and create thyrotoxicosis symptoms. *Subacute thyroiditis (de Quervain's thyroiditis)* is inflammation of thyroid gland, which is generally preceded by an upper respiratory tract infection. Patients generally have painful thyroid gland on examination, as well as fever and elevated levels of serum acute phase reactants. Unlike hyperthyroidism, radioiodine uptake level remains low. *Hashimoto's thyroiditis* often results in hypothyroidism, however initial gland destruction can result in thyrotoxicosis as well, which is called Hashitoxicosis. *Silent thyroiditis* and *postpartum thyroiditis* are the other thyroiditis types that can create thyrotoxicosis.

Hypothyroidism

Hypothyroidism is defined as decreased functioning of thyroid gland leading to insufficient thyroid hormone production. As thyroid hormones are necessary for function of various body system, thyroid hormone insufficiency results in many different symptoms, including weight gain, fatigue, cold intolerance, constipation, irritability, depression, memory problems, coarse hair and dry skin, hair loss and irregularity in menstrual cycle. In hypothyroidism metabolic rate is decreased and patients often have bradycardia, decreased cardiac output, increased level of triglycerides, cholesterol and low-density lipoproteins, anemia and decreased kidney functions. Congenital hypothyroidism results in delay in physical and mental development of the fetus, a condition called cretinism.

Causes of Hypothyroidism

The most common cause of hypothyroidism in countries with adequate iodine in diet is *Hashimoto's thyroiditis (chronic lymphocytic thyroiditis)*. Hashimoto's thyroiditis is an autoimmune disease, in which thyroid gland is destroyed due to presence of antibodies against thyroid gland structures, including TSH receptors, thyroid peroxidase (TPO) and thyroglobulin (Tg).

In iodine-deficient areas, *endemic goiter* is the most common cause of hypothyroidism. Iodine is an essential mineral for thyroid hormone synthesis, therefore in state of iodine-deficiency thyroid gland cannot produce enough thyroid hormone, leading to elevated TSH values, which creates thyroid gland enlargement. Iodine deficiency in infants and children as well as maternal iodine deficiency during pregnancy lead to endemic cretinism and mental retardation in affected children. *Riedel's thyroiditis* is another autoimmune disorder, where thyroid tissue is replaced by fibrous tissue, leading to thyroid cell loss and impaired thyroid hormone synthesis. Other diseases associated with *thyroiditis*, including acute suppurative thyroiditis and subacute thyroiditis can cause transient of permanent hypothyroidism.

Congenital defects in thyroid hormone synthesis, *lingual thyroid*, *hypopituitarism* leading to lack of TSH stimulus or *defects in hypothalamic TRH synthesis and action* can lead to hypothyroidism. Also, *drugs* interfering with thyroid hormone synthesis, including lithium, amiodarone and iodine can also create hypothyroidism. *External radiation exposure, radioiodine therapy* with I-131 and *thyroidectomy* are the other causes of hypothyroidism. *Infiltrative disorders*, such as amyloidosis, sarcoidosis, hemochromatosis and cystinosis can also create hypothyroidism [38].

Subclinical hypothyroidism is defined as elevated serum TSH levels with normal serum free T_3 and free T_4 levels. Although serum free thyroid hormone levels are within normal limits, subclinical hypothyroidism can be associated with hypothyroid symptoms, including elevated diastolic blood pressure [39].

Subclinical hyperthyroidism is defined as low serum TSH levels in the presence of normal serum free T_3 and free T_4 levels. Patients with subclinical hyperthyroidism generally have few or no signs of thyrotoxicosis, however it can also be associated with overt symptoms of hyperthyroidism, including atrial fibrillation, increased cardiac contractility and bone resorption. Despite the presence of cardiovascular disorders associated with subclinical hyperthyroidism, it was shown to be not associated with changes in blood pressure or incident hypertension [40, 41].

PATHOGENESIS OF THYROID DISEASE RELATED HYPERTENSION

Thyroid hormones affect all physiological systems and thyroid dysfunction has adverse effects on cardiovascular system and blood pressure regulation. Although thyroid disorders are generally considered as a rare cause of endocrine related hypertension, thyroid dysfunction is common in the population and thyroid disease related hypertension, which is reversible if early and adequate therapy is given, has to be excluded in hypertensive patients.

Blood pressure is created by cardiac output and total peripheral vascular resistance, both of which are influenced by thyroid hormones. Both hypothyroidism and hyperthyroidism can cause hypertension using different mechanisms of action: Hyperthyroidism generally causes increased cardiac output, resulting in systolic hypertension, whereas hypothyroidism is associated with increased peripheral vascular resistance, resulting in mainly diastolic hypertension. The prevalence of hypertension is three times higher in hypothyroid patients compared to euthyroid group [42].

Effects on Vascular System and Blood Volume

Although the exact mechanism of thyroid hormone on vascular system is still not clear, thyroid hormones have been shown to induce vasodilation by mediating relaxation of vascular smooth muscle cells and by enhancing endothelial nitric oxide production [43 - 46]. D1, D2, and D3 enzymes and TR were all shown to be expressed in endothelial microvascular cultured cell model [47]. D2 enzyme, which converts T_4 to T_3 is thought to mediate vasodilation and decrease peripheral vascular resistance [48]. Thyroid hormones enhance endothelial nitric oxide production, which mediates vasodilation possibly through phosphatidylinositol 3-kinase/Akt pathway and this effect is impaired when endothelial nitric oxide release is competitively inhibited [44, 45]. Several other mechanisms for T_3-induced vasodilation have also been proposed: In vitro studies on vascular smooth muscle cells showed that T_3 induces adrenomedullin expression, which is a potent vasorelaxant and antioxidant peptide [49, 50]. T_3 also increases adenosine monophosphate (AMP) hydrolysis to yield adenosine, through induction of ecto-5'-nucleotidase enzyme [51]. Similar to nitric oxide and adrenomedullin, adenosine also acts as a local vasodilator peptide on vascular smooth muscle cells. Another mechanism for vasodilation is downregulation of angiotensin II type-1 receptor expression in high serum T_3 concentrations [52]. Angiotensin II is a potent vasoconstrictor peptide, also promoting aldosterone synthesis and secretion, vasopressin secretion, cardiac hypertrophy and contractility, peripheral noradrenergic activity, vascular smooth muscle cell proliferation and renal tubular sodium reabsorption, all of which increase blood pressure [53]. In vascular smooth muscle cells, T_3 also increases matrix Gla protein, which is an inhibitor of vascular calcification [54]. Thus, atherosclerotic changes on vasculature can also be prevented by thyroid hormones.

In hypothyroid state, decreased level of T_3 is associated with vasoconstriction and increased peripheral vascular resistance [43]. The incidence of atherosclerosis is also increased in hypothyroid patients, which was postulated to be created by hypercholesterolemia, hypertension and endothelial dysfunction [46]. In the presence of hypothyroidism, activity of D2 enzyme present on coronary artery and aortic smooth muscle cells was shown to be increased, which possibly has a protective role on human vessels from local T_3 deficiency [48]. On contrary, D2 mRNA expression is inhibited when thyroid hormones are replaced, and the potency of inhibitory effect was found as $T_3 > T_4 > rT_3$ [48]. Hypothyroidism is also associated with arterial stiffness, changes in arterial wall elasticity and increased radial wall thickness and adequate thyroid hormone replacement therapy can reverse these effects [55 - 58]. On contrast, peripheral vascular resistance generally decreases in hyperthyroid state, due to vasodilatory effect of thyroid hormones on vasculature.

In addition to effects of thyroid hormones on vascular system, blood volume is also affected by thyroid hormone status. Blood volume is decreased in hypothyroidism, whereas in the presence of hyperthyroidism blood volume is increased, as a result of decreased vascular resistance, leading to activation of renin-angiotensin-aldosterone system and stimulation of renal sodium reabsorption [59, 60].

Effects on Cardiac Function

The primary thyroid hormone that acts on cardiomyocytes is T_3, which can enter the cells via diffusion due to its lipophilic nature and act on TR promoting transcription of several cardiac genes encoding important structural and regulatory proteins on myocardium, such as myosin heavy chain-α (MHC-α), sarco/endoplasmic reticulum Ca^{2+}-ATPase (SERCA), Na^+/K^+ ATPase, Na^+/Ca^{2+} exchanger, some voltage gated K^+ channels, β-adrenergic receptor, cardiac troponin I, protein kinases and atrial natriuretic peptide [61 - 66]. Thyroid hormones can also downregulate transcription of some other genes, such as myosin heavy chain-β (MHC-β) and phospholamban. Thyroid hormones upregulate expression of SERCA, which transfers Ca^{2+} from cytosol to the sarcoplasmic reticulum and enable muscle relaxation during diastole. On the other hand, thyroid hormones also repress phospholamban expression, which is a reversible inhibitor of SERCA [61, 67]. Besides SERCA, thyroid hormones also regulate other ion channels, which are Na^+/K^+ ATPase, Na^+/Ca^{2+} exchanger, some voltage gated K^+ channels, thereby coordinate cardiac electrochemical and mechanical responses [61, 68, 69]. Thyroid hormones effect action potential duration, which is prolonged in hypothyroid state compared to euthyroid cardiomyocytes [70]. T_3 stimulates the expression of β_1-adrenergic receptors, which increase heart rate, cardiomyocyte contractility and automaticity [71]. T_3 and T_4 can also exhibit non-genomic effects on actin polymerization, plasma membrane calcium ATPase, adenine nucleotide translocase of the inner mitochondrial membrane, adenylate cyclase and glucose transporters [35, 72].

Long term hyperthyroidism increases cardiac workload causing myocardial hypertrophy, especially in the left ventricle. Heart rate, cardiac contractility, diastolic function and venous blood return is increased in hyperthyroidism, which result in increased cardiac ejection fraction and cardiac output. Hyperthyroidism is characterized by decreased diastolic blood pressure, as a result of decreased vascular resistance and increased systolic blood pressure, which results from increased cardiac output. Thyroid hormone excess also stimulates cardiomyocyte automaticity, which results in atrial fibrillation [60].

On the other hand, in hypothyroid state, cardiac output is reduced, as a result of decreased myocardial contractility, heart rate and ejection fraction [35, 60, 71].

Renal Dysfunction

Thyroid hormones play role in kidney development and maturation. Congenital hypothyroidism results in decreased kidney volume and congenital renal abnormalities, including dysplastic kidney, hydronephrosis and renal agenesis [33, 73]. Thyroid hormones act on various ion channels and transporters in kidney via genomic or non-genomic alterations, including Na^+/K^+ ATPase, $Na^+/K^+/2Cl^-$ cotransporter, Na^+/Ca^{2+} exchanger, Na^+/H^+ exchanger, Cl^- channel and aquaporin [33].

In hypothyroidism, renal dysfunction occurs due to combination of both decreased cardiac output, which results in decreased renal blood flow and glomerular filtration rate, and dysfunction of renal ion channels and transporters. Hyponatremia is the most common electrolyte abnormality in hypothyroidism and it is due to impaired water excretion and reduced sodium reabsorption [74]. Despite electrolyte imbalance, creatinine levels can remain within normal limits, as a result of decreased creatinine production, therefore creatinine is not a reliable indicator of renal dysfunction in hypothyroidism [75, 76]. In addition to electrolyte imbalance, reduced expression of renal vasodilators, like vascular endothelial growth factor (VEGF), and insulin-like growth factor-1 (IGF-1) also contribute to hypertension in hypothyroid state [74].

In hyperthyroidism, activation of renal ion channels and transporters lead to increased Na^+ reabsorption. Increased cardiac output, renal blood flow and glomerular filtration rate downregulate aquaporin, which in turn increases water excretion leading to polyuria in hyperthyroidism [74, 77]. Increased chloride reabsorption activates renin-angiotensin-aldosterone system. In hyperthyroid state, dysfunction of kidneys leads to impaired urine concentration and decreased total body water [23, 74].

Effects on Blood Pressure Regulation

Renin-Angiotensin-Aldosterone System

Renin-angiotensin-aldosterone system (RAAS) is one of the main hormonal regulator of blood pressure. Renin is synthesized and secreted from renal juxtaglomerular apparatus, which is very sensitive to low blood pressure. Renin enables conversion of hepatic angiotensinogen to angiotensin I, which is subsequently converted to angiotensin II by angiotensin converting enzyme (ACE) in lungs. Angiotensin II has many effects on body systems mediating increased blood pressure, including renal Na^+, Cl^- and water reabsorption together with increased adrenal aldosterone secretion, arteriolar vasoconstriction, posterior pituitary gland ADH secretion and increased sympathetic activity.

Thyroid hormones increase renin synthesis and secretion, aldosterone production and hepatic angiotensinogen production [35]. Decreased systemic vascular resistance mediated by thyroid hormones also contribute to increased renin secretion in hyperthyroidism. As a result of RAAS activation, renal tubular Na^+ and Cl^- reabsorption, water retention and pituitary gland ADH secretion are increased, all of which mediate increased cardiac preload and cardiac output, resulting in systolic hypertension [78]. On the other hand, in hypothyroidism, many components of RAAS, including renal renin secretion, hepatic angiotensinogen production, serum angiotensin converting enzyme (ACE) activity and adrenal aldosterone production are decreased, which result in hyponatremia together with low serum renin values [60, 78].

Natriuretic Peptides

Atrial natriuretic peptide (ANP) and brain natriuretic peptide (BNP) are produced and secreted by cardiac atrium, which contains volume receptors and are activated when atrial blood volume is increased. Both target kidney glomerulus, distal tubules and collecting duct, increase glomerular filtration rate and promote Na^+ and water excretion, which result in reduced extracellular fluid volume and decreased blood pressure [79]. Expression of natriuretic peptide prohormone gene is regulated by thyroid hormones and plasma natriuretic peptide levels change depending on thyroid hormone state [35, 80 - 82].

Antidiuretic Hormone (Vasopressin)

Antidiuretic hormone (ADH) is synthesized as a prohormone in hypothalamus and transferred to posterior pituitary gland, where they are released into circulation in response to increased osmolarity. ADH targets kidney and arterioles, promoting both water reabsorption and vasoconstriction leading to increased blood pressure. Plasma ADH levels and related hyponatremia were reported in many hypothyroid patients, which is mainly attributed to decreased cardiac output in hypothyroidism [83, 84].

Catecholamines

Catecholamines, including adrenaline (epinephrine), noradrenaline (norepinephrine) are mainly synthesized in adrenal gland medulla in response to adrenergic stimuli, but also from postganglionic fibers of the sympathetic nervous system. Catecholamines are stress-hormones and regulate body response in case of disturbance of normal body equilibrium, including hypovolemia, hypoglycemia, psychosocial stress and trauma [85]. Catecholamines elevate blood pressure by increasing cardiac output, peripheral vasoconstriction and sodium retention. There are different types of adrenergic receptors in various tissues: α_1 and β_2-adrenergic receptors are expressed in heart and vascular smooth muscles, α_2-adrenergic receptors are on vascular smooth muscle and β_1-adrenergic receptors are on atria and ventricles [35, 86].

Thyroid hormones regulate several β-adrenergic system on cardiomyocytes, including β_1-adrenergic receptors, guanine nucleotide regulatory proteins and adenylate cyclase, which cause β-adrenergic symptoms despite normal or low serum catecholamine levels in hyperthyroidism [18, 71]. Beta-blockers are therefore often used for treatment of cardiac symptoms, including tachycardia and hypertension in hyperthyroidism.

Adrenomedullin

Adrenomedullin is a vasodilator peptide produced by many organs and tissues including endothelial and smooth muscle cells. Besides vasodilation, it also enhances natriuresis and nitric oxide production and it has anti-apoptotic effects [87]. Relationship between adrenomedullin and thyroid hormones is controversial: In vitro studies have shown T_3 induced adrenomedullin mRNA expression in endothelial and vascular smooth muscle cells, whereas in vivo human studies could not confirm the relationship between plasma adrenomedullin concentration and peripheral vascular resistance [50, 76, 88, 89].

Erythropoietin

Erythropoietin is synthesized and secreted from kidneys in response to hypoxia and induces erythropoiesis in bone marrow. Thyroid hormones increase erythropoietin secretion, which leads to increase in erythrocyte production, total blood volume and blood pressure [78, 90].

DIAGNOSIS OF THYROID DISORDERS

Serum TSH measurement is the most common laboratory test for diagnosis of thyroid disorders. A normal serum TSH value is generally a strong indicator of euthyroid state. Hyperthyroidism is generally presented with low serum TSH levels and high serum free T_3 and free T_4 levels, whereas in hypothyroidism serum TSH value is generally elevated and serum T_4 value is generally low. However, these combinations of TSH and free T_3 and T_4 values are not valid for each thyroid disease or patient and low TSH values can also be seen in other conditions, such as non-thyroidal illness, central hypothyroidism and early pregnancy [91]. In TSH-secreting pituitary adenomas, serum TSH levels are elevated. Patients with central hypothyroidism TSH value can be within normal limits or elevated. Also, patients with generalized thyroid hormone resistance can have elevated TSH and free T_4 levels [92].

Apart from TSH and free thyroid hormone level measurement, other laboratory tests are also used for differential diagnosis of thyroid disorder. In Hashimoto's thyroiditis, serum level of anti-TPO antibodies and/or anti-Tg antibodies are elevated. TRAB measurement can be helpful to diagnose Graves' disease and to detect disease activation on follow-up. In subacute thyroiditis, acute phase reactants, including C-reactive protein level, sedimentation rate and leukocyte count are elevated.

Thyroid ultrasonography (USG) is the first line imaging tool for diagnosis of thyroid disorders, which can aid measurement of thyroid volume and detection of thyroid nodules and presence of thyroiditis. Thyroid scintigraphy and radioiodine uptake test also help differentiating toxic adenomas, toxic multinodular goiter, Graves' disease and thyroiditis. Scintigraphic imaging with Tc-99m pertechnetate generally yields bilateral diffuse hyperplasia of the thyroid gland in Graves' disease, solitary nodular increased radiopharmaceutical uptake with/without suppression of the surrounding thyroidal tissue in toxic adenomas, multinodular hyperplasia of the thyroid gland with/without suppression of the surrounding thyroidal tissue in toxic multinodular goiter and reduced thyroidal radiopharmaceutical uptake in thyroiditis. Hashitoxicosis can scintigraphically mimic Graves' disease and be initially presented with diffuse increased radiopharmaceutical uptake. I-123 or I-131 uptake is generally elevated in hyperthyroidism and decreased in thyroiditis.

TREATMENT OF THYROID DISEASE RELATED HYPERTENSION

Hypertension secondary to thyroid disorders usually resolves after achievement of euthyroidism [78, 93]. Therefore, thyroid function tests are recommended for patients with resistant hypertension. However, treatment of the underlying thyroid pathology can take time and hypertension may be prolonged even after achievement of euthyroid state, therefore antihypertensive treatment may also be necessary.

Beta-blockers, like propranolol are commonly used for hyperthyroid patients with palpitations and tachycardia and aid reducing the systolic hypertension. Propranolol also reduce serum T_3 concentration by inhibition of peripheral conversion of T_4 to T_3. If beta-blockers are contra-indicated, for instance in asthmatic patients, either β_1-selective drugs, calcium channel blockers or ACE inhibitors are recommended for anti-hypertensive treatment [78].

Treatment alternatives for hyperthyroidism are anti-thyroid drugs, including propylthiouracil and methimazole, radioiodine therapy with I-131 or thyroidectomy operation. The optimal treatment modality can vary among patients and disease status. Generally anti-thyroid drugs are preferred for initial therapy of Graves' disease for 12-18 months, unless contra-indicated or indications for definitive treatment exist, like refractory disease despite anti-thyroid drugs, severe orbitopathy, liver or bone-marrow toxicity or suspicion for a malignant thyroid nodule [60]. In case of toxic adenoma or toxic multinodular goiter, radioiodine therapy is generally preferred as the first-line treatment, and anti-thyroid drugs are generally used until euthyroid state is established.

Treatment of hypothyroidism involves L-thyroxin replacement therapy, which was shown to reduce blood pressure after establishment of euthyroid state. Subclinical hypothyroidism can remain unnoticed leading to a challenge in patients with resistant hypertension and can be depicted easily after thyroid function tests. As many components of renin-angiotensin-aldosterone system are decreased in hypothyroidism, including renal renin secretion, hepatic angiotensinogen production, serum ACE activity and adrenal aldosterone production, hypothyroidism is typically associated with low serum renin values and hyponatremia [60, 78]. Yet, salt restriction in hypothyroid state was shown to lower blood pressure [78, 94]. Generally, calcium channel blockers and diuretics are recommended for anti-hypertensive treatment in hypothyroid patients [78].

CONCLUSION

Thyroid hormones affect several mechanisms regulating blood pressure by modulating gene expression of several hormones and regulatory proteins or by exhibiting non-genomic effects on plasma membrane and cytoplasmic proteins. The most profound effects of thyroid hormones are on metabolic rate and cardiovascular function, but effects of thyroid hormones can be seen on all body systems, including liver metabolism, kidney function and pulmonary system. Thyroid hormones induce vasodilation mainly by mediating relaxation of vascular smooth muscle cells and by enhancing endothelial nitric oxide production, but also by modulating expression of other regulatory proteins, including adrenomedullin, adenosine and angiotensin II. Thyroid hormones promote transcription of several cardiac genes encoding important structural and regulatory proteins on myocardium, thereby act on heart rate, cardiomyocyte contractility, automaticity and cardiac output. They also play role in kidney development and act on various ion channels and transporters in kidney, affecting blood pressure. Finally, thyroid hormones act on synthesis and secretion of several hormones regulating blood pressure, including renin-angiotensin-aldosterone system, natriuretic peptides, ADH and catecholamines.

Both hyperthyroidism and hypothyroidism can result in hypertension using different mechanisms of action: Hyperthyroidism generally causes increased cardiac output, resulting in systolic hypertension, whereas hypothyroidism is generally associated with increased peripheral vascular resistance, resulting in mainly diastolic hypertension.

Hypertension secondary to thyroid disorders usually resolves after achievement of euthyroidism. Therefore, screening for an underlying thyroid pathology is recommended in all patients with resistant hypertension in order to give the appropriate treatment.

CONSENT FOR PUBLICATION

Not applicable.

CONFLICT OF INTEREST

The authors declare no conflict of interest, financial or otherwise.

ACKNOWLEDGEMENT

Declare none.

REFERENCES

[1]   Gereben B, Zavacki AM, Ribich S, *et al.* Cellular and molecular basis of deiodinase-regulated thyroid hormone signaling. Endocr Rev 2008; 29(7): 898-938.
[http://dx.doi.org/10.1210/er.2008-0019] [PMID: 18815314]

[2]   Wu Y, Koenig RJ. Gene regulation by thyroid hormone. Trends Endocrinol Metab 2000; 11(6): 207-11.
[http://dx.doi.org/10.1016/S1043-2760(00)00263-0] [PMID: 10878749]

[3]   Yen PM, Ando S, Feng X, Liu Y, Maruvada P, Xia X. Thyroid hormone action at the cellular, genomic and target gene levels. Mol Cell Endocrinol 2006; 246(1-2): 121-7.
[http://dx.doi.org/10.1016/j.mce.2005.11.030] [PMID: 16442701]

[4]   Bianco AC, Salvatore D, Gereben B, Berry MJ, Larsen PR. Biochemistry, cellular and molecular biology, and physiological roles of the iodothyronine selenodeiodinases. Endocr Rev 2002; 23(1): 38-89.
[http://dx.doi.org/10.1210/edrv.23.1.0455] [PMID: 11844744]

[5]   Buettner C, Harney JW, Larsen PR. The role of selenocysteine 133 in catalysis by the human type 2 iodothyronine deiodinase. Endocrinology 2000; 141(12): 4606-12.
[http://dx.doi.org/10.1210/endo.141.12.7831] [PMID: 11108274]

[6]   Berry MJ, Banu L, Larsen PR. Type I iodothyronine deiodinase is a selenocysteine-containing enzyme. Nature 1991; 349(6308): 438-40.
[http://dx.doi.org/10.1038/349438a0] [PMID: 1825132]

[7]   Rhee CM, Ravel VA, Streja E, *et al.* Thyroid functional disease and mortality in a national peritoneal dialysis cohort. J Clin Endocrinol Metab 2016; 101(11): 4054-61.
[http://dx.doi.org/10.1210/jc.2016-1691] [PMID: 27525529]

[8]   Fonseca TL, Correa-Medina M, Campos MP, *et al.* Coordination of hypothalamic and pituitary T3 production regulates TSH expression. J Clin Invest 2013; 123(4): 1492-500.
[http://dx.doi.org/10.1172/JCI61231] [PMID: 23524969]

[9]   Larsen PR. Thyroid-pituitary interaction: feedback regulation of thyrotropin secretion by thyroid hormones. N Engl J Med 1982; 306(1): 23-32.
[http://dx.doi.org/10.1056/NEJM198201073060107] [PMID: 7031472]

[10]   Reed HL. Environmental influences upon thyroid hormone regulation. Werner & Ingbar's the thyroid: a fundamental and clinical text. 9th ed. Philadelphia, Penn.; London: Lippincott Williams & Wilkins 2004; pp. 219-29.

[11]   Malik R, Hodgson H. The relationship between the thyroid gland and the liver. QJM 2002; 95(9): 559-69.
[http://dx.doi.org/10.1093/qjmed/95.9.559] [PMID: 12205333]

[12]   Visser TJ. Pathways of thyroid hormone metabolism. Acta Med Austriaca 1996; 23(1-2): 10-6.
[PMID: 8767510]

[13]   Mullur R, Liu YY, Brent GA. Thyroid hormone regulation of metabolism. Physiol Rev 2014; 94(2): 355-82.
[http://dx.doi.org/10.1152/physrev.00030.2013] [PMID: 24692351]

[14]   Yen PM. Genomic and nongenomic actions of thyroid hormones. Werner & Ingbar's the thyroid: a fundamental and clinical text. 9th ed. Philadelphia, Penn.; London: Lippincott Williams & Wilkins 2004; pp. 135-50.

[15]   Brent GA. Mechanisms of thyroid hormone action. J Clin Invest 2012; 122(9): 3035-43.
[http://dx.doi.org/10.1172/JCI60047] [PMID: 22945636]

[16]   Chi HC, Chen CY, Tsai MM, Tsai CY, Lin KH. Molecular functions of thyroid hormones and their clinical significance in liver-related diseases. BioMed Res Int 2013; 2013 601361.

[http://dx.doi.org/10.1155/2013/601361] [PMID: 23878812]

[17] Oppenheimer JH, Schwartz HL, Mariash CN, Kinlaw WB, Wong NC, Freake HC. Advances in our understanding of thyroid hormone action at the cellular level. Endocr Rev 1987; 8(3): 288-308.
[http://dx.doi.org/10.1210/edrv-8-3-288] [PMID: 3308445]

[18] Klein I, Ojamaa K. Thyroid hormone and the cardiovascular system. N Engl J Med 2001; 344(7): 501-9.
[http://dx.doi.org/10.1056/NEJM200102153440707] [PMID: 11172193]

[19] Kim B. Thyroid hormone as a determinant of energy expenditure and the basal metabolic rate. Thyroid: Official journal of the American Thyroid Association 2008; 18(2): 141-4.
[http://dx.doi.org/10.1089/thy.2007.0266]

[20] Warner A, Mittag J. Thyroid hormone and the central control of homeostasis. J Mol Endocrinol 2012; 49(1): R29-35.
[http://dx.doi.org/10.1530/JME-12-0068] [PMID: 22586142]

[21] Williams GR. Actions of thyroid hormones in bone. Endokrynol Pol 2009; 60(5): 380-8.
[PMID: 19885809]

[22] Kawa MP, Grymula K, Paczkowska E, *et al.* Clinical relevance of thyroid dysfunction in human haematopoiesis: biochemical and molecular studies. Eur J Endocrinol 2010; 162(2): 295-305.
[http://dx.doi.org/10.1530/EJE-09-0875] [PMID: 19903799]

[23] Basu G, Mohapatra A. Interactions between thyroid disorders and kidney disease. Indian J Endocrinol Metab 2012; 16(2): 204-13.
[http://dx.doi.org/10.4103/2230-8210.93737] [PMID: 22470856]

[24] Hume R, Richard K, Kaptein E, Stanley EL, Visser TJ, Coughtrie MW. Thyroid hormone metabolism and the developing human lung. Biol Neonate 2001; 80 (Suppl. 1): 18-21.
[http://dx.doi.org/10.1159/000047172] [PMID: 11359040]

[25] Cheng SY, Leonard JL, Davis PJ. Molecular aspects of thyroid hormone actions. Endocr Rev 2010; 31(2): 139-70.
[http://dx.doi.org/10.1210/er.2009-0007] [PMID: 20051527]

[26] Brent GA. The molecular basis of thyroid hormone action. N Engl J Med 1994; 331(13): 847-53.
[http://dx.doi.org/10.1056/NEJM199409293311306] [PMID: 8078532]

[27] Bianco AC, Kim BW. Deiodinases: implications of the local control of thyroid hormone action. J Clin Invest 2006; 116(10): 2571-9.
[http://dx.doi.org/10.1172/JCI29812] [PMID: 17016550]

[28] Peeters RP, Debaveye Y, Fliers E, Visser TJ. Changes within the thyroid axis during critical illness. Crit Care Clin 2006; 22(1): 41-55.
[http://dx.doi.org/10.1016/j.ccc.2005.08.006] [PMID: 16399019]

[29] Martino E, Bartalena L, Bogazzi F, Braverman LE. The effects of amiodarone on the thyroid. Endocr Rev 2001; 22(2): 240-54.
[PMID: 11294826]

[30] Huang SA, Tu HM, Harney JW, *et al.* Severe hypothyroidism caused by type 3 iodothyronine deiodinase in infantile hemangiomas. N Engl J Med 2000; 343(3): 185-9.
[http://dx.doi.org/10.1056/NEJM200007203430305] [PMID: 10900278]

[31] Alexander EK, Marqusee E, Lawrence J, Jarolim P, Fischer GA, Larsen PR. Timing and magnitude of increases in levothyroxine requirements during pregnancy in women with hypothyroidism. N Engl J Med 2004; 351(3): 241-9.
[http://dx.doi.org/10.1056/NEJMoa040079] [PMID: 15254282]

[32] Huang SA, Dorfman DM, Genest DR, Salvatore D, Larsen PR. Type 3 iodothyronine deiodinase is highly expressed in the human uteroplacental unit and in fetal epithelium. J Clin Endocrinol Metab

2003; 88(3): 1384-8.
[http://dx.doi.org/10.1210/jc.2002-021291] [PMID: 12629133]

[33]   Mariani LH, Berns JS. The renal manifestations of thyroid disease. J Am Soc Nephrol 2012; 23(1): 22-6.
[http://dx.doi.org/10.1681/ASN.2010070766] [PMID: 22021708]

[34]   Biondi B, Palmieri EA, Lombardi G, Fazio S. Effects of thyroid hormone on cardiac function: the relative importance of heart rate, loading conditions, and myocardial contractility in the regulation of cardiac performance in human hyperthyroidism. J Clin Endocrinol Metab 2002; 87(3): 968-74.
[http://dx.doi.org/10.1210/jcem.87.3.8302] [PMID: 11889145]

[35]   Danzi S, Klein I. Thyroid hormone and blood pressure regulation. Curr Hypertens Rep 2003; 5(6): 513-20.
[http://dx.doi.org/10.1007/s11906-003-0060-7] [PMID: 14594573]

[36]   Grais IM, Sowers JR. Thyroid and the heart. Am J Med 2014; 127(8): 691-8.
[http://dx.doi.org/10.1016/j.amjmed.2014.03.009] [PMID: 24662620]

[37]   Prabhakar BS, Bahn RS, Smith TJ. Current perspective on the pathogenesis of Graves' disease and ophthalmopathy. Endocr Rev 2003; 24(6): 802-35.
[http://dx.doi.org/10.1210/er.2002-0020] [PMID: 14671007]

[38]   Singer PA. Primary Hypothyroidism due to other causes. Werner & Ingbar's the thyroid: a fundamental and clinical text. 9th ed. Philadelphia, Penn.; London: Lippincott Williams & Wilkins 2004; pp. 745-53.

[39]   Polat Canbolat I, Belen E, Bayyigit A, Helvaci A, Kilickesmez K. Evaluation of daily blood pressure alteration in subclinical hypothyroidism. Acta Cardiol Sin 2017; 33(5): 489-94.
[PMID: 28959101]

[40]   Völzke H, Alte D, Dörr M, *et al.* The association between subclinical hyperthyroidism and blood pressure in a population-based study. J Hypertens 2006; 24(10): 1947-53.
[http://dx.doi.org/10.1097/01.hjh.0000244942.57417.8e] [PMID: 16957553]

[41]   Völzke H, Ittermann T, Schmidt CO, *et al.* Subclinical hyperthyroidism and blood pressure in a population-based prospective cohort study. Eur J Endocrinol 2009; 161(4): 615-21.
[http://dx.doi.org/10.1530/EJE-09-0376] [PMID: 19581285]

[42]   Saito I, Saruta T. Hypertension in thyroid disorders. Endocrinol Metab Clin North Am 1994; 23(2): 379-86.
[http://dx.doi.org/10.1016/S0889-8529(18)30103-8] [PMID: 8070428]

[43]   Ojamaa K, Klemperer JD, Klein I. Acute effects of thyroid hormone on vascular smooth muscle. Thyroid: Official journal of the American Thyroid Association 1996; 6(5): 505-12.
[http://dx.doi.org/10.1089/thy.1996.6.505]

[44]   Napoli R, Biondi B, Guardasole V, *et al.* Impact of hyperthyroidism and its correction on vascular reactivity in humans. Circulation 2001; 104(25): 3076-80.
[http://dx.doi.org/10.1161/hc5001.100621] [PMID: 11748103]

[45]   Hiroi Y, Kim HH, Ying H, *et al.* Rapid nongenomic actions of thyroid hormone. Proc Natl Acad Sci USA 2006; 103(38): 14104-9.
[http://dx.doi.org/10.1073/pnas.0601600103] [PMID: 16966610]

[46]   Ichiki T. Thyroid hormone and atherosclerosis. Vascul Pharmacol 2010; 52(3-4): 151-6.
[http://dx.doi.org/10.1016/j.vph.2009.09.004] [PMID: 19808101]

[47]   Sabatino L, Lubrano V, Balzan S, Kusmic C, Del Turco S, Iervasi G. Thyroid hormone deiodinases D1, D2, and D3 are expressed in human endothelial dermal microvascular line: effects of thyroid hormones. Mol Cell Biochem 2015; 399(1-2): 87-94.
[http://dx.doi.org/10.1007/s11010-014-2235-8] [PMID: 25304215]

[48]   Mizuma H, Murakami M, Mori M. Thyroid hormone activation in human vascular smooth muscle cells: expression of type II iodothyronine deiodinase. Circ Res 2001; 88(3): 313-8.
[http://dx.doi.org/10.1161/01.RES.88.3.313] [PMID: 11179199]

[49]   Isumi Y, Shoji H, Sugo S, *et al.* Regulation of adrenomedullin production in rat endothelial cells. Endocrinology 1998; 139(3): 838-46.
[http://dx.doi.org/10.1210/endo.139.3.5789] [PMID: 9492011]

[50]   Imai T, Hirata Y, Iwashina M, Marumo F. Hormonal regulation of rat adrenomedullin gene in vasculature. Endocrinology 1995; 136(4): 1544-8.
[http://dx.doi.org/10.1210/endo.136.4.7895664] [PMID: 7895664]

[51]   Tamajusuku AS, Carrillo-Sepúlveda MA, Braganhol E, *et al.* Activity and expression of ecto-5--nucleotidase/CD73 are increased by thyroid hormones in vascular smooth muscle cells. Mol Cell Biochem 2006; 289(1-2): 65-72.
[http://dx.doi.org/10.1007/s11010-006-9148-0] [PMID: 16718378]

[52]   Fukuyama K, Ichiki T, Takeda K, *et al.* Downregulation of vascular angiotensin II type 1 receptor by thyroid hormone. Hypertension 2003; 41(3): 598-603.
[http://dx.doi.org/10.1161/01.HYP.0000056524.35294.80] [PMID: 12623965]

[53]   Catt KJ, Mendelsohn FA, Millan MA, Aguilera G. The role of angiotensin II receptors in vascular regulation. J Cardiovasc Pharmacol 1984; 6 (Suppl. 4): S575-86.
[http://dx.doi.org/10.1097/00005344-198406004-00004] [PMID: 6083400]

[54]   Sato Y, Nakamura R, Satoh M, *et al.* Thyroid hormone targets matrix Gla protein gene associated with vascular smooth muscle calcification. Circ Res 2005; 97(6): 550-7.
[http://dx.doi.org/10.1161/01.RES.0000181431.04290.bd] [PMID: 16100044]

[55]   Dagre AG, Lekakis JP, Papaioannou TG, *et al.* Arterial stiffness is increased in subjects with hypothyroidism. Int J Cardiol 2005; 103(1): 1-6.
[http://dx.doi.org/10.1016/j.ijcard.2004.05.068] [PMID: 16061115]

[56]   Obuobie K, Smith J, Evans LM, John R, Davies JS, Lazarus JH. Increased central arterial stiffness in hypothyroidism. J Clin Endocrinol Metab 2002; 87(10): 4662-6.
[http://dx.doi.org/10.1210/jc.2002-020493] [PMID: 12364455]

[57]   Giannattasio C, Rivolta MR, Failla M, Mangoni AA, Stella ML, Mancia G. Large and medium sized artery abnormalities in untreated and treated hypothyroidism. Eur Heart J 1997; 18(9): 1492-8.
[http://dx.doi.org/10.1093/oxfordjournals.eurheartj.a015477] [PMID: 9458457]

[58]   Nagasaki T, Inaba M, Henmi Y, *et al.* Decrease in carotid intima-media thickness in hypothyroid patients after normalization of thyroid function. Clin Endocrinol (Oxf) 2003; 59(5): 607-12.
[http://dx.doi.org/10.1046/j.1365-2265.2003.01893.x] [PMID: 14616885]

[59]   Resnick LM, Laragh JH. PLasma renin activity in syndromes of thyroid hormone excess and deficiency. Life Sci 1982; 30(7-8): 585-6.
[http://dx.doi.org/10.1016/0024-3205(82)90273-9] [PMID: 7040894]

[60]   Spitzweg C, Reincke M. Thyroid diseases and hypertension. Der Internist 2010; 51(5): 603-4.

[61]   Mishra P, Samanta L. Oxidative stress and heart failure in altered thyroid States. ScientificWorldJournal 2012; 2012741861
[http://dx.doi.org/10.1100/2012/741861] [PMID: 22649319]

[62]   Tsika RW, Bahl JJ, Leinwand LA, Morkin E. Thyroid hormone regulates expression of a transfected human alpha-myosin heavy-chain fusion gene in fetal rat heart cells. Proc Natl Acad Sci USA 1990; 87(1): 379-83.
[http://dx.doi.org/10.1073/pnas.87.1.379] [PMID: 2296592]

[63]   Zarain-Herzberg A, Marques J, Sukovich D, Periasamy M. Thyroid hormone receptor modulates the expression of the rabbit cardiac sarco (endo) plasmic reticulum Ca(2+)-ATPase gene. J Biol Chem

1994; 269(2): 1460-7.
[PMID: 8166809]

[64]   Orlowski J, Lingrel JB. Thyroid and glucocorticoid hormones regulate the expression of multiple
        Na,K-ATPase genes in cultured neonatal rat cardiac myocytes. J Biol Chem 1990; 265(6): 3462-70.
        [PMID: 1689303]

[65]   Bahouth SW. Thyroid hormones transcriptionally regulate the beta 1-adrenergic receptor gene in
        cultured ventricular myocytes. J Biol Chem 1991; 266(24): 15863-9.
        [PMID: 1651924]

[66]   Fullerton MJ, Stuchbury S, Krozowski ZS, Funder JW. Altered thyroidal status and the in vivo
        synthesis of atrial natriuretic peptide in the rat heart. Mol Cell Endocrinol 1990; 69(2-3): 227-33.
        [http://dx.doi.org/10.1016/0303-7207(90)90016-2] [PMID: 2139421]

[67]   MacLennan DH, Kranias EG. Phospholamban: a crucial regulator of cardiac contractility. Nat Rev
        Mol Cell Biol 2003; 4(7): 566-77.
        [http://dx.doi.org/10.1038/nrm1151] [PMID: 12838339]

[68]   Gick GG, Melikian J, Ismail-Beigi F. Thyroidal enhancement of rat myocardial Na,K-ATPase:
        preferential expression of alpha 2 activity and mRNA abundance. J Membr Biol 1990; 115(3): 273-82.
        [http://dx.doi.org/10.1007/BF01868642] [PMID: 2165172]

[69]   Ojamaa K, Sabet A, Kenessey A, Shenoy R, Klein I. Regulation of rat cardiac Kv1.5 gene expression
        by thyroid hormone is rapid and chamber specific. Endocrinology 1999; 140(7): 3170-6.
        [http://dx.doi.org/10.1210/endo.140.7.6776] [PMID: 10385411]

[70]   Sun ZQ, Ojamaa K, Coetzee WA, Artman M, Klein I. Effects of thyroid hormone on action potential
        and repolarizing currents in rat ventricular myocytes. Am J Physiol Endocrinol Metab 2000; 278(2):
        E302-7.
        [http://dx.doi.org/10.1152/ajpendo.2000.278.2.E302] [PMID: 10662715]

[71]   Klein I, Danzi S. Thyroid disease and the heart. Circulation 2007; 116(15): 1725-35.
        [http://dx.doi.org/10.1161/CIRCULATIONAHA.106.678326] [PMID: 17923583]

[72]   Davis PJ, Davis FB. Nongenomic actions of thyroid hormone on the heart. Thyroid: Official journal of
        the American Thyroid Association 2002; 12(6): 459-66.
        [http://dx.doi.org/10.1089/105072502760143827]

[73]   Kumar J, Gordillo R, Kaskel FJ, Druschel CM, Woroniecki RP. Increased prevalence of renal and
        urinary tract anomalies in children with congenital hypothyroidism. J Pediatr 2009; 154(2): 263-6.
        [http://dx.doi.org/10.1016/j.jpeds.2008.08.023] [PMID: 18823909]

[74]   Iglesias P, Bajo MA, Selgas R, Díez JJ. Thyroid dysfunction and kidney disease: An update. Rev
        Endocr Metab Disord 2017; 18(1): 131-44.
        [http://dx.doi.org/10.1007/s11154-016-9395-7] [PMID: 27864708]

[75]   Panciera DL, Lefebvre HP. Effect of experimental hypothyroidism on glomerular filtration rate and
        plasma creatinine concentration in dogs. J Vet Intern Med 2009; 23(5): 1045-50.
        [http://dx.doi.org/10.1111/j.1939-1676.2009.0371.x] [PMID: 19678885]

[76]   Stabouli S, Papakatsika S, Kotsis V. Hypothyroidism and hypertension. Expert Rev Cardiovasc Ther
        2010; 8(11): 1559-65.
        [http://dx.doi.org/10.1586/erc.10.141] [PMID: 21090931]

[77]   Wang W, Li C, Summer SN, Falk S, Schrier RW. Polyuria of thyrotoxicosis: downregulation of
        aquaporin water channels and increased solute excretion. Kidney Int 2007; 72(9): 1088-94.
        [http://dx.doi.org/10.1038/sj.ki.5002475] [PMID: 17700641]

[78]   Mazza A, Beltramello G, Armigliato M, *et al.* Arterial hypertension and thyroid disorders: what is
        important to know in clinical practice? Ann Endocrinol (Paris) 2011; 72(4): 296-303.
        [http://dx.doi.org/10.1016/j.ando.2011.05.004] [PMID: 21777903]

[79]   Goetz KL. Physiology and pathophysiology of atrial peptides. Am J Physiol 1988; 254(1 Pt 1): E1-E15.
[PMID: 2962513]

[80]   Argentin S, Drouin J, Nemer M. Thyroid hormone stimulates rat pro-natriodilatin mRNA levels in primary cardiocyte cultures. Biochem Biophys Res Commun 1987; 146(3): 1336-41.
[http://dx.doi.org/10.1016/0006-291X(87)90796-0] [PMID: 2956954]

[81]   Ladenson PW, Bloch KD, Seidman JG. Modulation of atrial natriuretic factor by thyroid hormone: messenger ribonucleic acid and peptide levels in hypothyroid, euthyroid, and hyperthyroid rat atria and ventricles. Endocrinology 1988; 123(1): 652-7.
[http://dx.doi.org/10.1210/endo-123-1-652] [PMID: 2968239]

[82]   Kohno M, Horio T, Yasunari K, et al. Stimulation of brain natriuretic peptide release from the heart by thyroid hormone. Metabolism 1993; 42(8): 1059-64.
[http://dx.doi.org/10.1016/0026-0495(93)90023-H] [PMID: 8345811]

[83]   Hanna FW, Scanlon MF. Hyponatraemia, hypothyroidism, and role of arginine-vasopressin. Lancet 1997; 350(9080): 755-6.
[http://dx.doi.org/10.1016/S0140-6736(05)62563-9] [PMID: 9297992]

[84]   Liamis G, Filippatos TD, Liontos A, Elisaf MS. Management of endocrine disease: Hypothyroidism-associated hyponatremia: mechanisms, implications and treatment. Eur J Endocrinol 2017; 176(1): R15-20.
[http://dx.doi.org/10.1530/EJE-16-0493] [PMID: 27484454]

[85]   Ranabir S, Reetu K. Stress and hormones. Indian J Endocrinol Metab 2011; 15(1): 18-22.
[http://dx.doi.org/10.4103/2230-8210.77573] [PMID: 21584161]

[86]   Rockman HA, Koch WJ, Lefkowitz RJ. Cardiac function in genetically engineered mice with altered adrenergic receptor signaling. Am J Physiol 1997; 272(4 Pt 2): H1553-9.
[PMID: 9139936]

[87]   Wong HK, Cheung TT, Cheung BM. Adrenomedullin and cardiovascular diseases. JRSM Cardiovasc Dis 2012; 1(5)cvd.2012.012003
[http://dx.doi.org/10.1258/cvd.2012.012003] [PMID: 24175071]

[88]   Diekman MJ, Harms MP, Endert E, Wieling W, Wiersinga WM. Endocrine factors related to changes in total peripheral vascular resistance after treatment of thyrotoxic and hypothyroid patients. Eur J Endocrinol 2001; 144(4): 339-46.
[http://dx.doi.org/10.1530/eje.0.1440339] [PMID: 11275942]

[89]   Nagasaki S, Fukui M, Asano S, et al. Induction of adrenomedullin 2/intermedin expression by thyroid stimulating hormone in thyroid. Mol Cell Endocrinol 2014; 395(1-2): 32-40.
[http://dx.doi.org/10.1016/j.mce.2014.07.008] [PMID: 25102228]

[90]   Klein I, Levey GS. Unusual manifestations of hypothyroidism. Arch Intern Med 1984; 144(1): 123-8.
[http://dx.doi.org/10.1001/archinte.1984.00350130143025] [PMID: 6229226]

[91]   Ladenson PW. Management of thyrotoxicosis. In: Braverman LE, Cooper D, Eds. Werner & Ingbar's the thyroid: A fundamental and clinical text. 9th ed. Philadelphia, Penn.; London: Lippincott Williams & Wilkins 2004; pp. 659-64.

[92]   Ladenson PW. Management of hypothyroidism. In: Braverman LE, Cooper D, Eds. Werner & Ingbar's the thyroid: A fundamental and clinical text. 9th ed. Philadelphia, Penn.; London: Lippincott Williams & Wilkins 2004; pp. 857-63.

[93]   Osman F, Franklyn JA, Holder RL, Sheppard MC, Gammage MD. Cardiovascular manifestations of hyperthyroidism before and after antithyroid therapy: a matched case-control study. J Am Coll Cardiol 2007; 49(1): 71-81.
[http://dx.doi.org/10.1016/j.jacc.2006.08.042] [PMID: 17207725]

[94]   Marcisz C, Jonderko G, Kucharz EJ. Influence of short-time application of a low sodium diet on blood pressure in patients with hyperthyroidism or hypothyroidism during therapy. Am J Hypertens 2001; 14(10): 995-1002.
[http://dx.doi.org/10.1016/S0895-7061(01)02186-0] [PMID: 11710792]

CHAPTER 6

Arterial Hypertension in Type 2 Diabetes: Pathogenesis and Treatment

Mustafa Kanat[1,*], Abdulhalim Senyigit[2] and Muhammad A Abdul-Ghani[3]

[1] *Division of Diabetes, Department of Internal Medicine, University of Istanbul Medeniyet, Goztepe Training and Research Hospital, Istanbul, Turkey*

[2] *Department of Internal Medicine, Istanbul Biruni University, Istanbul, Turkey*

[3] *Division of Diabetes, University of Texas Health Science Center at San Antonio, San Antonio, TX, USA*

Abstract: Diabetes and hypertension are increasing worldwide as an important public health problem. There is a fairly common ground that combines diabetes and hypertension. Especially insulin resistance is very important in this respect. Epidemiological data and randomized clinical trials indicate that appropriate treatment of diabetes and hypertension provides a significant reduction in cardiovascular events. For this reason, it is extremely important that these two diseases be handled separately. ACE inhibitors, ARB blockers, calcium channel blockers and thiazide diuretics are the preferred agents in these patients. For patients with albuminuria, ARB or ACEI should be preferred for renoprotective effects. In patients with resistant hypertension, aldosterone antagonists therapy may be added to present therapy.

Keywords: Aldosterone antagonists therapy, Albuminuria, Arterial hypertension, ACE inhibitors, ARB blockers, Calcium channel blockers, Insulin resistance, Resistant hypertension, Type 2 diabetes, Thiazide diuretics.

INTRODUCTION

Diabetes, Hypertension and their Coexistence

The prevalence of type 2 diabetes (T2DM) and hypertension is dramatically increasing worldwide over the past few decades. Globally, an estimated 430 million adults are living with T2DM, representing 9% of all adults and 1.39 billion persons are living with hypertension, representing 30% of all adults [1, 2]. Diabetes and hypertension which are two component of metabolic syndrome freq-

---

* **Corresponding author Mustafa Kanat:** Division of Diabetes, Department of Internal Medicine, University of Istanbul Medeniyet, Goztepe Training and Research Hospital, Istanbul, Turkey; Tel: + 90- 216- 566-40 00; Fax: + 90-216-566-4023; E-mail: mustafa.kanat@medeniyet.edu.tr

Hafize Uzun & Pınar Atukeren (Eds.)

uently accompany each other. Only one third of T2DM patients have normal blood pressure and only fifty percent of patients with hypertension have normal glucose tolerance [3, 4]. There is strong evidence suggesting that many common pathophysiological mechanisms (genetic factors, obesity, insülin resistance, hyperinsulinemia, renin-angiotensin-aldosterone axis activation) are responsible for this association. Systolic hypertension, an independent risk factor for cardiovascular death, is more frequent in T2DM than in non-diabetics In addition, the INTERHEART Study has clearly shown that the combination of diabetes and hypertension poses a particular high risk for MI [5].

Diabetes and Hypertension: What do They Share in Common?

A growing body of scientific evidence demonstrates that the link between diabetes and hypertension is insulin resistance. The close relationship between insulin resistance and essential hypertension is explained by several mechanisms: i) hyperinsuinemia ii) sympathetic nervous system overactivity, iii) nitric-oxide pathway, iv) Na/H^+ ion transport overactivity v) renin-angiotensin-aldosterone system (RAAS) activation, vi) increased sodium glucose co-transporter 2 (SGLT2) activity viii) stimulation of growth factors (Fig. **1**).

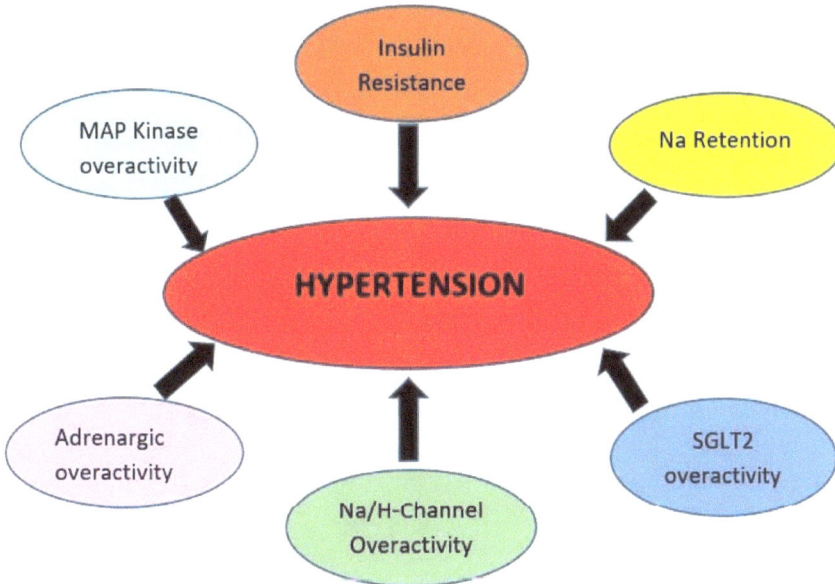

Fig. (1). Possible pathophysiological mechanisms leading to hypertension in diabetes.

Increased Renal Sodium Retention

Total body Na content is increased in obese people with hypertension [6]. In contrast, weight loss results in decreased blood pressure and insulin resistance. All these observations shed light on the significant role of hyperinsulinemia in sodium and water retention in obese subjects with insulin resistance [7]. The relationship between plasma insulin concentration and renal Na excretion has been extensively studied. Even physiologic elevation in plasma insulin levels have greatly reduced urinary Na excretion [8]. Even elevations of 30-40 µU/ml in plasma insulin concentrations are sufficient to start the antinatriuretic effect [9]. As a result, compensatory hyperinsulinemic response to insulin resistance causes Na and fluid retention in the kidneys, leading to hypertension.

Sympathetic Nervous System (SNS) Overactivity

The second mechanism that links hyperinsulinemia and hypertension is over-stimulation of the sympathetic nervous system (SNS). SNS activity is closely related to plasma insulin levels. Although hyperglycemia has no effect on plasma norepinephrine, pulse and blood pressure, insulin has a positive effect on all three. Insulin increases plasma norepinephrine levels [10]. Increased plasma norepinephrine levels lead to increased pulse rate and blood pressure. The increased SNS activity, on the one hand, leads to increased renal Na absorption and volume expansion peripheral vasoconstriction and increased cardiac output leading to hypertension [11].

Nitric-Oxide Pathway, MAPK Overactivity, and Enhanced Growth Factors

The third mechanism to explain the association of diabetes and hypertension is the decrease in nitric-oxide (NO) production and the increase in growth factor activity. Insulin acts mainly by the pathways of Ras-mitogen-activated protein kinase (MAPK) and phosphatidylinositol-3-kinase (PI3K). The PI3K pathway controls endothelium-derived NO, glycogen, lipid and protein synthesis. The MAPK pathway controls cell growth, proliferation and differentiation, the synthesis of transcription factors, and the production of matrix proteins [12]. Both of these pathways play a critical role in insulin vascular endothelial effects. Under physiological conditions, the antiatherogenic and atherogenic effects of insulin are balanced; However, this balance shifts to the atherogenic side in diabetics. This condition results from diminished insulin response through the PI3K pathway, rather than increased activity in MAPK pathway. Since the PI3K pathway activity is reduced and the MAPK pathway remains intact, the predominant effect of insulin will be on the MAPK pathway. Eventually, factors that play a crucial role in atherosclerosis such as vascular smooth muscle cell proliferation and collagen, growth factor and inflammatory cytokine production are augmented. In diabetic patients, however, NO-induced vasodilatation is reduced in both arterial and venous systems [13, 14]. The consequence of all of these is peripheral vasoconstriction, hypertrophy of vascular wall smooth muscle cells, narrowing of lumen, atherosclerosis and systemic blood pressure increase [15] (Figs. **2** and **3**).

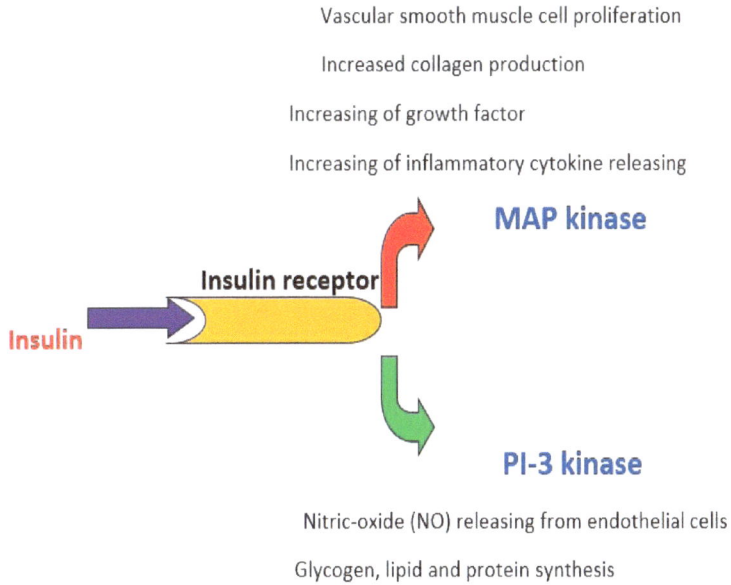

Vascular smooth muscle cell proliferation

Increased collagen production

Increasing of growth factor

Increasing of inflammatory cytokine releasing

MAP kinase

Insulin receptor

Insulin

PI-3 kinase

Nitric-oxide (NO) releasing from endothelial cells

Glycogen, lipid and protein synthesis

Fig. (2). Two major signaling pathways that antiatherogenic (PI-3 kinase pathway) and atherogenic (MAP kinase pathway) effects of insulin have a balance in healthy individuals (reproduced from Kanat [15]).

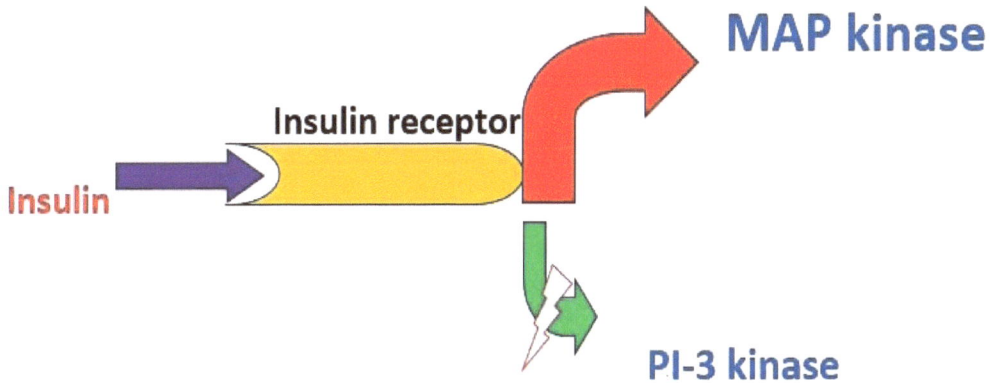

MAP kinase

Insulin receptor

Insulin

PI-3 kinase

Fig. (3). The MAPK pathway becomes relatively dominant due to insulin resistance in the PI-3 kinase signaling pathway in diabetics (reproduced from Kanat [15]).

Sodium-Glucose Cotransporter 2 (SGLT2) Overactivity

The fourth possible mechanism to explain the association of hypertension in patients with diabetes is sodium-glucose cotransporter 2 (SGLT2) overactivity. Renal tubular regulation of glucose reabsorption depends on SGLT1 and SGLT2. Interestingly, in diabetic patients SGLT2 mRNA and protein expression are increased in proportion to hyperglycemia. As a result of increased SGLT2 activity, increased sodium uptake in the proximal tubule in diabetic individuals is expected to accompany increased glucose reabsorption. It can be assumed that increased sodium reabsorption may lead to extracellular volume expansion and increased blood pressure. Studies have shown that inhibition of SGLT2 in experimental animals results in a two to three fold increase in sodium excretion [16, 17]. Randomized clinical trials have clearly demonstrated that inhibition of SGLT2 leads to both systolic and diastolic blood pressure decline [17].

Altered Cellular Ion Pumps Activity and Increased pH

Finally, the increase in Na / H and Na/K pumps activity and the change in cellular electrolyte composition can be mentioned. Na / H pump activity, which is normally found in arterial smooth muscle cells as in each cell, is regulated by insulin. Hyperinsulinemia leads to an increase in Na / H pump activity. This will lead to intracellular accumulation of sodium, which will sensitize the resulting smooth muscle cells to the effects of norepinephrine and angiotensin II [18]. It has been shown that Na / H pump depends on Ca exchange and plays a critical role in maintaining intracellular pH. Intracellular accumulation of Na and Ca is expected to increase the sensitivity of norepinephrine and angiotensin. Increased Na / H pump activity will also lead to an increase in cell pH. Intracellular alkalosis leads to protein synthesis, cell proliferation and smooth muscle hypertrophy.

In summary, there is much evidence to support that hyperinsulinemia may play a critical role in the development of hypertension in diabetic patients. Insulin can elevate blood pressure through various mechanisms: renal Na retention, SGLT2 overactivity, sympathetic nervous system hyperactivity, increased Na and Ca ions in vascular smooth muscle cells, increased cell pH and proliferation of arteriolar smooth muscle cells [11, 19].

Blood Pressure Control in Patients with Diabetes

Hypertension itself is an important risk factor for both atherosclerotic cardiovascular disease (ASCVD) and microvascular complications. The INTERHEART Study has shown that in the presence of diabetes this risk is more than triple [5]. Antihypertensive therapy reduces ASCVD and microvascular complications in patients with T2DM regardless of the agent utilized. Therefore, blood pressure should be measured at every visit in patients with diabetes. The blood pressure should be measured with the appropriate cuff size, after at least 5 minutes of rest in sitting position. Blood pressure measurements should be repeated multiple times in patients with high blood pressure ($\geq$ 140/90) to confirm the diagnosis of hypertension.

Blood Pressure Goal in Patients with T2DM

Epidemiological data and randomized clinical trials suggest that blood pressure less than 140/90 mmHg in patients with diabetes reduces ASCVD and microvascular events [20, 21]. Most patients with diabetes and hypertension should be treated with a target of <140/90 mmHg systolic and diastolic blood pressure, respectively [22]. Although there is no strong scientific evidence in this regard, lower systolic and diastolic blood pressure targets may be appropriate in individuals with a high risk of cardiovascular disease.

What did We Learn from Randomized Clinical Trials?

The UKPDS trial showed that tight control of blood pressure (BP target ≤150 / 85 mmHg, achieved 144/82 mmHg) reduced microvascular and macrovascular complications in patients with T2DM (32% in death, 44% in strokes, 37% in microvacular endpoints) [20]. One of the most serious studies evaluating the effect of intensive blood pressure control on ASCVD in type 2 diabetic patients is the Action to Control Cardiovascular Disease in Diabetes-Blood Pressure (ACCORD-BP) study. In 4733 patients with type 2 diabetes, the intensive treatment group with a systolic blood pressure target of <120 mm Hg and the standard treatment group with a systolic blood pressure target of <140 mm Hg were compared. The primary combined cardiovascular disease outcome (cardio vascular death, non-fatal myocardial infarction, or non-fatal stroke) was not significantly reduced in the intensive-treatment group compared with the standard treatment group [23]. Another hypertension study conducted in patients with diabetes is the Action in Diabetes and Vascular Disease: Preterax and Diamicron Modified-Release Controlled Evaluation (ADVANCE) trial [24]. There was no specific blood pressure target in the ADVANCE study. In the intensive treatment group (achieved 136/73 mmHg *vs.* 142/75 mmHg), the combination of thiazide diuretic and ACEi did not significantly reduce the composite macrovascular outcome. Diastolic blood pressure targets(80 mmHg *vs.* 90 mmHg) are aimed at the Hypertension Optimal Treatment (HOT) study. There was no CV benefit in intensive arm. However, CV events in the diabetic subpopulation have decreased significantly in the HOT study [25]. An important recent study in non-diabetic patients is the SPRINT study [26]. In the intensive treatment group, the target for systolic blood pressure was below 120 mmHg, while for standard treatment this target was less than 140 mmHg. Among patients at high risk for cardiovascular events but without diabetes, intensive treatment resulted in lower rates of fatal and nonfatal major cardiovascular events and death from any cause. Based on all these studies, antihypertensive treatment appears to be beneficial when mean baseline blood pressure is ≥140/90 mmHg (Table **1**).

Table 1. Randomised controlled trials evaluating blood pressure goals in hypertensive patients with diabetes (ACCORD BP, ADVANCE BP, HOT, and UKPDS) and without diabetes (SPRINT).

Clinical Trial (Ref.)	Population (n)	Duration (year)	Intensive Arm	Standard Arm	Outcomes (Risk Reduction)
ACCORD BP [23]	n=4733 patients with T2DM plus CVD or multiple cardiovascular risk factors	4.7	Systolic BP target <120 mmHg, Achieved 119/64 mmHg	Systolic BP target <130-140 mmHg Achieved 134/71 mmHg	No reduction in primary end point: composite of nonfatal MI, nonfatal stroke, and CVD death. Stroke (-41%) with intensive control
ADVENCE BP [24]	n=11.140 patients with T2DM plus CVD or multiple cardiovascular risk factors	4.3	Achieved 136/73 mmHg	Achieved 142/75 mmHg	Primary composite end point of major macovascular and microvascular events (-9%) Death from CVD (-18%)
HOT [25]	n=18790 1501 patients with T2DM	3	Diastolic BP target ≤ 80 mmHg Achieved 144/81 mmHg	Diastolic BP target ≤ 90 mmHg Achieved 148/85 mmHg	There was no CV benefit in intensive arm. In the diabetic subpopulation CVD events (-51%)
UKPDS [20]	n=1148 patients with T2DM	8.4	BP target ≤150/85 mmHg Achieved 144/82 mmHg	Achieved 154/87 mmHg	Death (-32%) Stroke (-44%)
SPRINT [26]	n=9361 patients without diabetes	3.3	Systolic BP target <120 mmHg, Achieved 121 mmHg	Systolic BP target <140 mmHg Achieved 136 mmHg	Primary end point (-25%) including: MI, ACS, stroke, heart failure, death from CVD

BP=blood pressure. CVD=cardiovascular disease. CHD=coronary heart disease. CV=cardiovascular. ACS= acute coronary syndrome MI=myocardial infarction CVA=cerebrovascular accident ACCORD-BP=Action to Control Cardiovascular Risk in Diabetes-Blood Pressure trial. ADVANCE BP= Action in Diabetes and Vascular Disease: Preterax and Diamicron MR Controlled Evaluation-Blood Presure. HOT=Hypertension Optimal Treatment trial. UKPDS=UK Prospective Diabetes Study. SPRINT= Systolic Blood Pressure Intervention Trial

Treatment of Hypertension in Diabetic Patients

Once hypertension is diagnosed (defined as a sustained blood pressure ≥ 140/90 mmHg), the treatment, including lifestyle intervention and pharmacological therapy should be started.

Lifesytle Intervention

Lifestyle intervention includes weight loss in overweight patients, reduction of dietary sodium intake (<2.3 g/day), increased potassium intake, and increased physical activity. These lifestyle interventions should be initiated in addition to pharmacologic treatment when hypertension is diagnosed ($\geq$140/90 mmHg) in people with diabetes and slightly elevated blood pressure (=120/80 mmHg).

Pharmacological Therapy

It is suggested that treatment with a pharmacologic agent should be started as soon as possible in addition to the lifestyle change in confirmed blood pressure elevated patients ($\geq$140/90 mmHg). In patients with higher blood pressure ($\geq$ 160/100 mmHg), it is recommended to start treatment with 2 pharmacological agents as soon as possible in addition to lifestyle. Angiotensin-receptor blockers, ACE inhibitors, thiazide-type diuretics,, and dihidropyridine calcium channel blockers (DCCB) appear to be initially considered as antihypertensive drugs for diabetic patients. Combinations of these drugs may also be preferred. However, combinations of ACE inhibitors and ARB should not be used together [26].

Albuminuria as a Guide for the Selection of Antihypertensive Drugs

In the absence of albuminuria, ARB or ACEI treatment have not demonstrated superiority to thiazide diuretics and DCCB in terms of cardioprotection. On the other hand, RAS-blockers have renoprotective effects in patients with diabetes, for patients with albuminuria initial treatment should include an ACE inhibitor or ARB in order to reduce the risk of progressive renal disease.

Treatment of Hypertension with Chronotherapy

Disappearance of nocturnal blood pressure dipping is closely associated with ASCVD. Clinical trials show that nighttime antihypertensive therapy reduces the incidence of ASCVD events. Therefore, it is considered that it may be beneficial to take at least one antihypertensive agent at bedtime in a patient who needs multiple antihypertensive treatment [27, 28].

Treatment of Resistant Hypertension

Despite triple therapy (including a diuretic), if the blood pressure is still high, it is called resistant hypertension. In these patients, mineralocorticoid receptor antagonists may be added to existing combinations of antihypertensive therapy (ARB, ACEi, DCCB, thiazide diuretics). Patients receiving the mineralocorticoid receptor antagonist and ARB or ACEI combination should be closely monitored for hyperkalemia.

CONCLUDING REMARKS

Type 2 diabetes and hypertension has increased dramatically worldwide over the past few decades. Coexistence of these two diseases exponentially increases the risk of ASCVD. There is strong evidence that many common pathophysiological mechanisms (genetic factors, obesity, insulin resistance, hyperinsulinemia, renin-angiotensin-aldosterone axis activation, SNS overactivity, NO pathway) are responsible for this association. Antihypertensive treatment reduces ASCVD and microvascular complications in T2DM patients independently of the agent. Randomized clinical trials suggest that blood pressure less than 140/90 mmHg in diabetics reduces ASCVD and microvascular events. Therefore, diabetes and hypertension should be treated with a target of <140/90 mmHg. If the patient is not accompanied by albuminuria, any antihypertensive agent of ARB, ACEI, NCCB, thiazide diuretics may be preferred. In patients with albuminuria, ARB or ACEI should be preferred due to renoprotective effects. In the case of resistant hypertension, addition of a mineralocorticoid receptor antagonist would be appropriate (Fig. **4** and Table **2**).

Table 2. Striking features of antihypertensive drugs used in diabetes.

Drug Categories	Drug Name	Dose (mg)	The Most Remarkable Features
Angiotensin-Receptor Blockers (ARB)	Candesartan Valsartan Losartan Olmesartan Telmisartan	8-32 80-320 50-100 20-40 20-80	Cough Hyperkalemia Losartan lowers uric acid levels Reduces proteinuria
Angiotensin-Converting Enzyme inhibitors (ACEi)	Ramipril Lisinopril Fosinopril Benazapril Quinapril Trandolapril Perindopril	5-10 10-40 10-40 10-40 10-40 2-8	Cough Angioedema Hyperkalemia Reduces proteinuria
Diuretics	Hydrochlorothiazide Chlorthalidone Indapamide Triamterene Spironolactone Furosemide	12.5-50 12.5-25 1.25-2,5 100 25-50 20-80	Spironolactone causes gynecomastia and hyperkalamia Monitor potassium level
Calcium Channel Blockers (CCB)	Dihydropyridines: Amlodipine Nifedipide ER Non-dihydropyridine: Diltiazem ER Verapamil ER	5-10 30-90 180-360 240-480	Edema, dihydropyridines may be safely combined with beta-blockers Non-dihydropyridines reduce heart rate and preteinuria

(Table 2) cont.....

	Metoprolol	50-100	Propronalol bid
Beta-Blockers (BB)	Nebivolol	5-10	Carvedilol bid
	Propranolol	40-120	Labetolol bid
	Carvedilol	6.25-25	Not first line agents
	Bisoprolol	5-10	Reserve for post MI/CHF
	Labetolol	100-300	Cause bronchospasm
			Mask hypoglycemic awareness

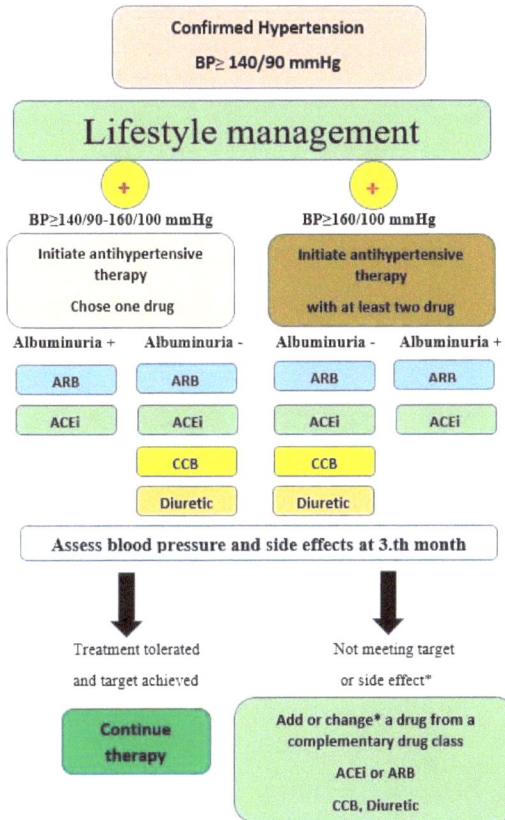

Treatment Algorithm for Hypertension in Patients with T2DM

Fig. (4). Treatment algorithm for hypertension in patients with T2DM.
BP= Blood pressure, **ARB**= Angiotensin-Receptor Blockers, **ACEi**= Angiotensin-Converting Enzyme inhibitors, **CCB**= Calcium Channel Blockers. **Note:** ARB and ACEi should not be used together.

CONSENT FOR PUBLICATION

Not applicable.

CONFLICT OF INTEREST

The authors declare no conflict of interest, financial or otherwise.

ACKNOWLEDGEMENT

Declare none.

REFERENCES

[1]   Mathers CD, Loncar D. Projections of global mortality and burden of disease from 2002 to 2030. PLoS Med 2006; 3(11) e442.
[http://dx.doi.org/10.1371/journal.pmed.0030442] [PMID: 17132052]

[2]   Bloch MJ. Worldwide prevalence of hypertension exceeds 1.3 billion. J Am Soc Hypertens 2016; 10(10): 753-4.
[http://dx.doi.org/10.1016/j.jash.2016.08.006] [PMID: 27660007]

[3]   Cheung BM. The hypertension-diabetes continuum. J Cardiovasc Pharmacol 2010; 55(4): 333-9.
[http://dx.doi.org/10.1097/FJC.0b013e3181d26430] [PMID: 20422737]

[4]   Ferrannini E, Cushman WC. Diabetes and hypertension: the bad companions. Lancet 2012; 380(9841): 601-10.
[http://dx.doi.org/10.1016/S0140-6736(12)60987-8] [PMID: 22883509]

[5]   Yusuf S, Hawken S, Ounpuu S, *et al.* Effect of potentially modifiable risk factors associated with myocardial infarction in 52 countries (the INTERHEART study): case-control study. Lancet 2004; 364(9438): 937-52.
[http://dx.doi.org/10.1016/S0140-6736(04)17018-9] [PMID: 15364185]

[6]   Dustan HP. Mechanisms of hypertension associated with obesity. Ann Intern Med 1983; 98(5 Pt 2): 860-4.
[http://dx.doi.org/10.7326/0003-4819-98-5-860] [PMID: 6342497]

[7]   DeFronzo RA. The effect of insulin on renal sodium metabolism. A review with clinical implications. Diabetologia 1981; 21(3): 165-71.
[http://dx.doi.org/10.1007/BF00252649] [PMID: 7028550]

[8]   DeFronzo RA, Cooke CR, Andres R, Faloona GR, Davis PJ. The effect of insulin on renal handling of sodium, potassium, calcium, and phosphate in man. J Clin Invest 1975; 55(4): 845-55.
[http://dx.doi.org/10.1172/JCI107996] [PMID: 1120786]

[9]   DeFronzo RA, Goldberg M, Agus ZS. The effects of glucose and insulin on renal electrolyte transport. J Clin Invest 1976; 58(1): 83-90.
[http://dx.doi.org/10.1172/JCI108463] [PMID: 932211]

[10] Rowe JW, Young JB, Minaker KL, Stevens AL, Pallotta J, Landsberg L. Effect of insulin and glucose infusions on sympathetic nervous system activity in normal man. Diabetes 1981; 30(3): 219-25.
[http://dx.doi.org/10.2337/diab.30.3.219] [PMID: 7009270]

[11] DeFronzo RA, Ferrannini E. Insulin resistance. A multifaceted syndrome responsible for NIDDM, obesity, hypertension, dyslipidemia, and atherosclerotic cardiovascular disease. Diabetes Care 1991; 14(3): 173-94.
[http://dx.doi.org/10.2337/diacare.14.3.173] [PMID: 2044434]

[12] Saltiel AR, Kahn CR. Insulin signalling and the regulation of glucose and lipid metabolism. Nature 2001; 414(6865): 799-806.
[http://dx.doi.org/10.1038/414799a] [PMID: 11742412]

[13] Hsueh WA, Law RE. Insulin signaling in the arterial wall. Am J Cardiol 1999; 84(1A): 21J-4J.

[http://dx.doi.org/10.1016/S0002-9149(99)00353-7] [PMID: 10418854]

[14]   Dandona P, Chaudhuri A, Aljada A. Endothelial dysfunction and hypertension in diabetes mellitus. Med Clin North Am 2004; 88(4): 911-931, x-xi.
[http://dx.doi.org/10.1016/j.mcna.2004.04.006] [PMID: 15308385]

[15]   Kanat M. Is daytime insulin more physiologic and less atherogenic than bedtime insulin? Med Hypotheses 2007; 68(6): 1228-32.
[http://dx.doi.org/10.1016/j.mehy.2006.10.037] [PMID: 17145138]

[16]   Thomson SC, Rieg T, Miracle C, *et al.* Acute and chronic effects of SGLT2 blockade on glomerular and tubular function in the early diabetic rat. Am J Physiol Regul Integr Comp Physiol 2012; 302(1): R75-83.
[http://dx.doi.org/10.1152/ajpregu.00357.2011] [PMID: 21940401]

[17]   Abdul-Ghani MA, Norton L, DeFronzo RA. The role of SGLT2 inhibitors in the treatment of type 2 diabetes. Endocr Rev 2011; 32(4): 515-31.
[http://dx.doi.org/10.1210/er.2010-0029] [PMID: 21606218]

[18]   Blaustein MP. Sodium ions, calcium ions, blood pressure regulation, and hypertension: a reassessment and a hypothesis. Am J Physiol 1977; 232(5): C165-73.
[http://dx.doi.org/10.1152/ajpcell.1977.232.5.C165] [PMID: 324293]

[19]   Bakris GL, Tarif N, Balck HR. Arterial Hypertension in Diabetes: Etiology and Treatment. In: DeFronzo R, Ferrannini E, Keen H, Zimmet P, Eds. International Textbook of Diabetes Mellitus. New Jersey: John Wiley & Sons, Ltd 2004; pp. 1473-88.

[20]   UK Prospective Diabetes Study Group. Tight blood pressure control and risk of macrovascular and microvascular complications in type 2 diabetes: UKPDS 38. BMJ 1998; 317(7160): 703-13.
[http://dx.doi.org/10.1136/bmj.317.7160.703] [PMID: 9732337]

[21]   Emdin CA, Rahimi K, Neal B, Callender T, Perkovic V, Patel A. Blood pressure lowering in type 2 diabetes: a systematic review and meta-analysis. JAMA 2015; 313(6): 603-15.
[http://dx.doi.org/10.1001/jama.2014.18574] [PMID: 25668264]

[22]   Brunström M, Carlberg B. Effect of antihypertensive treatment at different blood pressure levels in patients with diabetes mellitus: systematic review and meta-analyses. BMJ 2016; 352: i717.
[http://dx.doi.org/10.1136/bmj.i717] [PMID: 26920333]

[23]   Cushman WC, Evans GW, Byington RP, *et al.* Effects of intensive blood-pressure control in type 2 diabetes mellitus. N Engl J Med 2010; 362(17): 1575-85.
[http://dx.doi.org/10.1056/NEJMoa1001286] [PMID: 20228401]

[24]   Patel A, MacMahon S, Chalmers J, *et al.* Effects of a fixed combination of perindopril and indapamide on macrovascular and microvascular outcomes in patients with type 2 diabetes mellitus (the ADVANCE trial): a randomised controlled trial. Lancet 2007; 370(9590): 829-40.
[http://dx.doi.org/10.1016/S0140-6736(07)61303-8] [PMID: 17765963]

[25]   Hansson L, Zanchetti A, Carruthers SG, *et al.* Effects of intensive blood-pressure lowering and low-dose aspirin in patients with hypertension: principal results of the Hypertension Optimal Treatment (HOT) randomised trial. Lancet 1998; 351(9118): 1755-62.
[http://dx.doi.org/10.1016/S0140-6736(98)04311-6] [PMID: 9635947]

[26]   Wright JT Jr, Williamson JD, Whelton PK, *et al.* A randomized trial of intensive versus standard blood-pressure control. N Engl J Med 2015; 373(22): 2103-16.
[http://dx.doi.org/10.1056/NEJMoa1511939] [PMID: 26551272]

[27]   Standards of medical care in diabetes. Diabetes Care 2018; 41 (Suppl. 1): S1-2.
[PMID: 29222369]

[28]   Hermida RC, Ayala DE, Mojón A, Fernández JR. Influence of time of day of blood pressure-lowering treatment on cardiovascular risk in hypertensive patients with type 2 diabetes. Diabetes Care 2011; 34(6): 1270-6.
[http://dx.doi.org/10.2337/dc11-0297] [PMID: 21617110]

CHAPTER 7

Hypertension in Pregnancy-Preeclampsia

Karolin Yanar and **Pınar Atukeren**[*]

Department of Medical Biochemistry, Cerrahpaşa Faculty of Medicine, Istanbul University-Cerrahpaşa, İstanbul, Turkey

Abstract: Hypertensive disorders are heterogeneous, multifactorial disorders. They affect more than 10% pregnancies worldwide. Hypertensive disorders in pregnancy are divided into four groups such as chronic hypertension, gestational hypertension, white coat hypertension and preeclampsia. The underlying mechanism is still unclear. Inflammation, impaired redox balance, vasoactive substances, changes in renin-angiotensin system and genetic factors play a role in the development of hypertensive disorders. Screening methods are important for early detection of hypertensive disorders because of further undesirable outcomes. Therapies of diseases are important for mother and fetus. Some of the drugs are used for first line therapy and the others for second line therapy. However, existing therapies are not fully successful due to adverse effects of drugs. Today some of the drugs such as, small molecules, antioxidants and vitamins used for experimental research are focused on halt proposal pathobiochemical mechanisms however, further studies are needed to clarify the underlying mechanisms and preventive therapy. This chapter summarizes risk factors and their related mechanisms, screening methods and proposal therapies of hypertensive disorders in pregnancy.

Keywords: Antihypertensive drugs, Alternative treatment, Blood pressure, Carbon monoxide, Chronic hypertension, Endoglin, Endothelial dysfunction, Gestational hypertension, Growth factors, HELLP syndrome, Inflammation, Maternal genes, Nitric oxide, Paternal genes, Polymorphism, Placental ischemia, Preeclampsia, Pregnancy, Redox balance, Vitamin D.

INTRODUCTION

Pregnancy, also known as gestation, is the special physiological period of carrying a developing embryo or fetus within the female body [1]. It is conventionally divided into three trimesters, each approximately lasting three months. For nurturing and develop the fetus during pregnancy, significant hemodynamic, anat-

---

[*] **Corresponding author Pınar Atukeren:** Department of Medical Biochemistry, Cerrahpaşa Faculty of Medicine, Istanbul University-Cerrahpaşa, İstanbul, Turkey; Tel: +902124143056; Fax: +902126332987; E-mail: p_atukeren@yahoo.com

Hafize Uzun & Pınar Atukeren (Eds.)

omical and physiological changes are seen in the endocrine, renal, respiratory, and cardiac system for supply to the growing fetus [2 - 4]. A healthy pregnancy is characterized by a decrease in blood pressure (BP) in early pregnancy until 24 weeks due to a decrease in vascular resistance, which increases after 24 weeks until birth, due to an increase in stroke volume and after birth, it increases again 3-4 days postpartum [5].

Pregnancy-specific/ induced hypertensive disorders which are heterogeneous disorders affect more than 10% pregnancies worldwide [6, 7]. They are responsible for 14% maternal and neonatal morbidity and mortality [8]. On the other hand, maternal death falling almost 44% globally due to undertaken efforts between 1990 to 2015 [9]. The International Society for the Study of Hypertension in Pregnancy (ISSHP) divided hypertensive disorders during pregnancy into four groups as [7];

• Chronic hypertension
• Gestational hypertension
• de novo or superimposed on chronic hypertension or white coat hypertension
• Preeclampsia-eclampsia

Chronic Hypertension

Chronic hypertension in pregnancy is defined by the American College of Obstetrics and Gynecology as blood pressure equal or more than 140 mm Hg systolic and 90 mm Hg diastolic observed at the booking visit or before 20 weeks' gestation, or if the patient is already taking antihypertensive medication. Chronic hypertension affects 1%-5% of pregnancies. Obesity, advancing age and advanced fertility techniques lead to the development of chronic hypertension [10].

Gestational Hypertension

Gestational hypertension affects approximately 6% of pregnancies. It occurs after 20 weeks' gestation without proteinuria, and it is a transient condition [10]. Nulligravida, black or Hispanic ethnicity, multiple pregnancies, and obesity are the major risk factors. Studies showed that in gestational hypertension, changes in angiogenic factors and also placental pathologies are different from preeclampsia. Thus, controversial to gestational hypertension, preeclampsia is characterized by an anti-angiogenic milieu [11].

De Novo or Superimposed on Chronic Hypertension or White Coat Hypertension

Adrenergic transient response to the stressful condition such as measuring the BP in the physician's office leads to white coat hypertension [12].

Preeclampsia-Eclampsia

Preeclampsia is generally defined as the *de Novo* hypertension of at least 140/90 mmHg on two separate occasions ≥4 hours apart, occurring after 20 weeks of gestation accompanied by substantial proteinuria of at least 300 mg/24 hour of urine or >30 mg/mmol protein/creatinine ratio, and maternal multiorgan dysfunction (Fig. **1**) [13, 14].

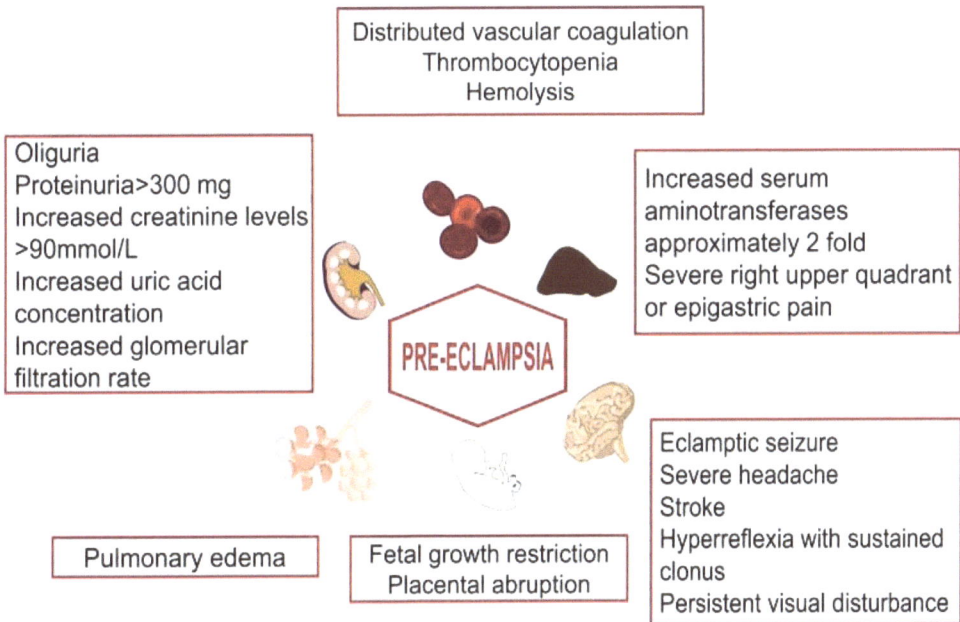

Fig. (1). Features of preeclampsia.

Preeclampsia is divided into subtypes as early onset (placental), and late onset (maternal) [13, 14]. Maternal systolic blood pressure equal or more than 160 mm Hg or/and diastolic blood pressure equal or more than 110 mm Hg is defined as severe preeclampsia [15]. On the other hand, HELLP syndrome is a variant of preeclampsia. Its name comes from an abbreviation of (H)emolysis, (EL)evated liver enzymes such as transaminases and (L)ow (P)latelet count.

Preeclampsia affects approximately 3-5% of pregnancies worldwide, being the second cause/major contributor to mortality after hemorrhage [16, 17]. It is responsible for 70000 maternal and 500000 infant deaths annually [18]. In high-income countries, this prevalence is much lower than low-income countries [16]. The leading cause of preeclampsia remains mostly unknown. Environmental and genetic factors lead to preeclampsia.

Risk Factors of Preeclampsia

Risk factors of preeclampsia are given in Table **1** [19].

Table 1. Risk factors of preeclampsia.

Risk Factors	
Preeclampsia history	Live in high altitude
Family history	Fetal gender
Previous hypertension in pregnancy, Preexisting hypertension	Assisted reproductive technology
New paternity	Elevated transferrin, ferritin and reduced unsaturated iron binding capacity
First pregnancy /primigravida	Undernutrition
Pregnancy interval greater than ten years	Deficiency of vitamin D
Multiple pregnancy	Infections
Limited sperm exposure	Antiphospholipid Antibody Syndrome
Maternal age $\geq$ 40	Systemic lupus erythematosus
Body mass index (BMI) $\geq$ 35 kg/m^2	Renal disease
Ethnicity	Polycystic ovarian syndrome
Education, income	Genetic factors

Preeclampsia History

Preeclampsia history alone and with maternal susceptibility genes play an essential role in preeclampsia development [20, 21].

Family History

Family (maternal or sister) history is one of the significant risk factors of severe preeclampsia [22].

Previous Hypertension in Pregnancy, Preexisting Hypertension

These factors are related to preeclampsia [10, 15].

New Paternity

The prevalence of preeclampsia is higher in new paternity [23]. It is associated with immune maladaptation theory of preeclampsia. T helper (TH) TH1/TH2 balance in a pregnant woman affects the reaction against foreign antigens. T helper-2 cell cytokines can reduce the production of TH1 cytokines which are harmful to pregnancy [24, 25].

First Pregnancy /Primigravida

Higher circulating soluble fms-like tyrosine kinase-1 (sFlt-1) levels and sFlt1/PlGF ratios are observed in the first pregnancy as compared to the second [26]. Higher placental secretion of sFlt-1 (the antiangiogenic factor) antagonizes the effects of proangiogenic placental growth factor (PlGF) and vascular endothelial growth factor (VEGF), leading to abnormal placentation during pregnancy [21]. Multiparity has a protective effect against preeclampsia only in case of same partner [27, 28].

Pregnancy Interval Greater than 10 Years

The number of paternal antigen-specific regulatory T (Treg) cells may diminish [29]. The decreased number of Treg cells may lead to preeclampsia.

Multiple Pregnancy

Twin pregnancy is associated with an increased ratio of protein in the urine. Proteinuria is thought to derive from the placental production of high levels of sFlt-1, which results in an inhibition of free vascular endothelial growth factor on podocytes and glomerular endotheliosis. BMI is also formerly linked with an enhanced risk of proteinuria in pregnancy, and uncomplicated twin pregnancies represent higher protein-creatinine ratios [30].

Limited Sperm Exposure

Women treated with intracytoplasmic sperm injection with ejaculated sperm and *in vitro* fertilization, have enhanced risk of preeclampsia due to loss of stimulation of paternal antigen-specific Treg cells by seminal plasma [31].

Maternal Age ≥ 40

Women more than 40 old age have more significant risk than young ones because of placental senescence which affects small arteries of kidney and uterus and leading to the progression of atherosclerosis [32].

BMI ≥ 35 kg/m²

Increased BMI is a risk factor for the development of various disorders such as diabetes mellitus, insulin resistance, gestational diabetes mellitus, late preeclampsia and autoimmune diseases [33, 34]. Each of them increases the risk of preeclampsia *via* reactive oxygen species (ROS) and increases systemic inflammation response [35]. For example, hyperglycemia may inhibit endothelium-dependent vasorelaxation *via* activation of nicotinamide adenine dinucleotide phosphate (NADPH) oxidase and lead to increased ROS production. Increased ROS levels reduce the nitric oxide (NO) levels and affected eNOS glutathionylation turnover and activity of glutaredoxin-1 [36]. Increased inflammatory parameters such as a toll-like receptor (TLR)-4, monocyte chemoattractant protein, and interleukin-1β and also leptin levels are associated with preeclampsia [37].

Furthermore, hyperlipidemia, hyperinsulinemia, and hyperleptinemia may be linked with the disruption of cytotrophoblast migration and placental uterovascular morphogenesis. Oxidized low-density lipoprotein can decrease extravillous cytotrophoblast migration and advocate trophoblast apoptosis [37]. Oxysterols, inhibit first- trimester trophoblast cell function and reduce glial cell missing-1 [38], which play a role in the fusion of syncytiotrophoblasts and the formation of the maternal-fetal interface. Increased free fatty acid levels can also induce the nuclear receptor peroxisome proliferator-activated receptor-γ (PPAR-γ) and lead to inhibition of the invasiveness of trophoblast cells. Leptin reduces cytotrophoblast proliferation and PlGF production, and also activates hypoxia-inducible factor (HIF)-1α [39]. On the other hand, decreased adipokine levels may lead to preeclampsia *via* increased expression levels of adhesion molecules and cytokines by macrophages.

Ethnicity

Non-Hispanic black women have shown more tendency to severe disease, while Asian/Pacific Islanders and Hispanic women have an overall reduced risk compared to non-Hispanic whites. There may be similar pathways, and risk factors between preeclampsia and cardiovascular disease which depend on ethnicity [40]. Preeclampsia is more widely observed in blacks than whites [41].

Education, Income

Socioeconomic disadvantages are related to maternal complications [42]. In low-income countries, frailty in the care, erroneous diagnosis, insufficient lab evaluation, heterogeneity practices, inadequate registration, and an absence of a therapeutic plan may result in the development of preeclampsia [43]. Education is also a risk factor of preeclampsia development [44].

Live in High Altitude

Cytokines such as interleukin (IL) IL-6, IL-8, IL-1ra play an essential role in altitude-induced preeclampsia [45].

Fetal Gender

Female fetal gender carries more risk than male fetal gender. Enhanced regulatory cytokines especially IL-10 are associated with preeclampsia [46].

Assisted Reproductive Technology

Supraphysiologic estrogen associated with hyperestrogenic ovarian stimulation [47].

Elevated Transferrin, Ferritin And Reduced Unsaturated Iron Binding Capacity

Increased levels of transferrin, ferritin and decreased levels of unsaturated iron binding capacity are seen in preeclampsia [48]. Their mechanisms are related to impaired redox homeostasis *via* decreasing serum antioxidant buffering against redox-active iron [48].

Undernutrition

Undernutrition may lead to epigenetic modification. Calcium, vitamin A, zinc, magnesium, potassium, and iodine are necessary for maternal and fetal health [49, 50]. Calcium is transferred to the fetus *via* the placenta. In pregnancy, the requirement of calcium is high. Inadequate calcium supplementation leads to preeclampsia *via* decreased uterine blood flow and increased blood pressure and also increased pressor effects of angiotensinogen II [51]. Calcium supplementation reduces half the risk of development of preeclampsia [52]. Magnesium serves as a cofactor for many enzymes that regulate protein synthesis and water balance [52]. Magnesium serves as a cofactor for many enzymes that regulate protein synthesis and water balance [53]. Both of them are vital in vascular smooth muscle tone and contraction, and they play a crucial role in blood pressure regulation [54]. Zinc and iodine are antioxidant trace metals, and their deficiency may lead to loss of Cu, Zn superoxide dismutase (Cu, Zn-SOD) activity and increase in lipid peroxidation, an imbalance between thromboxane and prostacyclin [55, 56]. Impaired redox balance can trigger apoptosis. Increased apoptosis may release inflammatory mediators into the maternal circulation and lead to abnormal placentation and endothelial cell dysfunction [55].

Deficiency of Vitamin D

Immunomodulator properties of vitamin D and its relation to calcium play a key role in the immunological tolerance in pregnancy and the presence of a sufficient level of vitamin D has a role in the prevention of PE [57]. Deficiency of vitamin D may lead to multiple comorbidities such as preeclampsia [58, 59]. A decrease in the level of vitamin D disrupts the balance between Th1 and Th2 and leads to excess activity of Th1 cytokines [60]. Vitamin D may play the role of a robust endocrine suppressor in renin biosynthesis for the regulation of the renin-angiotensin system (RAS) [61]. Vitamin D also serves as a significant signal and plays a role in gene regulations in the development of placental trophoblasts during the placental growth phase. Insufficient vitamin D levels have been related with higher IL-6 concentrations through stress induced kinase, inhibition of p38 inactivation, and inflammatory cytokines such as tumor necrosis factor alpha (TNF-α) [62]. Vitamin D plays an important role in calcium homeostasis. Vitamin D increase the levels of calcium. Calcitriol binds to vitamin D receptor and increases the production of the antimicrobial peptide cathelicidin in macrophages. Deficiency of vitamin D leads to reduced levels of cathelicidin. Reduced placental vitamin D production may increase susceptibility to infections at the maternal-fetal interface [51].

Infections

Bacterial (Helicobacter pylori, Chlamydia pneumonia), viral (human immunodeficiency virus, herpes simplex virus type-2), and parasitic (Plasmodium spp. and *Toxoplasma gondii*) infections play a role in the development of preeclampsia [63].

Immune Maladaptation

Macrophage, T cell and Natural killer cells play essential roles in vascular remodeling of the spiral artery. Saito *et al.* showed that effector Treg cells diminished and exhausted Treg cells enhanced in peripheral blood of preeclampsia. The expression of Bcl-2 in Treg cells reduced, and the expression of Bax in Treg cells enhanced [64].

Antiphospholipid Antibody Syndrome

Obstetrical antiphospholipid syndrome is an acquired thrombophilia that is related to antiphospholipid antibodies (aPLs) with preeclampsia. aPLs are the member of a heterogeneous family of antibodies directed against phospholipid binding proteins and are involved in anticardiolipin, lupus anticoagulant, immunoglobulin G and immunoglobulin M as well as antiβ2GP1 antibody IgG and IgM which are associated with preeclampsia [65].

Polycystic Ovarian Syndrome

A connection between polycystic ovarian syndrome (PCOs) and preeclampsia may relate to obesity and more common usage of assisted reproductive technology by women with PCOs [66].

Renal Disease

Uterine artery ligation leads to ischemia and ischemia results in preeclampsia [67].

Systemic Lupus Erythematosus

It is a systemic autoimmune disease that primarily affects women in their reproductive years [68].

Genetic Factors

Preeclampsia is known as a multifactorial disease. Not only changes in intra and extra environmental factors but also genetic effects or each of them result in the onset or progression of preeclampsia. However, there is no specific gene directly associated with preeclampsia. Preeclampsia may be diagnosed by genetic susceptibility [69]. Thus, genetic polymorphism might be a useful tool to determine the risk of preeclampsia. Some of the candidate genes and gene polymorphism may play a role in the development of preeclampsia. According to genetic conflict theory, maternal, fetal genes and paternal genes and their interactions are partially associated with preeclampsia development (Fig. **2**).

Fetal genes lead to increase the transfer of nutrients to the fetus; maternal genes reduce the excessive transfer to maintaining optimal conditions. This theory anticipates that fetal genes with placenta act adverse with maternal genes and serve to increase maternal blood pressure. More than one maternal gene locus on chromosomes 1,2,3,4,9,10,11,12,15,17,18,22 is related to preeclampsia. Preeclampsia related candidate maternal genetic factors are given in Fig. (**3**).

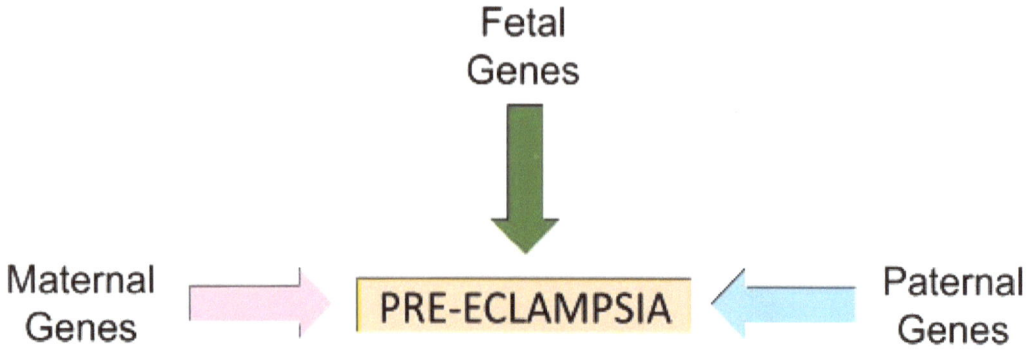

Fig. (2). Genetic factors of preeclampsia.

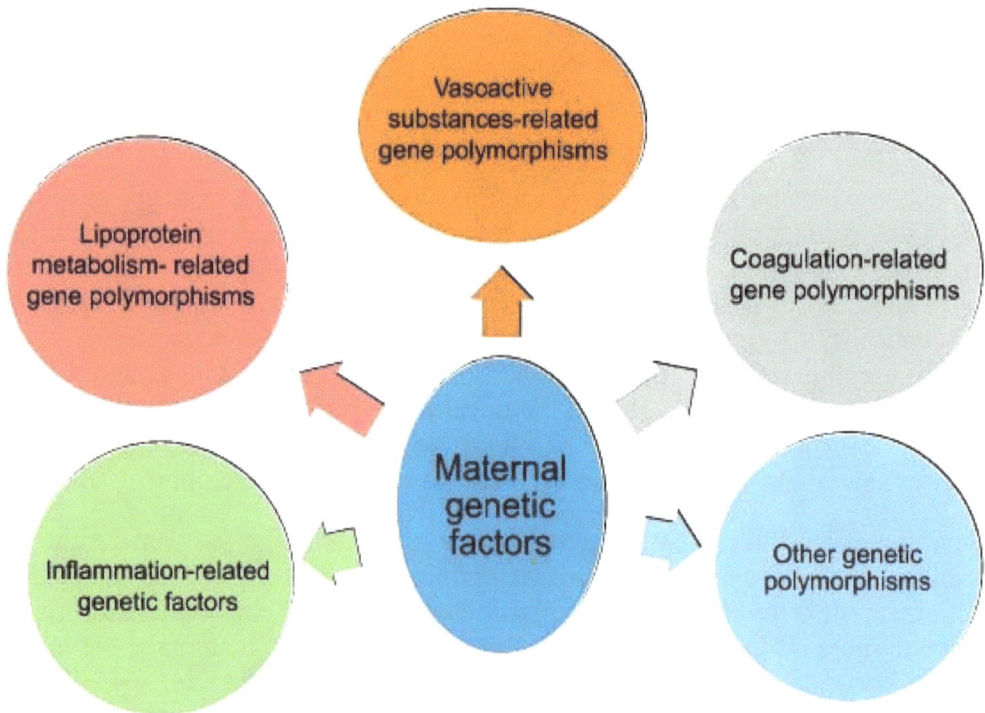

Fig. (3). Maternal genetic factors related with preeclampsia.

Vasoactive Substances -Related Gene Polymorphism

Vasoactive substances- related gene polymorphisms are summarized in Table **2**.

Table 2. Vasoactive substances-related gene polymorphism.

Gene	Genotype	Location	Consequence
Angiotensinogen	rs699	Chromosome 1 (1q42-43), exon 2 [70]	Increases angiotensinogen, higher blood pressure [71], increases in Angiotensin II production, and leads to vascular tone and vascular hypertrophy, positively correlates with increased BMI [72]
	rs4762	In exon 2	Higher blood pressure [73]
Angiotensin-converting enzyme	rs1799752	Intron, chromosome 17	Increases Angiotensin- converting enzyme [44, 74] related with atherosclerosis, ischemic heart disease [75]
	rs4646994	Intron	[76]
Angiotensin II receptor type 1	rs5186	In the 3'untranslated region [77]	Increases response to angiotensin [76]
eNOS	rs1799983	Exon 7 7q35–36 [78, 79]	Hypoxia, decreases placental perfusion
	rs2070744	In the promoter region [79]	Hypoxia, decreases placental perfusion, decreases eNOS gene promotor activity [76]
	27bp-VNTR	In an intron 4 [79]	Changes nitrate and nitrite levels [76]
	rs1799983	In the promoter region	Reduces nitrate and nitrite nitric oxide production [76]
Vascular endothelial growth factor (VEGF)	rs3025039	3′ untranslated region [80]	Decreases levels of VEGF
	rs2010963	5′ untranslated region [81]	

Coagulation Factors- Related Gene Polymorphism

Coagulation factors-related gene polymorphisms are summarized in Table **3**.

Table 3. Coagulation factors-related gene polymorphism.

Gene	Genotype	Location	Consequence
Prothrombin	rs1799963	In the 3' untranslated region [82]	Increases in prothrombin levels
Factor V	rs6020	1q23	Diminishes response to activated protein C [76]
Serine	rs1799889	In the promotor region [83]	Increases plasminogen activator inhibitor-1 levels

Inflammation-Related Gene Polymorphisms

Inflammation-related gene polymorphisms are summarized in Table **4**.

Table 4. Inflammation-related gene polymorphisms.

Gene	Genotype	Location	Consequence
TNF-α	rs1800629	5' upstream promoter region [84]	Increases TNF-α gene expression
Interleukin-10 (IL10)	rs1800896	1q31 and 1q32 promoter region [85]	Changes IL10 levels
Interferon gamma (IFN-γ)	rs2430561	Intron 1 [86]	Inhibits the projection of trophoblast cells and synergistically excites the programmed death of primary villous trophoblast cells [87]
CTLA4	rs231775	exon 1 [88]	Increases T cell activation and proliferation
FoxP3	rs4824747	Xp11.23	Changes development and functioning of regulator T cells and regulation of TH1/TH2 balance [89]
FAS ligand	670G		Reduces Fas production in activated T cells, diminishes T cell apoptosis, enhances destruction of cytotrophoblast, defective invasion of spiral arteries [69]

Lipoprotein Metabolism-Related Gene Polymorphism

Lipoprotein metabolism-related gene polymorphisms are summarized in Table **5**.

Table 5. Lipoprotein metabolism-related gene polymorphisms.

Gene	Genotype	Location	Consequence
Lipoprotein lipase (LPL)	rs268	8p22	Lower LPL activity and dyslipidemia. dyslipidemia can contribute to endothelial cell dysfunction [90].
	rs429358	Chromosome 19	Hyperlipoproteinemia [76], dyslipidemia
Apoenzyme-E	rs7412	Chromosome 19	Hyperlipoproteinemia [76]

Other Maternal Gene Polymorphism

Other preeclampsia related gene polymorphisms are summarized in Table **6**.

Table 6. Other preeclampsia related gene polymorphism.

Gene	Genotype	Location	Consequence
Methylenetetrahydrofolate reductase (MTHR)	rs1801133	1p36.3, exon 4	Higher plasma homocysteine levels and lower folate levels. Reduces activity of MTHR, increases chromosomal aberrations risk, alters the balance DNA synthesis, repair and methylation
Sialic acid binding Ig- like lectin 6(Siglec-6)		19q13.3	Placental expression of the encoded protein is upregulated in preeclampsia [91]
CORIN * only in Caucasian Women	rs2271036 rs2271037	4p12-p13	Uterine levels of Corin mRNA and protein were significantly lower. Corin associated with atrial natriuretic peptide (ANP) [92]. ANP regulates blood pressure [93].

Fetal genes may play a role in the development of preeclampsia. Especially, the homozygote inhibitory killer, immunoglobulin-like receptor AA haplotypes and human leukocyte antigen class II haplotype associated with preeclampsia [3]. On the other hand, paternal family history increases the risk of development preeclampsia [3].

Pathophysiologic and Pathobiochemical Mechanisms of Preeclampsia

The terminal branches of the uterine arteries are called spiral arteries that supply blood to the endometrium in non-pregnant women. These arteries are quite characteristic, small, muscular arteries, richly innervated and sensitive to neural and humoral signals [94]. Between 10 and 20 weeks of gestation in a healthy pregnancy, these arteries undergo physiologic remodelings such as an increase in terminal luminal diameter, removal of smooth muscle and internal elastic lamina components and these changes result in structural changes in vessels that became a flaccid dilated tube. These changes extend upto the inner third of the myometrium resulting in a failure in condensation of vascular smooth muscle adjacent to the myometrial decidual junction. The segment of vascular smooth muscle serves as a functional sphincter. This sphincter is accountable for finishing blood flow at the time of menses. In placental ischemia, this process is not complete. The terminal dilatation is not as thorough, and the elimination of smooth muscle is not complete and does not extend beyond the decidua leaving the functional vascular sphincter intact. These incomplete processes result in inadequate placental perfusion [95].

Although exact unclarified nature of preeclampsia, one of the proposal pathophysiologic mechanisms that probably explain that preeclampsia has two stages as placental ischemia and endothelial dysfunction (Fig. **2**). In the first stage, environmental factors, diets, some diseases such as diabetes mellitus, obesity, systemic lupus erythematosus, genetic factors such as maternal-fetal and paternal genes and their polymorphism and also immunologic factors such as infection or immune maladaptation may result in abnormal placentation and placental ischemia. Placental ischemia leads to an alteration in vasoactive substances. In healthy pregnancy, these vasoactive substances are in balance (Fig. **4**).

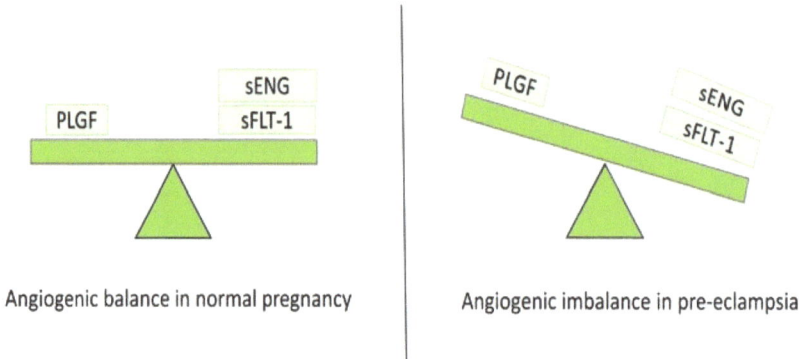

Angiogenic balance in normal pregnancy   Angiogenic imbalance in pre-eclampsia

Fig. (4). Angiogenic balance.

Altered Vasoactive Substances

VEGF, Sflt-1, PLGF, Arginine, Testosterone

VEGF plays a role in vascular homeostasis, regulation of endothelial cell proliferation and normal placentation process [3]. It leads to an increase in intracellular free calcium levels. Increased free calcium levels result in calmodulin binding to eNOS. Thus, VEGF indirectly acts as a vasodilator and induces NO production *via* interaction with sflt-1 [3]. NO upregulates both the expression and activities of matrix metalloproteinase 2 and matrix metalloprotease 9 which are necessary for invasion during embryo implantation. In preeclampsia, the half-life of NO is reduced and rapidly degrades to peroxynitrite. eNOS promotes the production of superoxide anion. Intracellular levels of arginine regulate relative amounts of NO and superoxide anion. In preeclamptic women, arginine levels are lower as a consequence of arginase II activity which is stimulated by testosterone [96]. VEGF might have a signal chain. VEGF activates sflt-1. It comprises an extracellular domain with seven immunoglobulin-like domains, a membrane domain, and a cytoplasmic tyrosine kinase domain. Sflt-1, an antiangiogenic factor, serves as a scavenger of VEGF and PLGF (angiogenic factor) *via* high binding affinity, leads to decrease both VEGF and also PLGF, inhibits their interaction with endothelial receptors, disrupts endothelial cells and leads to endotheliosis and microvascular obstruction. Increased levels of Sflt-1 result in increased production of free radicals and exaggerated vasoconstriction. Sflt-1 levels are not only used for diagnosis of preeclampsia but also are useful in determining the severity of the disease [97].

Endoglin

Endoglin is a homodimeric transmembrane glycoprotein and serves as an antiangiogenic protein that leads to the inhibition of anti-inflammatory vasodilator growth factor signaling [3, 96, 97]. Reduced transforming growth factor (TGF-β1) levels result in vasoconstriction, overexpression of adhesion molecules and decreased T cells [97]. Endoglin is localized on cell surfaces and acts as a co-receptor for TGF-β1 and TGF-β3. It not only maintains vascular tone *via* the regulation of nitric oxide-dependent vasodilatation but also may control placental implantation and spiral artery remodeling during pregnancy [96]. Especially in HELLP syndrome, endoglin with sflt-1 induces endothelial dysfunction.

Endotelin-1, Cytokines

TNF-α, IL-6 and IL-8 levels enhance in preeclampsia. TNF-α leads to an increase in endotelin-1 levels which lead to vasoconstriction, inflammation and proteinuria [98]. TNF- α also induces impaired redox homeostasis *via*increased lipid peroxidation [3].

Hypoxia Inducible Factor

HIF-1 activates the expression of VEGF, leptin Endotelin-1, and TGF-β3. In normoxic conditions, induces HIF-1 hydroxylation and HIF-1 undergoes polyubiquitination and proteasomal degradation [99]. Hypoxic condition activates HIF-1 [3]. HIF-1 alters trophoblast transcriptional regulation and promotes invasion [99].

Impaired Redox Homeostasis and Related Pathways

In preeclampsia, redox balance is impaired *via* the enhanced generation of reactive oxygen and nitrogen species such as superoxide anion, hydroxyl radicals, peroxynitrites *via* VEGF, sflt-1, sEng, eNOS and lipid peroxidation and also decreased levels of non-enzymatic and enzymatic antioxidant defense system such as thiol compounds, hem oxygenase, glutathione peroxidase (GPx), Cu, Zn- SOD, and catalase activity [100]. Excessive free radicals not only lead to vascular dysfunction *via* stimulation of some matrix metalloproteases but also induce extracellular calcium levels, reduce Ca^{2+}ATPase activity, stimulate inositol triphosphate-induced calcium release, and activate protein kinase C and vasoconstriction. Oxidative stress influences the regulation of transcription factors such as Nuclear factor-erythroid 2 (NF-E2)-related factor 2 (NRF2), forkhead box protein O1 (FoxO), CAMP-response element binding protein (CREB) and High-mobility group box 1 (HMG1) [100].

Nrf2 is a transcription factor that regulates the expression of antioxidant genes such as NAD(P)H: quinone oxidoreductase-1, GPX2, and heme oxygenase-1 (HO-1), by activating Nrf2-antioxidant response element pathway. Nrf2 is known as a multi-organ protector [100]. One of the preventive, therapeutic targets is Nrf2 activation.

FoxO is a transcriptional factor and serves role of a cellular regulator in cell cycle regulation, differentiation, proliferation, DNA repair, and metabolism and also plays a role in resistance to oxidative stress, apoptosis and placental morphogenesis [101].

CREB is a member of the basic region leucine zipper family of transcription factors that bind to the cAMP response element and promotes the expression of antioxidant genes such as peroxisome proliferator-activated receptor gamma coactivator-1α [102].

HMG is a non-histone protein, playing pivotal roles in the inflammatory responses. Extracellular HMGB1 secretes pro-inflammatory cytokine and induces pro-inflammatory responses. Also, it binds to the receptor for advanced glycation end-products (RAGE). RAGE is associated with oxidative stress *via* interaction between advanced glycation end products and nuclear factor-k β (NFK-β) [103]

Endoplasmic Reticulum Stress

Impaired redox balance is associated with unfolded proteins response which is called endoplasmic reticulum stress. Elevated ROS levels lead to a decrease in calcium stores and intracellular ATP, thereby, misfolded proteins accumulate. The cells undergo apoptosis if misfolded proteins excessively accumulate. As a result, syncytiotrophoblast microvillus membranes participate in maternal circulation and lead to endothelial dysfunction and preeclampsia [3]. Endothelial dysfunction affects the vascular system, kidney and brain and results in preeclampsia (Fig. **5**).

Outcomes of Preeclampsia on Fetus

Preeclampsia may cause adverse effects on fetus such as growth restriction, placental abruption, retinopathy of prematurity, sepsis, stillbirth, cerebral palsy, preterm delivery, and necrotizing enterocolitis [97].

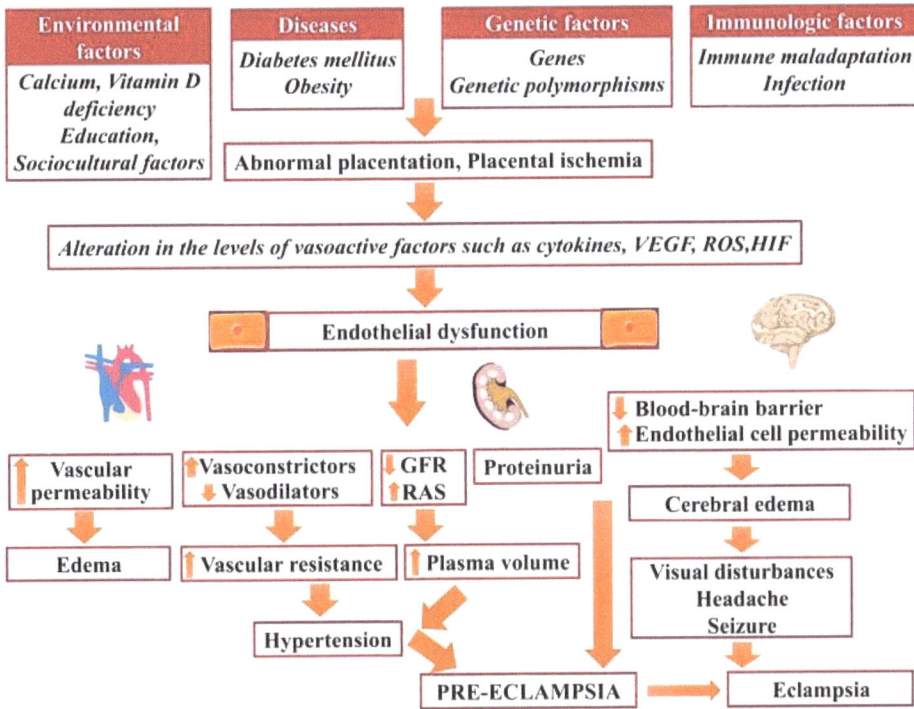

Fig. (5). Proposal pathophysiologic mechanism of preeclampsia.
GFR: Glomerular filtration rate, RAS: Renin-angiotensin system, ROS: Reactive oxygen species, system, VEGF: Vascular endothelial growth factor, HIF: Hypoxia inducible factor.

Outcomes of Preeclampsia on Mother

Adverse effects of preeclampsia on mother are summarized as hypertension, cardiovascular disease risk, future hypertension, kidney dysfunction, liver failure, central nervous system damage, stroke, seizure, diabetes mellitus, coronary artery disease, pulmonary edema and also death [97].

Screening Methods for Early Detection of Preeclampsia

Early detection of diseases is vital for their possible treatment and also for minimal therapeutic expenditure. Preeclampsia may categorize early detectable disease. Its screening methods are summarized in Table **7**.

Table 7. Screening methods for early detection of preeclampsia [104].

Screening Methods	
Maternal factors and history	Biomarkers; Proangiogenic biomarkers (PIGF), antiangiogenic biomarkers (sFlt-1, sEng), PAPP-A, inhibin-A, activin-A, PP-13, Disintegrin, MMP 12, cystatin C, pentraxin 3, P-selectin, fetal hemoglobin
Uterine artery doppler	Genetic evaluation
Placental volume and 3D power doppler	Cell-free DNA
Blood pressure and mean arterial pressure	microRNA

Prevention of Preeclampsia with Endogen Factors

Most of the researches focused on clarifying pathobiochemical pathways of preeclampsia *via* finding the accelerators. However, the deep mechanism may be located in endogenous protective pathways, in other words, the control switch of accelerators. Two endogen pathway may play a protective role in preeclampsia. One of them is the hem oxygenase-carbon monoxide pathway, and the other is the cystathionine-γ-lyase-hydrogen sulfide pathway. These pathway products inhibit sflt-1 and sEng release and protect against angiogenic imbalance [105].

Prevention of Preeclampsia with Environmental Factors

Smoking

Cigarette includes carbon monoxide. Smoking reduces the levels of endothelial and placental sflt-1 and induces the expression of hem oxygenase -1 hat exposure to carbon monoxide reduces endothelial and placental sVEGFR-1 and sEng release [105].

Summer Birth

In winter, preeclampsia risk is more than other seasons. Summer birth decreases the risk of preeclampsia. This preventive effect may relate with the levels of vitamin D and melatonin levels and the receptors which are decreased in pre-eclamptic women especially in winter births [15].

Management of Hypertensive Disorders with Therapeutics

According to 2013 ESH/ESC guidelines, antihypertensive treatment is recommended in pregnancy when blood pressure levels are ≥150/95 mmHg.

Initiation of antihypertensive treatment at values ≥140/90 mmHg is recommended in women with a) gestational hypertension, with or without proteinuria, b) pre-existing hypertension with the superimposition of gestational hypertension [106] or c) hypertension with asymptomatic organ damage or symptoms at any time during pregnancy. Treatment of pregnancy-related hypertensive disorders, is still a challenging problem in obstetrics because of their adverse effects. Antihypertensive drugs are summarized in Table **8**. On the other hand, there are some antioxidants, vitamins, smart molecules such as aspirin that are used for the alternative treatment of preeclampsia (Fig. **6**).

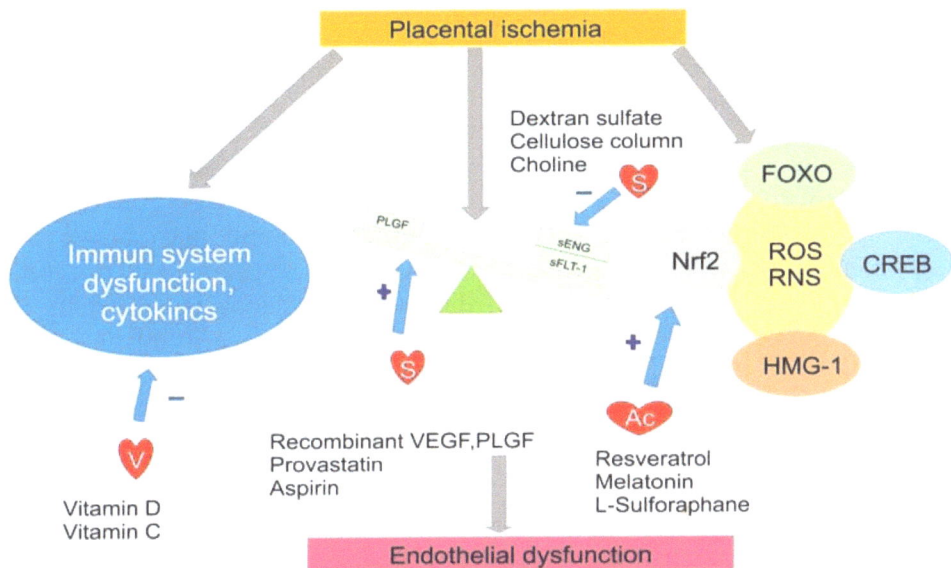

Fig. (6). Experimental treatment of hypertensive disorders.
VEGF; Vascular Endothelial Growth Factor, PLGF; Placental growth factor, sflt-1;soluble fms-like tyrosine kinase-1, sEng; soluble endoglin, Nrf2 Nuclear factor-erythroid 2 (NF-E2)-related factor,FOXO; forkhead box protein O1, CREB; CAMP-response element binding protein, HMG-1; High-mobility group box 1 ROS; reactive oxygen species, RNS; reactive nitrogen species, S; small molecules,V; vitamins Ac;activators.

Table 8. Antihypertensive drug and their adverse effects [107 - 109].

Drug	Adverse Effect
Methyldopa	Depression, hepatic disturbance, hemolytic anemia
Labetalol	Fetal growth restriction, neonatal hypoglycemia

(Table 8) cont.....

Drug	Adverse Effect
Hydralazine	Maternal
	polyneuropathy,
	lupus,
	neonatal lupus and
	thrombocytopenia
Nifedipine	Hypotension when used with magnesium
Aspirin	If its usage begins at the second trimester daily, it prevents preeclampsia. No harms were identified for short-term but long -term evidence was limited.

CONCLUDING REMARKS

Hypertensive disorders are a major contributor to mortality after hemorrhage, still the underlying mechanisms are not fully clarified because of multifactorial heterogeneous characteristics of these diseases. Genetic factors, environmental factors, immunologic factors, and their interaction could play a role in the development of hypertensive diseases. Because of non-negligible rate of mortality and morbidity rate of hypertensive disorders, early diagnosis is important. Early diagnosis and effective proposal therapies may prevent severity of diseases and improve the health of mothers and also fetus.

CONSENT FOR PUBLICATION

Not applicable.

CONFLICT OF INTEREST

The authors declare no conflict of interest, financial or otherwise.

ACKNOWLEDGEMENT

Declare none.

REFERENCES

[1] Sachdeva P, Patel BG, Patel BK. Drug use in pregnancy; A point to ponder. Indian J Pharm Sci 2009; 71(1): 1-7.
[http://dx.doi.org/10.4103/0250-474X.51941] [PMID: 20177448]

[2] Soma-Pillay P, Nelson-Piercy C, Tolppanen H, Mebazaa A, Tolppanen H, Mebazaa A. Physiological changes in pregnancy. Cardiovasc J Afr 2016; 27(2): 89-94.
[http://dx.doi.org/10.5830/CVJA-2016-021] [PMID: 27213856]

[3] M Reslan O, A Khalil R. Molecular and vascular targets in the pathogenesis and management of the hypertension associated with preeclampsia. Cardiovascular & Hematological Agents in Medicinal Chemistry (Formerly Current Medicinal Chemistry-Cardiovascular & Hematological Agents).

2010;8(4):204-26.

[4]   Jafar N, Hippalgaonkar N, Parikh N. Preeclampsia and Hypertension in Pregnancy. 2014.

[5]   Arulkumaran S, Collins S, Hayes K, Impey L, Jackson S. Oxford handbook of obstetrics and gynaecology. Oxford University Press 2008.

[6]   Roberts J, August P, Bakris G, Barton J, Bernstein I, Druzin M, *et al.* Hypertension in pregnancy. Report of the American college of obstetricians and gynecologists' task force on hypertension in pregnancy. Obstet Gynecol 2013; 122(5): 1122-31.
        [PMID: 24150027]

[7]   Ryan RM, McCarthy FP. Hypertension in pregnancy. Obstetrics, Gynaecol Reprod Med 2018; 28(5): 141-7.
        [http://dx.doi.org/10.1016/j.ogrm.2018.03.003]

[8]   Sutton ALM, Harper LM, Tita ATN. Hypertensive disorders in pregnancy. Obstet Gynecol Clin North Am 2018; 45(2): 333-47.
        [http://dx.doi.org/10.1016/j.ogc.2018.01.012] [PMID: 29747734]

[9]   Alkema L, Chou D, Hogan D, *et al.* Global, regional, and national levels and trends in maternal mortality between 1990 and 2015, with scenario-based projections to 2030: A systematic analysis by the UN Maternal Mortality Estimation Inter-Agency Group. Lancet 2016; 387(10017): 462-74.
        [http://dx.doi.org/10.1016/S0140-6736(15)00838-7] [PMID: 26584737]

[10]   Leslie D, Collis RE. Hypertension in pregnancy. BJA Educ 2016; 16(1): 33-7.
        [http://dx.doi.org/10.1093/bjaceaccp/mkv020]

[11]   Melamed N, Ray JG, Hladunewich M, Cox B, Kingdom JC. Gestational hypertension and preeclampsia: are they the same disease? J Obstet Gynaecol Can 2014; 36(7): 642-7.
        [http://dx.doi.org/10.1016/S1701-2163(15)30545-4] [PMID: 25184984]

[12]   Shahbazian N, Shahbazian H, Mohammadjafari R, Mousavi M. Ambulatory monitoring of blood pressure and pregnancy outcome in pregnant women with white coat hypertension in the third trimester of pregnancy. J Nephropharmacol 2013; 2(1): 5-9.
        [PMID: 28197434]

[13]   Davey DA, MacGillivray I. The classification and definition of the hypertensive disorders of pregnancy. Am J Obstet Gynecol 1988; 158(4): 892-8.
        [http://dx.doi.org/10.1016/0002-9378(88)90090-7] [PMID: 3364501]

[14]   Steegers EA, von Dadelszen P, Duvekot JJ, Pijnenborg R. Pre-eclampsia. Lancet 2010; 376(9741): 631-44.
        [http://dx.doi.org/10.1016/S0140-6736(10)60279-6] [PMID: 20598363]

[15]   Zeng K, Gao Y, Wan J, *et al.* The reduction in circulating levels of melatonin may be associated with the development of preeclampsia. J Hum Hypertens 2016; 30(11): 666-71.
        [http://dx.doi.org/10.1038/jhh.2016.37] [PMID: 27251079]

[16]   Firoz T, Sanghvi H, Merialdi M, von Dadelszen P. Pre-eclampsia in low and middle income countries. Best Pract Res Clin Obstet Gynaecol 2011; 25(4): 537-48.
        [http://dx.doi.org/10.1016/j.bpobgyn.2011.04.002] [PMID: 21592865]

[17]   Moroz LA, Simpson LL, Rochelson B, Eds. Management of severe hypertension in pregnancy Seminars in perinatology. Elsevier 2016.

[18]   Peres GM, Mariana M, Cairrão E. Pre-Eclampsia and eclampsia: An update on the pharmacological treatment applied in portugal. J Cardiovasc Dev Dis 2018; 5(1): 3.
        [http://dx.doi.org/10.3390/jcdd5010003] [PMID: 29367581]

[19]   English FA, Kenny LC, McCarthy FP. Risk factors and effective management of preeclampsia. Integr Blood Press Control 2015; 8: 7-12.
        [PMID: 25767405]

[20] Harutyunyan A, Armenian H, Petrosyan V. Interbirth interval and history of previous preeclampsia: A case-control study among multiparous women. BMC Pregnancy Childbirth 2013; 13(1): 244.
[http://dx.doi.org/10.1186/1471-2393-13-244] [PMID: 24373629]

[21] Wolf M, Shah A, Lam C, *et al.* Circulating levels of the antiangiogenic marker sFLT-1 are increased in first versus second pregnancies. Am J Obstet Gynecol 2005; 193(1): 16-22.
[http://dx.doi.org/10.1016/j.ajog.2005.03.016] [PMID: 16021053]

[22] Endeshaw M, Abebe F, Bedimo M, Asrat A, Gebeyehu A, Keno A. Family history of hypertension increases risk of preeclampsia in pregnant women: a case-control study. Universa Medicina 2016; 35(3): 181-91.
[http://dx.doi.org/10.18051/UnivMed.2016.v35.181-191]

[23] Hercus A, Dekker G, Leemaqz S. Primipaternity and birth interval; Independent risk factors for preeclampsia. J Matern Fetal Neonatal Med 2018; 1-4.
[http://dx.doi.org/10.1080/14767058.2018.1489794] [PMID: 29914280]

[24] Tubbergen P, Lachmeijer AM, Althuisius SM, Vlak ME, van Geijn HP, Dekker GA. Change in paternity: A risk factor for preeclampsia in multiparous women? J Reprod Immunol 1999; 45(1): 81-8.
[http://dx.doi.org/10.1016/S0165-0378(99)00040-6] [PMID: 10660264]

[25] North RA, McCowan LM, Dekker GA, *et al.* Clinical risk prediction for pre-eclampsia in nulliparous women: development of model in international prospective cohort. BMJ 2011; 342: d1875.
[http://dx.doi.org/10.1136/bmj.d1875] [PMID: 21474517]

[26] Bdolah Y, Elchalal U, Natanson-Yaron S, *et al.* Relationship between nulliparity and preeclampsia may be explained by altered circulating soluble fms-like tyrosine kinase 1. Hypertens Pregnancy 2014; 33(2): 250-9.
[http://dx.doi.org/10.3109/10641955.2013.858745] [PMID: 24304210]

[27] Feeney JG, Scott JS. Pre-eclampsia and changed paternity. Eur J Obstet Gynecol Reprod Biol 1980; 11(1): 35-8.
[http://dx.doi.org/10.1016/0028-2243(80)90051-9] [PMID: 7193608]

[28] Trupin LS, Simon LP, Eskenazi B. Change in paternity: a risk factor for preeclampsia in multiparas. Epidemiology 1996; 7(3): 240-4.
[http://dx.doi.org/10.1097/00001648-199605000-00004] [PMID: 8728435]

[29] Saito S, Sakai M, Sasaki Y, Nakashima A, Shiozaki A. Inadequate tolerance induction may induce pre-eclampsia. J Reprod Immunol 2007; 76(1-2): 30-9.
[http://dx.doi.org/10.1016/j.jri.2007.08.002] [PMID: 17935792]

[30] Macdonald-Wallis C, Lawlor DA, Heron J, Fraser A, Nelson SM, Tilling K. Relationships of risk factors for pre-eclampsia with patterns of occurrence of isolated gestational proteinuria during normal term pregnancy. PLoS One 2011; 6(7)e22115
[http://dx.doi.org/10.1371/journal.pone.0022115] [PMID: 21789220]

[31] Shima T, Inada K, Nakashima A, *et al.* Paternal antigen-specific proliferating regulatory T cells are increased in uterine-draining lymph nodes just before implantation and in pregnant uterus just after implantation by seminal plasma-priming in allogeneic mouse pregnancy. J Reprod Immunol 2015; 108: 72-82.
[http://dx.doi.org/10.1016/j.jri.2015.02.005] [PMID: 25817463]

[32] Cox LS, Redman C. The role of cellular senescence in ageing of the placenta. Placenta 2017; 52: 139-45.
[http://dx.doi.org/10.1016/j.placenta.2017.01.116] [PMID: 28131318]

[33] Mrema D, Lie RT, Østbye T, Mahande MJ, Daltveit AK. The association between pre pregnancy body mass index and risk of preeclampsia: a registry based study from Tanzania. BMC Pregnancy Childbirth 2018; 18(1): 56.
[http://dx.doi.org/10.1186/s12884-018-1687-3] [PMID: 29466949]

[34]   Sohlberg S, Stephansson O, Cnattingius S, Wikström AK. Maternal body mass index, height, and risks of preeclampsia. Am J Hypertens 2012; 25(1): 120-5.
[http://dx.doi.org/10.1038/ajh.2011.175] [PMID: 21976280]

[35]   Shao Y, Qiu J, Huang H, *et al.* Pre-pregnancy BMI, gestational weight gain and risk of preeclampsia: a birth cohort study in Lanzhou, China. BMC Pregnancy Childbirth 2017; 17(1): 400.
[http://dx.doi.org/10.1186/s12884-017-1567-2] [PMID: 29191156]

[36]   Karimi Galougahi K, Liu CC, Garcia A, *et al.* β3 Adrenergic stimulation restores nitric oxide/redox balance and enhances endothelial function in hyperglycemia. J Am Heart Assoc 2016; 5(2) e002824.
[http://dx.doi.org/10.1161/JAHA.115.002824] [PMID: 26896479]

[37]   Spradley FT, Palei AC, Granger JP. Increased risk for the development of preeclampsia in obese pregnancies: weighing in on the mechanisms. Am J Physiol Regul Integr Comp Physiol 2015; 309(11): R1326-43.
[http://dx.doi.org/10.1152/ajpregu.00178.2015] [PMID: 26447211]

[38]   Aye IL, Waddell BJ, Mark PJ, Keelan JA. Oxysterols inhibit differentiation and fusion of term primary trophoblasts by activating liver X receptors. Placenta 2011; 32(2): 183-91.
[http://dx.doi.org/10.1016/j.placenta.2010.12.007] [PMID: 21208656]

[39]   Gonzalez-Perez RR, Xu Y, Guo S, Watters A, Zhou W, Leibovich SJ. Leptin upregulates VEGF in breast cancer *via* canonic and non-canonical signalling pathways and NFkappaB/HIF-1α activation. Cell Signal 2010; 22(9): 1350-62.
[http://dx.doi.org/10.1016/j.cellsig.2010.05.003] [PMID: 20466060]

[40]   Ghosh G, Grewal J, Männistö T, *et al.* Racial/ethnic differences in pregnancy-related hypertensive disease in nulliparous women. Ethn Dis 2014; 24(3): 283-9.
[PMID: 25065068]

[41]   Bryant AS, Seely EW, Cohen A, Lieberman E. Patterns of pregnancy-related hypertension in black and white women. Hypertens Pregnancy 2005; 24(3): 281-90.
[http://dx.doi.org/10.1080/10641950500281134] [PMID: 16263600]

[42]   Choe S-A, Min H-S, Cho S-I. The income-based disparities in preeclampsia and postpartum hemorrhage: a study of the Korean National Health Insurance cohort data from 2002 to 2013. Springerplus 2016; 5(1): 895.
[http://dx.doi.org/10.1186/s40064-016-2620-8] [PMID: 27386343]

[43]   Bordinoski LF, da Silva KS, de Sousa FLP, Fonseca VM, Dias MAB. 124 Evaluation of the hospital management of preeclampsia and eclampsia leading to maternal death: Preeclampsia in low and middle income countries. Pregnancy Hypertension: An International Journal of Women's Cardiovascular Health 2016; 6(3): 240-1.
[http://dx.doi.org/10.1016/j.preghy.2016.08.206]

[44]   Zhang H, Li YX, Peng WJ, *et al.* The Gene Variants of Maternal/Fetal Renin-Angiotensin System in Preeclampsia: A Hybrid Case-Parent/Mother-Control Study. Sci Rep 2017; 7(1): 5087.
[http://dx.doi.org/10.1038/s41598-017-05411-z] [PMID: 28698595]

[45]   Dávila RD, Julian CG, Browne VA, *et al.* Role of cytokines in altitude-associated preeclampsia. Pregnancy Hypertens 2012; 2(1): 65-70.
[http://dx.doi.org/10.1016/j.preghy.2011.11.001] [PMID: 22247821]

[46]   Taylor BD, Ness RB, Klebanoff MA, *et al.* The impact of female fetal sex on preeclampsia and the maternal immune milieu. Pregnancy Hypertens 2018; 12: 53-7.
[http://dx.doi.org/10.1016/j.preghy.2018.02.009] [PMID: 29674199]

[47]   Martin AS, Monsour M, Kawwass JF, Boulet SL, Kissin DM, Jamieson DJ. Risk of Preeclampsia in Pregnancies After Assisted Reproductive Technology and Ovarian Stimulation. Matern Child Health J 2016; 20(10): 2050-6.
[http://dx.doi.org/10.1007/s10995-016-2067-0] [PMID: 27400915]

[48]   Bandaru AK. Comparative Study of Iron status between Toxemia of pregnancy and Normal pregnancy. Journal of Investigational Biochemistry 2015; 4(1): 18-22.
[http://dx.doi.org/10.5455/jib.20150413025836]

[49]   Black RE, Victora CG, Walker SP, *et al.* Maternal and child undernutrition and overweight in low-income and middle-income countries. Lancet 2013; 382(9890): 427-51.
[http://dx.doi.org/10.1016/S0140-6736(13)60937-X] [PMID: 23746772]

[50]   Lopez-Jaramillo P, Gomez-Arbelaez D, Sotomayor-Rubio A, Mantilla-Garcia D, Lopez-Lopez J. Maternal undernutrition and cardiometabolic disease: A Latin American perspective. BMC Med 2015; 13(1): 41.
[http://dx.doi.org/10.1186/s12916-015-0293-8] [PMID: 25858591]

[51]   Aiko A, Ito M, Okamura H, Araki H, Nishi K. Effect of a low calcium intake on the vascular sensitivity to angiotensin II in normotensive pregnant rats. Artery 1992; 19(4): 199-210.
[PMID: 1520073]

[52]   Kanagal DV, Rajesh A, Rao K, *et al.* Levels of serum calcium and magnesium in pre-eclamptic and normal pregnancy: A study from Coastal India. J Clin Diagn Res 2014; 8(7): OC01-4.
[http://dx.doi.org/10.7860/JCDR/2014/8872.4537] [PMID: 25177604]

[53]   Sissi C, Palumbo M. Effects of magnesium and related divalent metal ions in topoisomerase structure and function. Nucleic Acids Res 2009; 37(3): 702-11.
[http://dx.doi.org/10.1093/nar/gkp024] [PMID: 19188255]

[54]   Walsh SB, Zdebik AA, Unwin RJ, Eds. Magnesium: the disregarded cation. Mayo Clinic Proceedings. Elsevier 2015.

[55]   Jauniaux E, Poston L, Burton GJ. Placental-related diseases of pregnancy: Involvement of oxidative stress and implications in human evolution. Hum Reprod Update 2006; 12(6): 747-55.
[http://dx.doi.org/10.1093/humupd/dml016] [PMID: 16682385]

[56]   Cuellar-Rufino S, Navarro-Meza M, García-Solís P, Xochihua-Rosas I, Arroyo-Helguera O. Iodine levels are associated with oxidative stress and antioxidant status in pregnant women with hypertensive disease. Nutr Hosp 2017; 34(3): 661-6.
[http://dx.doi.org/10.20960/nh.460] [PMID: 28627204]

[57]   Xu L, Lee M, Jeyabalan A, Roberts JM. The relationship of hypovitaminosis D and IL-6 in preeclampsia. American journal of obstetrics and gynecology. 2014;210(2):149. e1-e7.

[58]   Mol R, Kansu AD, Cebe T, *et al.* High versus moderate dosage of daily and weekly administration of vitamin d supplements in the form of oil drop in nursing home residents. J Coll Physicians Surg Pak 2018; 28(8): 618-22.
[http://dx.doi.org/10.29271/jcpsp.2018.08.618] [PMID: 30060791]

[59]   Purswani JM, Gala P, Dwarkanath P, Larkin HM, Kurpad A, Mehta S. The role of vitamin D in pre-eclampsia: a systematic review. BMC Pregnancy Childbirth 2017; 17(1): 231.
[http://dx.doi.org/10.1186/s12884-017-1408-3] [PMID: 28709403]

[60]   Behjat Sasan S, Zandvakili F, Soufizadeh N, Baybordi E. The effects of Vitamin D supplement on prevention of recurrence of preeclampsia in pregnant women with a history of preeclampsia. Obstetrics and gynecology international. 2017;2017.

[61]   Ullah MI, Koch CA, Tamanna S, Rouf S, Shamsuddin L. Vitamin D deficiency and the risk of preeclampsia and eclampsia in Bangladesh. Horm Metab Res 2013; 45(9): 682-7.
[http://dx.doi.org/10.1055/s-0033-1345199] [PMID: 23733167]

[62]   Bakacak M, Serin S, Ercan O, *et al.* Comparison of Vitamin D levels in cases with preeclampsia, eclampsia and healthy pregnant women. Int J Clin Exp Med 2015; 8(9): 16280-6.
[PMID: 26629145]

[63]   Nourollahpour Shiadeh M, Behboodi Moghadam Z, Adam I, Saber V, Bagheri M, Rostami A. Human

infectious diseases and risk of preeclampsia: an updated review of the literature. Infection 2017; 45(5): 589-600.
[http://dx.doi.org/10.1007/s15010-017-1031-2] [PMID: 28577241]

[64]   Saito S, Shiozaki A, Nakashima A, Nakabayashi Y, Molvarec A, Rigó J Jr. STA55. Pathophysiology of preeclampsia from the view point of immunology. Pregnancy Hypertens 2015; 5(3): 222.
[http://dx.doi.org/10.1016/j.preghy.2015.07.033]

[65]   Marchetti T, de Moerloose P, Gris JC. Antiphospholipid antibodies and the risk of severe and non-severe pre-eclampsia: the NOHA case-control study. J Thromb Haemost 2016; 14(4): 675-84.
[http://dx.doi.org/10.1111/jth.13257] [PMID: 26782635]

[66]   Yu H-F, Chen H-S, Rao D-P, Gong J. Association between polycystic ovary syndrome and the risk of pregnancy complications: A PRISMA-compliant systematic review and meta-analysis. Medicine (Baltimore) 2016; 95(51) e4863.
[http://dx.doi.org/10.1097/MD.0000000000004863] [PMID: 28002314]

[67]   Makris A, Yeung KR, Lim SM, *et al.* Placental growth factor reduces blood pressure in a uteroplacental ischemia model of preeclampsia in nonhuman primates. Hypertension 2016; 67: 1263-72.
[http://dx.doi.org/10.1161/HYPERTENSIONAHA.116.07286]

[68]   Miyamoto T, Hoshino T, Hayashi N, *et al.* Preeclampsia as a manifestation of new-onset systemic lupus erythematosus during pregnancy: a case-based literature review. AJP Rep 2016; 6(1): e62-7.
[PMID: 26929873]

[69]   Ciarmela P, Boschi S, Bloise E, *et al.* Polymorphisms of FAS and FAS ligand genes in preeclamptic women. Eur J Obstet Gynecol Reprod Biol 2010; 148(2): 144-6.
[http://dx.doi.org/10.1016/j.ejogrb.2009.10.026] [PMID: 19926197]

[70]   Moon J-Y. Recent update of renin-angiotensin-aldosterone system in the pathogenesis of hypertension. Electrolyte Blood Press 2013; 11(2): 41-5.
[http://dx.doi.org/10.5049/EBP.2013.11.2.41] [PMID: 24627703]

[71]   Makuc J, Šeruga M, Završnik M, Cilenšek I, Petrovič D. Angiotensinogen (AGT) gene missense polymorphisms (rs699 and rs4762) and diabetic nephropathy in Caucasians with type 2 diabetes mellitus. Bosn J Basic Med Sci 2017; 17(3): 262-7.
[http://dx.doi.org/10.17305/bjbms.2017.1823] [PMID: 28488548]

[72]   Zitouni H, Ben Ali Gannoum M, Raguema N, *et al.* Contribution of angiotensinogen M235T and T174M gene variants and haplotypes to preeclampsia and its severity in (North African) Tunisians. J Renin Angiotensin Aldosterone Syst 2018; 19(1)1470320317753924
[http://dx.doi.org/10.1177/1470320317753924] [PMID: 29366364]

[73]   Purkait P, Halder K, Thakur S, *et al.* Association of angiotensinogen gene SNPs and haplotypes with risk of hypertension in eastern Indian population. Clin Hypertens 2017; 23(1): 12.
[http://dx.doi.org/10.1186/s40885-017-0069-x] [PMID: 28361007]

[74]   Kalita J, Misra UK, Bindu IS, Kumar B, Mittal B. Angiotensin-converting enzyme (rs4646994) and α ADDUCIN (rs4961) gene polymorphisms' study in primary spontaneous intracerebral hemorrhage. Neurol India 2011; 59(1): 41-6.
[http://dx.doi.org/10.4103/0028-3886.76856] [PMID: 21339657]

[75]   Sugawara J, Oe Y, Wagata M. Genetic Background of Preeclampsia Preeclampsia. Springer 2018; pp. 29-43.

[76]   Buurma AJ, Turner RJ, Driessen JH, *et al.* Genetic variants in pre-eclampsia: a meta-analysis. Hum Reprod Update 2013; 19(3): 289-303.
[http://dx.doi.org/10.1093/humupd/dms060] [PMID: 23300202]

[77]   Plummer S, Tower C, Alonso P, *et al.* Haplotypes of the angiotensin II receptor genes AGTR1 and AGTR2 in women with normotensive pregnancy and women with preeclampsia. Hum Mutat 2004;

24(1): 14-20.
[http://dx.doi.org/10.1002/humu.20050] [PMID: 15221785]

[78] Zeng F, Zhu S, Wong MC-S, *et al.* Associations between nitric oxide synthase 3 gene polymorphisms and preeclampsia risk: a meta-analysis. Sci Rep 2016; 6: 23407.
[http://dx.doi.org/10.1038/srep23407] [PMID: 26997284]

[79] Luizon MR, Palei AC, Cavalli RC, Sandrim VC. Pharmacogenctics in the treatment of pre-eclampsia: current findings, challenges and perspectives. Pharmacogenomics 2017; 18(6): 571-83.
[http://dx.doi.org/10.2217/pgs-2016-0198] [PMID: 28358601]

[80] Amosco MD, Villar VAM, Naniong JMA, David-Bustamante LMG, Jose PA, Palmes-Saloma CP. VEGF-A and VEGFR1 SNPs associate with preeclampsia in a Philippine population. Clin Exp Hypertens 2016; 38(7): 578-85.
[http://dx.doi.org/10.3109/10641963.2016.1174252] [PMID: 27668980]

[81] Shadrina AS, Smetanina MA, Sokolova EA, *et al.* Allele rs2010963 C of the VEGFA gene is associated with the decreased risk of primary varicose veins in ethnic Russians. Phlebology 2018; 33(1): 27-35.
[http://dx.doi.org/10.1177/0268355516683611] [PMID: 27932624]

[82] Li C, Ren H, Chen H, *et al.* Prothrombin G20210A (rs1799963) polymorphism increases myocardial infarction risk in an age-related manner: A systematic review and meta-analysis. Sci Rep 2017; 7(1): 13550.
[http://dx.doi.org/10.1038/s41598-017-13623-6] [PMID: 29051591]

[83] Morgan JA, Bombell S, McGuire W. Association of plasminogen activator inhibitor-type 1 (-675 4G/5G) polymorphism with pre-eclampsia: systematic review. PLoS One 2013; 8(2) e56907.
[http://dx.doi.org/10.1371/journal.pone.0056907] [PMID: 23457639]

[84] Liu ZH, Ding YL, Xiu LC, *et al.* A meta-analysis of the association between TNF-α -308G>A polymorphism and type 2 diabetes mellitus in Han Chinese population. PLoS One 2013; 8(3) e59421.
[http://dx.doi.org/10.1371/journal.pone.0059421] [PMID: 23527193]

[85] Lin M-T, Storer B, Martin PJ, *et al.* Relation of an interleukin-10 promoter polymorphism to graft-versus-host disease and survival after hematopoietic-cell transplantation. N Engl J Med 2003; 349(23): 2201-10.
[http://dx.doi.org/10.1056/NEJMoa022060] [PMID: 14657427]

[86] Lee S-W, Chuang T-Y, Huang H-H, *et al.* Interferon gamma polymorphisms associated with susceptibility to tuberculosis in a Han Taiwanese population. J Microbiol Immunol Infect 2015; 48(4): 376-80.
[http://dx.doi.org/10.1016/j.jmii.2013.11.009] [PMID: 24529854]

[87] Pinheiro MB, Gomes KB, Ronda CR, *et al.* Severe preeclampsia: association of genes polymorphisms and maternal cytokines production in Brazilian population. Cytokine 2015; 71(2): 232-7.
[http://dx.doi.org/10.1016/j.cyto.2014.10.021] [PMID: 25461403]

[88] Tu Y, Fan G, Dai Y, *et al.* Association between rs3087243 and rs231775 polymorphism within the cytotoxic T-lymphocyte antigen 4 gene and Graves' disease: a case/control study combined with meta-analyses. Oncotarget 2017; 8(66): 110614-24.
[http://dx.doi.org/10.18632/oncotarget.22702] [PMID: 29299173]

[89] Norouzian M, Rahimzadeh M, Rajaee M, Arabpour F, Naderi N. FoxP3 gene promoter polymorphism affects susceptibility to preeclampsia. Hum Immunol 2016; 77(12): 1232-8.
[http://dx.doi.org/10.1016/j.humimm.2016.09.001] [PMID: 27614018]

[90] Spracklen CN, Saftlas AF, Triche EW, *et al.* Genetic predisposition to dyslipidemia and risk of preeclampsia. Am J Hypertens 2015; 28(7): 915-23.
[http://dx.doi.org/10.1093/ajh/hpu242] [PMID: 25523295]

[91] Rumer KK, Uyenishi J, Hoffman MC, Fisher BM, Winn VD. Siglec-6 expression is increased in

placentas from pregnancies complicated by preterm preeclampsia. Reprod Sci 2013; 20(6): 646-53.
[http://dx.doi.org/10.1177/1933719112461185] [PMID: 23171684]

[92]   Hod T, Cerdeira AS, Karumanchi SA. Molecular mechanisms of preeclampsia. Cold Spring Harb
       Perspect Med 2015; 5(10) a023473.
       [http://dx.doi.org/10.1101/cshperspect.a023473] [PMID: 26292986]

[93]   Stepanian A, Alcaïs A, de Prost D, *et al.* Highly significant association between two common single
       nucleotide polymorphisms in CORIN gene and preeclampsia in Caucasian women. PLoS One 2014;
       9(12)e113176
       [http://dx.doi.org/10.1371/journal.pone.0113176] [PMID: 25474356]

[94]   Burton GJ, Woods AW, Jauniaux E, Kingdom JC. Rheological and physiological consequences of
       conversion of the maternal spiral arteries for uteroplacental blood flow during human pregnancy.
       Placenta 2009; 30(6): 473-82.
       [http://dx.doi.org/10.1016/j.placenta.2009.02.009] [PMID: 19375795]

[95]   Roberts JM, Ed. Pathophysiology of ischemic placental disease Seminars in perinatology. Elsevier
       2014.

[96]   Nikuei P, Rajaei M, Malekzadeh K, Nejatizadeh A, Mohseni F, AtashAbParvar A. AtashAbParvar A.
       Accuracy of soluble endoglin for diagnosis of preeclampsia and its severity. Iran Biomed J 2017;
       21(5): 312-30.
       [http://dx.doi.org/10.18869/acadpub.ibj.21.5.312] [PMID: 28558439]

[97]   Armaly Z, Jadaon JE, Jabbour A, Abassi ZA. Preeclampsia: Novel mechanisms and potential
       therapeutic approaches. Front Physiol 2018; 9: 973.
       [http://dx.doi.org/10.3389/fphys.2018.00973] [PMID: 30090069]

[98]   Bakrania B, Duncan J, Warrington JP, Granger JP. The endothelin type a receptor as a potential
       therapeutic target in preeclampsia. Int J Mol Sci 2017; 18(3): 522.
       [http://dx.doi.org/10.3390/ijms18030522] [PMID: 28264495]

[99]   Highet AR, Khoda SM, Buckberry S, *et al.* Hypoxia induced HIF-1/HIF-2 activity alters trophoblast
       transcriptional regulation and promotes invasion. Eur J Cell Biol 2015; 94(12): 589-602.
       [http://dx.doi.org/10.1016/j.ejcb.2015.10.004] [PMID: 26531845]

[100] Aouache R, Biquard L, Vaiman D, Miralles F. Oxidative stress in preeclampsia and placental diseases.
       Int J Mol Sci 2018; 19(5): 1496.
       [http://dx.doi.org/10.3390/ijms19051496] [PMID: 29772777]

[101] Sheridan R, Belludi C, Khoury J, Stanek J, Handwerger S. FOXO1 expression in villous trophoblast of
       preeclampsia and fetal growth restriction placentas. Histol Histopathol 2015; 30(2): 213-22.
       [PMID: 25202916]

[102] Lee B, Cao R, Choi YS, *et al.* The CREB/CRE transcriptional pathway: Protection against oxidative
       stress-mediated neuronal cell death. J Neurochem 2009; 108(5): 1251-65.
       [http://dx.doi.org/10.1111/j.1471-4159.2008.05864.x] [PMID: 19141071]

[103] Zhu L, Zhang Z, Zhang L, *et al.* HMGB1-RAGE signaling pathway in severe preeclampsia. Placenta
       2015; 36(10): 1148-52.
       [http://dx.doi.org/10.1016/j.placenta.2015.08.006] [PMID: 26303759]

[104] Park HJ, Shim SS, Cha DH. Combined screening for early detection of preeclampsia. Int J Mol Sci
       2015; 16(8): 17952-74.
       [http://dx.doi.org/10.3390/ijms160817952] [PMID: 26247944]

[105] Ahmed A, Ramma W. Unravelling the theories of pre-eclampsia: are the protective pathways the new
       paradigm? Br J Pharmacol 2015; 172(6): 1574-86.
       [http://dx.doi.org/10.1111/bph.12977] [PMID: 25303561]

[106] Kintiraki E, Papakatsika S, Kotronis G, Goulis DG, Kotsis V. Pregnancy-induced hypertension.
       Hormones (Athens) 2015; 14(2): 211-23.

[http://dx.doi.org/10.14310/horm.2002.1582] [PMID: 26158653]

[107]   Burke SD, Karumanchi SA. Novel Therapies for Preeclampsia Preeclampsia. Springer 2018; pp. 227-37.

[108]   Brown CM, Garovic VD. Drug treatment of hypertension in pregnancy. Drugs 2014; 74(3): 283-96.
[http://dx.doi.org/10.1007/s40265-014-0187-7] [PMID: 24554373]

[109]   Henderson JT, Whitlock EP, O'Connor E, Senger CA, Thompson JH, Rowland MG. Low-dose aspirin for prevention of morbidity and mortality from preeclampsia: a systematic evidence review for the U.S. Preventive Services Task Force. Ann Intern Med 2014; 160(10): 695-703.
[http://dx.doi.org/10.7326/M13-2844] [PMID: 24711050]

CHAPTER 8

Endocrinal Hypertension and Hyperaldosteronism: Biochemical and Genetic Aspects of Adrenal Dependent Endocrinal Hypertension

Sinem Durmus and **Hafize Uzun**[*]

Department of Biochemistry, Cerrahpasa Faculty of Medicine, Istanbul University-Cerrahpasa, Istanbul, Turkey

Abstract: Endocrine causes of secondary hypertension include pheochromocytoma, hyperdeoxycorticosteronism, Cushing's syndrome, apparent mineralocorticoid excess/11ß-hydroxysteroid dehydrogenase deficiency and primary aldosteronism. They comprise of the 5-10% of the causes of secondary hypertension. The identification of the genetic determinants of hypertension has been most successful in endocrine forms of hypertension. Moreover, the latest discoveries in molecular pathogenesis of these disease will provide an important basis for future personalized therapy. A promising area for the application of genetic testing to personalized therapy is the prediction of responses and adverse reactions to antihypertensive drugs. Herein, we review the different forms of endocrine hypertension, with a focus on prevalence and human genetic studies of endocrine causes of secondary hypertension, focusing on the most prominent and latest discovered genes; and related biochemical pathways reported in the literature.

Keywords: Apparent mineralocorticoid excess/11ß-hydroxysteroid dehydrogenase deficiency Cushing's syndrome, Biochemical findings, Endocrinal Hyper-tension, Genetic testing, Hypertension, Hyperdeoxycorticosteronism, Pheochro-mocytoma, Primary aldosteronism, Prevalence, Secondary hypertension.

INTRODUCTION

Hypertension is an important disease worldwide because of its high prevalence, high mortality risk and concomitant risks of cardiovascular and renal disease. The global prevalence of hypertension is estimated to be 1 billion in 2010, and by 2025 this number will increase to reach 1.59 billion [1]. Hypertension is defined

---

[*] **Corresponding author Hafize Uzun:** Department of Medical Biochemistry, Cerrahpaşa Faculty of Medicine, Istanbul University-Cerrahpasa Istanbul, Turkey; Tel: +902124143056; Fax: +902126332987; E-mail: huzun59@hotmail.com

Hafize Uzun & Pınar Atukeren (Eds.)

as systolic blood pressure values ≥130 mmHg or diastolic blood pressure values ≥80 mmHg in adults, according to 2017 ACC/AHA/AAPA/ABC/ACPM/AGS/ APhA/ASH/ASPC/NMA/PCNA Guideline [2]. The vast majority of diagnosed cases have primary (idiopathic or essential) hypertension, which is caused by unknown causes, but approximately 15% of hypertensive patients develop as secondary disease and there are identifiable conditions that result in blood pressure elevation [3]. For this reason, the definition of secondary hypertension is very important in terms of showing the existence of a treatable problem [4]. The prevalence of secondary hypertension is around 30% in adults, while about half of hypertensive pediatric cases have secondary causes [5]. The secondary causes off hypertension include endocrine causes, renal causes and other possible causes such as sleep apnea [6].

The endocrine conditions causing secondary hypertension consist at least 15 endocrine disorders in which hypertension may be the initial clinical presentation and is caused by excessive hormone secretion due to a tumor or hyperplasia of endocrine organs and consequently abnormal hormonal mechanism [7 - 9]. Endocrine causes of hypertension, their clinical conditions and characteristics and also prevalence are shown in Table **1**.

Pheochromocytoma and Sympathetic Paraganglioma

Pheochromocytomas and paragangliomas (PHEOs/PGLs) are rare, and frequently heritable catecholamine-secreting vascular endocrine tumors; are originated from chromaffin cells of the adrenal medulla and neural crest progenitors located outside of the adrenal gland, respectively [10]. WHO defines pheochromocytomas as paragangliomas originating from the adrenal medulla, although some sources may be referred to as paragangliomas producing catecholamines, whether or not they are adrenal mediated [11]. Catecholamines, such as epinephrine, norepinephrine and dopamine, which are characteristically secreted from these tumors, cause sympathetic hyperactivity, hypertension, palpitations, and diaphoresis [12]. The most common of these symptoms (80-95% of patients) is hypertension; approximately 50% of patients develop sustained hypertension, 45% of them present paroxysmal hypertension, and 5-15% are normotensive [13].

Proper evaluation of the diagnosis and clinical presentations of pheochromocytoma requires a good understanding of catecholamine biosynthesis and metabolism. Until the year 2000, there was a rule namely the "10 percent rule" for PHEOs/PGLs -10% familial, 10% malignant, and 10% extra-adrenal-; however, with the detection of new susceptibility genes that contribute to tumorigenesis, this rule is no longer tenable.

Table 1. Endocrine causes of hypertension [14].

Etiology	Causes	Prevalence	Signs and Symptoms	Screening Test	Confirmatory Test
Adrenal dependent	Pheochromocytoma and sympathetic paraganglioma	0.1–0.6%	Hypertension (sustained and paroxysmal), postural hypotension, tachycardia, pallor, flushing (rare), weight loss, fasting hyperglycemia, decreased gastrointestinal motility, headaches, palpitations, excessive sweating, anxiety, tremulousness, pain in chest/abdomen, weakness, fatigue, nausea, vomiting, dizziness or faintness, paresthesia	24 h urinary fractionated metanephrines or plasma metanephrines under standard conditions (30' supine position with indwelling IV cannula)	CT or MRI scan of abdomen/pelvis
	Primary aldosteronism	8-20 %	Resistant hypertension, headache, muscle weakness and cramps, hypokalemia, metabolic alkalosis, incidentally discovered adrenal mass; obstructive sleep apnea; family history of early onset hypertension or stroke	Plasma aldosterone/ renin ratio	Oral sodium loading test (prior to 24 h urine aldosterone) or IV saline infusion test with plasma aldosterone at 4 h of infusion. Adrenal CT scan. Adrenal vein sampling. Trial of mineralocorticoid receptor blockers
	Hyperdeoxy-corticosteronism				
	1. Congenital adrenal hyperplasia	Rare	Hypertension and hypokalemia; virilization (11-beta-hydroxylase deficiency) [11-beta-OH]) incomplete masculinization in males and primary amenorrhea in females (17-alphahydroxylase deficiency) [17-alpha-OH])	Hypertension and hypokalemia with low or normal aldosterone and renin	11-beta-OH: elevated deoxycorticosterone (DOC), 11-deoxycortisol and androgens 17-alphaOH: decreased androgens and estrogen; elevated deoxycorticosterone and corticosterone
	2. Deoxycorticosterone-producing tumor				
	3. Primary cortisol resistance				
	Cushing syndrome	<0.1%	Fatigue, weight gain, round face, proximal myopathy, plethora, hirsutism, buffalo hump, central obesity	Overnight 1 mg dexamethasone suppression test	24 h urinary free cortisol excretion (preferably multiple); midnight salivary cortisol
	Apparent mineralocorticoid excess/11b-hydroxysteroid dehydrogenase deficiency	Rare	Virilization, tall stature, hirsutism, advanced bone age, amenorrhea; Early onset hypertension; resistant hypertension; hypokalemia or hyperkalemia	Low aldosterone and renin	Urinary cortisol metabolites; genetic testing

(Table 1) cont.....

Etiology	Causes	Prevalence	Signs and Symptoms	Screening Test	Confirmatory Test
Parathyroid-dependent	Hyperparathyroidism	Rare	Hypercalcemia	Serum calcium	Serum parathyroid hormone
Pituitary dependent	Acromegaly	Rare	Acral features, enlarging shoe, glove or hat size; headache, visual disturbances; diabetes mellitus	Serum growth hormone ≥1 ng/mL during oral glucose load	Elevated age- and sex-matched IGF-1 level; MRI scan of the pituitary
Thyroid-dependent	Hypothyroidism	<1%	Fatigue, cold intolerance, weight gain, periorbital puffiness; Dry skin; cold intolerance; constipation; hoarseness; weight gain	Thyroid stimulating hormone; free thyroxine	None
Thyroid-dependent	Hyperthyroidism	<1%	Tremor, tachycardia, AF, weight loss, goiter, ophthalmopathy; pretibial myxedema; Warm, moist skin; heat intolerance; nervousness; tremulousness; insomnia; weight loss; diarrhea; proximal muscle weakness	Thyroid stimulating hormone, free thyroxine	Radioactive iodine uptake and scan
Complex effects	Obstructive sleep apnea	25–50%	Resistant hypertension; snoringtful sleep; breathing pauses during sleep; daytime sleepiness	Berlin Questionnaire; Epworth Sleepiness Score; overnight oximetry	Polysomnography

Approximately 40% of all PHEOs/PGLs carry a germline mutations in one of at least 21 genes; and also, with the addition of somatic mutations, this rate is up to 60-65% [15 - 17]. Patients carrying germline mutations in predisposing genes often develop multiple, bilateral, and early onset PGLs [18]. Each of these genes is involved in regulating key biological processes, including cell development, proliferation, and growth; the cell's ability to respond to changes in nutrients, oxygen, and iron or energy; and cell transformation, including tumorigenesis and, ultimately, metastasis.

Until recent years, PHEOs/PGLs tumors have been generally examined in two major clusters and six subtypes based on driver mutation and transcription profiling as Cluster 1 (C1; C1-A and C1-B) and Cluster 2 (C2; C2-A, C2-B, C2-C and C2-D) [19]. In recent years, Fishbein *et al.* (as part of the Cancer Genome Atlas (TCGA) project) designed molecular classification for PGGLs based on tumor mRNA expression profiles, and have identified two new clusters in addition to known clusters, which were referred to as "WNT-altered" and "cortical admixture" clusters [20].

C1 cluster, or pseudo-hypoxic subtype, is associated with the activation of angiogenesis, pseudo-hypoxic pathway and reduced oxidative response, and can be divided into two groups: C1-A comprise tricarboxylic acid (TCA) cycle-related genes including loss-of-function and germline mutations in succinate dehydrogenase subunits (*SDHx*) and fumarate hydratase (*FH*); C1-B subtype include germline or somatic mutations in *VHL* and *EPAS1* [15, 21, 22]. C2 cluster, or the kinase signaling subtype, represent familial or sporadic mutations in *RET*, *NF1*, *TMEM127*, *HRAS*, *KIF1B*, and *MAX* are characterized by aberrant activation of kinase signaling pathways [12]. Although the signal pathways in these two clusters appear to be distinctly different, findings in recent years indicate that there may be significant existing links between signal pathways in both clusters. Major driver genes that have been proven to be involved in the pathogenesis of PHEOs/PGLs and their properties are shown in Table **2**.

The major signaling pathway in Cluster 1 is the pseudo-hypoxic pathway. Pseudo-hypoxia is a condition in which cells and tissues show a hypoxic phenotype even in the presence of oxygen. In the case of hypoxia or pseudohypoxia, cells activate a number of adaptive responses that are usually coordinated by various cellular pathways controlled by the hypoxia-inducible factor (HIF) transcription factor family, which regulate the expression of multiple genes involved in processes that direct the adaptation and progression of cancer cells [16, 23]. HIF is a heterodimeric transcription factor that composed of stable HIF-ß subunit and oxygen-sensitive HIF-α subunit that consist of three isoforms HIF-1α, HIF-2α and HIF-3α. HIF-1α and HIF-2α are similar, highly-conserved and act as transcription factor, and also are activated short periods and prolonged periods of hypoxia, respectively. HIF-3α acts as an inhibitor of HIF1 and shows a different characteristic than other isoforms [16].

Table 2. PHEOs/PGLs Clusters and Major Driver Genes [20, 24 - 26].

Cluster/Pathway	Gene	Official Full Name	Function	Locus	I	Gene Type	Biochemical Phenotype
C1-A (TCA cycle–related)/ Pseudohypoxia pathway	SDHA	Succinate dehydrogenase complex flavoprotein subunit A	Conversion of succinate to fumarate in TCA	5p15.33	G	T.S.	Unknown
	SDHB	Succinate dehydrogenase complex iron sulfur subunit B	Acts as intermediate in TCA	1p36.13	G	T.S.	MN, NMN, MTY, NS
	SDHC	Succinate dehydrogenase complex subunit C	Transfer of electrons to ubiquinone in TCA	1q23.3	G	T.S.	MN, NMN, NS
	SDHD	Succinate dehydrogenase complex subunit D	Transfer of electrons to ubiquinone in TCA	11q23.1	G	T.S.	MN, NMN, MTY, NS
	SDHAF2	Succinate dehydrogenase complex assembly factor 2	Flavination of SDHA in TCA	11q12.2	G	T.S.	Unknown
	FH	Fumarate hydratase	Hydration of fumarate to malate in TCA	1q42.1	G	T.S.	Unknown
C1-B (VHL/EPAS1-related) /Pseudohypoxia pathway	VHL	Von Hippel–Lindau tumor suppressor	Regulation of HIF	3p25.3	G/S	T.S.	NMN
C1-B (VHL/EPAS1-related) /Pseudohypoxia pathway	EGLN1 /PHD2	Prolyl hydroxylase domain 2	Regulate the stability of HIF1	1q42-q43	G/S	T.S.	Unknown
	EPAS1/ HIF2A	Endothelial PAS domain protein 1	Vasculogenesis and haematopoiesis during embryonic development	2p21	P/S	O.G.	Unknown

(Table 2) cont.....

	RET	Ret proto-oncogene	Cell growth and differentiation	10q11.2	G/S	O.G.	MN, NMN
	MAX	MYC-associated factor X	Regulation of cell proliferation, differentiation and death	14q23.3	G/S	T.S.	Unknown
C2 / **Kinase signaling**.	*TMEM127*	Transmembrane protein 127	Limits mTORC1 activation	2q11.2	G	T.S.	Unknown
	HRAS	HRas proto-oncogene, GTPase	Involved in signal transduction pathways	11p15.5	S	O.G.	Unknown
	NF1	Neurofibromin 1	Suppresses cell proliferation by converting RAS into its inactive form	17q11.2	G/S	T.S.	MN, NMN
-/ Wnt signaling	*CSDE1*	Cold shock domain containing E1	Decay interplay of the FOS mRNA mediated by the major coding-region determinant of instability (mCRD) domain.	1p13.2	S	T.S.	Unknown
	MAML3	Mastermind like transcriptional coactivator 3	Acts as a transcriptional coactivator for NOTCH proteins.	4q31.1	S	O.G., fusion	Unknown

I: Inheritance; G: Germline; S: Somatic; P: Postzygotic T.S.: Tumor supressor; O.G.: Oncogene; MN, metanephrine; MTY, metoxytyramine; NMN, normetanephrine; NS, nonsecreting, HIF: Hypoxia inducible factor

In normoxia, HIF-1α and HIF-2α are degraded via the ubiquitin-proteasome pathway. HIF degradation occurs in two stages. First, specific 2 prolyl residues of HIF-α are hydroxylated by prolyl hydroxylase domain proteins (PHDs) (requires oxygen and α-ketoglutarate as co-substrates and ferrous iron and ascorbate as cofactors for hydroxylation; and succinate and carbon dioxide are formed). The hydroxylated residues are then recognized by Von Hippel-Lindau tumor suppressor protein (pVHL), a complement of the E3 ubiquitin ligase complex, to direct the proteasome (Fig. **1A**) [16].

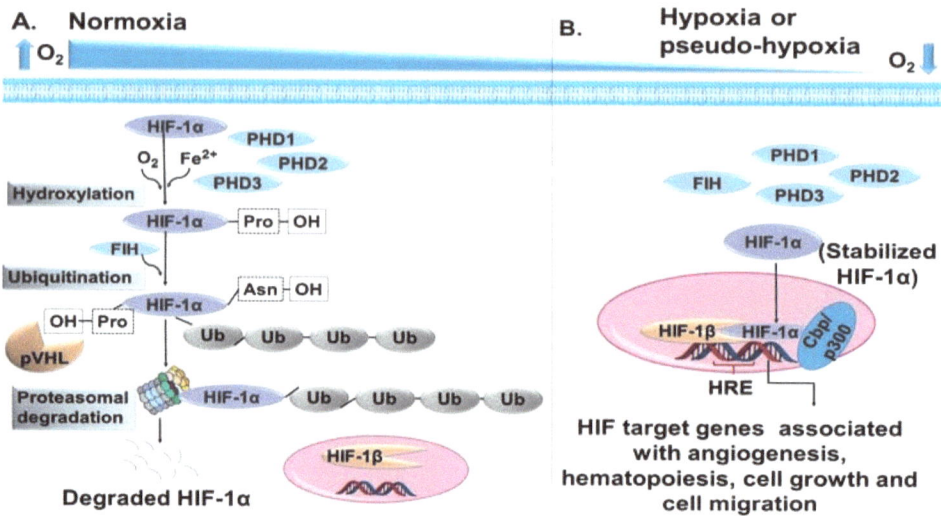

Fig. (1). HIF pathway in normoxic and hypoxic or pseudohypoxic conditions.
HIF: Hypoxia-inducible factor; pVHL: Von Hippel-Lindau tumor suppressor protein; PHD: Prolyl hydroxylase domain; HREs: hypoxia-responsive elements; Ub: Ubiquitin; Cbp/p300: CREB-binding protein (CBP) and its homologue p300 (transcriptional co- activators).

However, in hypoxic or pseudo-hypoxic conditions, HIF-α cannot undergo hydroxylation due to the absence of substrate and becomes stabilized, forms the heterodimer structure with the HIFß subunit, binds to the core DNA sequence at hypoxia-responsive elements (HREs) and so leads to activation of HIF target genes including those associated with angiogenesis, hematopoiesis, cell growth and cell migration (Fig. **1B**).

The major genes in Cluster 1A are *SDHx* and *FH*. SDH, is an enzyme found in the inner mitochondrial membrane which is part of both the Krebs's cycle (oxidizes succinate to fumarate) and electron transport chain (transports electrons to coenzyme Q in the electron transport chain). Mutations in the *SDHx* gene disrupt the enzyme's activity, causing succinate accumulation. Accumulated succinate leaks out into the cytosol, where it inhibits the activity of PHD enzyme by competes with α-ketoglutarate, and so causes HIF stabilization. The deficiency of SDH activity also inhibits succinate-ubiquinone activity; therefore, the electrons that have to be transferred to the ubiquinone pool are bound to the molecular oxygen to give the superoxide anion; ROS and oxidative stress occur. ROS exposure also inhibits the interaction of HIF-α and PHDs similar to the accumulation of succinate, and also leads to oxidative damage to DNA and genomic instability [27, 28]. Increased fumarate and succinate levels as a result of loss-of-function mutations in FH, another key enzyme in TCA, also causes HIF stabilization by inhibiting PHD activity in a similar manner to aforementioned mechanism [29].

More than 400 germline mutations have been found in the VHL gene according to the Human Gene Mutation Database (HGMD), and most of these mutations are associated with functional impairment of pVHL protein and loss of HIF1 inhibition [30, 31]. Also, HIF dysregulation due to PHD mutations plays role in PHEOs/PGLs because HIF-α subunits cannot be captured by pVHL and degraded due to the disruption in the hydroxylation step. Mutations in *HIF2A*, the other member gene of Cluster 1-B, cause stabilization by preventing HIF-2α from captured by pVHL [26].

Cluster 1 tumors show a noradrenergic phenotype and predominantly produce norepinephrine, resulting in high levels of norepinephrine and normetanephrine [10].

As a result of the mutation of the genes in Cluster 2 (*RET, NF1, H-RAS, KRAS, TMEM127, MAX, ATRX, and CSDE1*, BRAF, and NGFR), dysregulation occurs in the phosphatidyl inositol3-kinase/mechanistic target of rapamycin (PI3K/mTOR) pathway/receptor kinase signaling and RAS/mitogen activated protein kinases (MAPK) signaling pathways. Activation of PI3K/AKT and RAS/MAPK signaling regulates mechanisms of cell growth, proliferation, apoptosis, and chromatin remodeling; and is also involved in the metabolic switch toward glycolysis and glutaminolysis in cancer cells. Most PHEOs/PGLs in this cluster are adrenal and have a typical adrenergic phenotype compared with those in the Cluster 1 [32].

Cluster 2 tumors predominantly secrete methanephrine; and contains the PNMT enzyme which converts the norepinephrine to epinephrine. Since the PNMT enzyme is localized in the adrenal medulla, although the tumor is extra-adrenal (such as TMEMM127), the phenotype is called the adrenergic phenotype [10].

In the newly introduced cluster- Wnt signaling cluster, or cluster 3- also shows dysregulation of the Wnt and Hedgehog pathways as a result of somatic mutations in *CSDE1* and the mastermind like transcriptional coactivator 3 (*MAML3*) fusion genes [upstream binding transcription factor, RNA polymerase I (*UBTF*)–*MAML3* and transcription factor 4 (*TCF4*)–*MAML3*]. *MAML3* fusion-positive PHEOs display hypomethylating phenotype and increased Wnt and Hedgehog signaling. Wnt-altered tumors exhibit high expression of *CHGA*, a gene that encodes chromogranin A –a clinical marker of neuroendocrine tumors. The Wnt pathway regulates a variety of developmental processes such as cell proliferation, adhesion and motility, and cell polarity and differentiation [32].

Hyperdeoxycorticosteronism

Hyperdeoxycorticosteronism is divided into 3 subtypes: a) of congenital adrenal hyperplasia, b) Deoxycorticosterone-producing tumor and c) Primary cortisol resistance. The term of congenital adrenal hyperplasia (CAH) describes a group of autosomal recessive disorders resulting from mutations in genes encoding enzymes involved in the steroidogenic pathway. To date, 7 diseases are known to cause CAH and these diseases and defect genes are shown in Table **3** [33].

Among these diseases, 21-hydroxylase deficiency is the most common, and accounts for approximately 95% of CAH cases. As a result of the homozygous or compound heterozygous mutation in the *CYP21A2* gene, encoding steroid 21-hydroxylase, on chromosome 6p21, the functional enzyme cannot be transcribed, preventing the conversion of 17-hydroxyprogesterone to 11-deoxycortisol; results in decreased glucocorticoid and mineralocorticoid synthesis, increased in ACTH levels. The main characteristic of virtually observed is the increase in ACTH-stimulated androgen synthesis and the absence of cortisol to block [33]. 21-hydroxylase deficiency is divided into two classes as classical and non-classical CAH (NCCAH) (or late-onset) according to the severity of aldosterone deficiency. Also, classic form have two subtypes known as the salt-wasting and simple virilizing types according to the occurrence or not of a clinical salt loss in early infancy [34]. Gene encoding 21-hydroxylase exists in two highly homologous forms: *CYP21A2*, encoding the active enzyme and he inactive pseudogene *CYP21A1P*.

Table 3. Genetic causes and clinical features of the Steroidogenic Defects [33, 38].

Condition	Frequency	Affected Genes	Subtypes	Disorder of Sex Development	Biochemical Phenotype
21-hydroxylase deficiency	90-95%	*CYP21A2*	Salt wasting (Congenital), Simple virilizing (Congenital), Non-classic (Postnatal)	Salt wasting and Simple virilizing: 46,XX Non-classic: No	Common: Elevated 17-OHP, DHEA, and androstenedione Only in salt wasting: elevated K, low Na, CO_2 Only in simple virilizing: normal electrolytes

(Table 3) cont.....

11β-hydroxylase deficiency	0.2- 8%	*CYP11B1*	Classic CAH 11β-deficiency (Congenital), Non-classic CAH 11β-deficiency (Postnatal)	Classic: 46,XX Non-classic: No	Common: Elevated DOC, 11-deoxycortisol; androgens Only in classic type: low K, elevated Na, CO_2
17α-hydroxylase/ 17,20-lyase deficiency	rare	*CYP17A1*	17α-OH deficiency (Congenital), 17,20-Lyase deficiency (Congenital), Combined 17α-OH/17,20-lyase deficiency (Congenital or Postnatal)	46,XY	In 17α-OH deficiency: Normal or decreased androgens and estrogen, elevated DOC, corticosterone In 17,20-Lyase deficiency and Congenital Combined 17α-OH/17,20-lyase deficiency: Decreased androgens and estrogens In Postnatal Combined 17α-OH/17,20-lyase deficiency: Decreased follicular estradiol and increased progesterone
3β-hydroxy-steroid dehydrogenase type 2 deficiency	<5%	*HSD3B2*	Classic (Congenital), Non-classic (Postnatal)	Classic: 46,XY, 46,XX Non-classic: No	Common: Elevated DHEA, 17-pregnenolone, low androstenedione, testosterone, Only in classic type: elevated K, low Na, CO2
P450 oxidoreductase deficiency	rare	*POR*	-	46,XX, 46,XY	Partial, combined and variable defects of P450c21, P450c17 and P450aro activity
Lipoid adrenal hyperplasia	rare	*StAR*	Classic Non classic	46,XY	All steroid products low
Cholesterol side chain cleavage enzyme deficiency	rare	*CYP11A1*	Classic Non-classic	46,XY	All steroid products low

The recombination events between the active and inactive gene occur at a high rate and are responsible for a significant majority (estimated to be up to 95%) of the mutations in the active *CYP21A2* gene. More than 140 mutations have been described including deletions (10%), microconversions (75%), and macroconversions (10%). These are associated with the severity and phenotypes of the disease, causing 21-hydroxylase to undergo variable degrees of complete inactivation to partially functioning enzymes [35]. According to the most severe and least severe one is the following: salt-wasting, simple virilizing, and NCCAH; since the enzyme activity is completely destroyed in the salt-wasting type; while remains functional by 1-2% in simple virilizing and by 50% in NCCAH [33].

11β-hydroxylase enzyme catalyzes the conversion of 11-deoxycortisol to cortisol and 11-deoxycorticosterone to corticosterone; in the deficiency of the enzyme, increases in the substrate which are shunted into the androgen synthesis pathway, cause an increase in androstenedione [36]. Enzyme deficiency also causes hypertension from high 11-deoxycorticosterone and possibly other steroid precursors. The two homologous enzymes, 11β-hydroxylase and aldosterone synthase enzymes, are encoded by the *CYP11B1* and *CYP11B2* genes, respectively which both located on chromosome 8q21. However, unlike 21-hydroxylase, these two genes are also active, have distinct functions and do not have a pseudogene. More than 50 *CYP11B1*-inactivating mutations have been described including missense, nonsense, splice-site mutations, small deletions, small insertions, and complex rearrangements [37].

17-α-Hydroxylase deficiency (17OHD) is a rare form of CAH resulting from defective *CYP17A1* gene, located on chromosome 10. The *CYP17A1* enzyme is a microsomal P450 type II enzyme that catalyzes two different enzymatic reactions; 17-α hydroxylation of pregnenolone and progesterone, and the conversion of 17-hydroxypregnenolone to dehydroepiandrosterone and, with lesser efficiency, of 17-OHP to androstenedione through the 17,20 lyase reaction. Thus glucocorticoid and sex steroid deficiency, and impairments in both adrenal and gonadal function occurs due to a deficiency in the function of this enzyme, which can occur as a result of 70 *CYP17A1*-inactivating mutations. The accumulation of the corticosterone and 11-deoxycorticosterone exert glucocorticoid and mineralocorticoid activity respectively and lead to hypertension with hypokalemia. Among a group of diseases defined as CAH, those causing hypertension are only 11β-hydroxylase deficiency and 17α hydroxylase/17,20-lyase deficiency [37].

The membrane-bound enzyme 3β-Hydroxysteroid dehydrogenase/Δ5-4 isomerase is a key enzyme in the biosynthesis of all active steroid hormones, and catalyses 3β-hydroxysteroid dehydrogenation and Δ5- to Δ4-isomerisation of the Δ5-steroid precursors. This enzyme has two isoforms, type 1 and type 2, encoded by *HSD3B1* and *HSD3B2* respectively. The isoform of adrenal gland and gonads expressed is *HSD3B2*. Other forms of CAH are very rare, also their functions, genetic causes and biochemical phenotype have been shown in Table **3**.

Although deoxycorticosterone-producing adrenal tumors are known to be rare, large and malignant, patients with benign types have also been reported. In some of the patients, androgen and estrogen increase were found except deoxycorticosterone, and therefore it is reported that virilization cans be seen in women and feminization in men. Biochemical changes in patients, high levels of plasma deoxycorticosterone, aldosterone and renin low levels in blood, and hypokalemia [39, 40].

Primary cortisol resistance is the presence of cortisol secretion or plasma cortisol levels, although there are no signs of Cushing's syndrome. It is also known as glucocorticoid resistance and a rare familial syndrome. This syndrome occurs due to the defect in the glucocorticoid receptors and the steroid-receptor complex, and characterized by hypokalemic alkalosis, hypertension, increased plasma concentrations of deoxycorticosterone and increased adrenal androgen secretion. Hypertension and hypokalemia are the result of combined effects of excess deoxycorticosterone and cortisol, and due to increased effects of cortisol as a result of binding to mineralocorticoid receptors [41].

Cushing Syndrome

Cushing's syndrome is a syndrome caused by chronic exposure to endogenous or exogenous (pharmacological doses of corticosteroids) excess glucocorticoids. Among the endogenous causes of Cushing's syndrome, pituitary corticotroph adenoma over-secreting adrenocorticotropic hormone (ACTH) leading to excess cortisol secretion are the most common cause and constitute 70-80% of cases. Other endogenous causes include ectopic ACTH-producing neuroendocrine neoplasms or ACTH-independent adrenal cortisol hypersecretion. Cushing's syndrome, which is three times more common in women, has an estimated incidence of 0.2-0.5 per million people per year [42]. The clinical features of Cushing disease include central obesity, moon faces, 'buffalo hump', diabetes, hypertension, fatigue, easy bruising, depression, and reproductive disorders. Cushing disease is associated with increased morbidity and mortality, mainly due to cardiovascular or cerebrovascular disease and infections. Although the majority of Cushing's syndrome has sporadic origin as a result of specific germline and/or somatic gene defects, it can be seen as familial as part of various syndromes (Table **4**) [42 - 44]. In addition, researchers at the National Institutes of Health have found potential genetic cause of Cushing syndrome. They found some patients have mutant forms of *CABLES1* that do not respond to cortisol. CABLES1, the protein expressed by this gene, slows the division and growth of pituitary cells that produce the ACTH. Therefore, the loss-of function mutations in the *CABLES1* gene disrupt the tumor suppressor function in the pituitary gland by inhibiting ACTH negative feed-back regulation [45].

Apparent Mineralocorticoid Excess/11ß-Hydroxysteroid Dehydrogenase Deficiency

Apparent mineralocorticoid excess (AME) disease is an uncommon autosomal recessive disorder that is caused by a mutation in the gene encoding the kidney isoenzyme 11β-hydroxysteroid dehydrogenase type 2 (11β-HSD2) which located at 16q22.1 [46]. Most of these mutations are missense single point mutations. This enzyme is a microsomal enzyme complex responsible for the NAD+-dependent conversion of biologically active cortisol into inactive cortisone, and this reaction is thought to be necessary to protect the renal mineralocorticoid receptor from cortisol action, allowing aldosterone to regulate sodium homeostasis [47]. The clinical features of AME are hypertension, hypokalemia, low plasma renin activity, intrauterine growth retardation and postnatal failure to thrive. To date, 40 different mutations have been identified on this gene, causing to undergo complete inactivation or low enzymatic activation of the enzyme [46]. In conclusion, it has been shown that the half-life of cortisol is prolonged in patients with these mutations; and also urinary concentrations of cortisol metabolite (tetrahydrocortisol and allo-tetrahydrocortisol) increase (Fig. **2**) [48]. Therefore, the ratio of urinary concentrations of tetrahydrocortisol and allo-tetrahydrocortisol, to the concentration of tetrahydrocortisone ((THF + aTHF)/ THE) measurement is usually used as a diagnostic test [49].

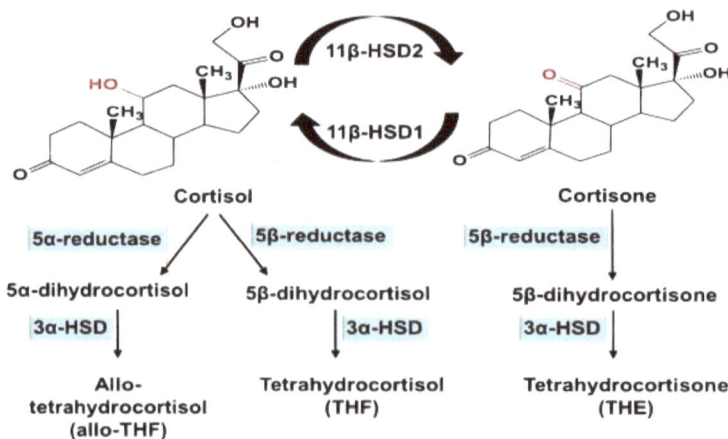

Fig. (2). The conversion of biologically active cortisol into inactive cortisone, and their metabolites. 3α-HSD: 3α-hydroxysteroid dehydrogenase; 11β-HSD1: 11β-hydroxysteroid dehydrogenase type 1; 11β-HSD2: 11β-hydroxysteroid dehydrogenase type 2.

In physiological conditions, aldosterone binds to cytosolic receptors and is transferred to the nucleus where it binds to nuclear receptors (mineralocorticoid receptor, abbreviated as "MR", or "type 1 steroid" receptor) and stimulate the transcription of specific genes, and directly or indirectly increasing activities of apical sodium (Na^+) channels and the basolateral sodium-potassium (Na^+/K) ATPase. Thus, aldosterone increases the absorption of sodium and potassium excretion into the tubular lumen. However, the sequence of these receptors is very similar to the glucocorticoid receptors, and in vitro the affinity of glucocorticoids and mineralocorticoids to this receptor is very close to each other. In normal conditions, blood concentrations of cortisol are 100-1000 fold higher than aldosterone. For this reason, in the 11β-HSD2 absence, elevated cortisol results in higher MR activation [50].

Table 4. Abnormalities in Gene and Protein Expression Levels in Cushing's Disease and Syndrome.

	Gene Mutations		
	Gene	**Function**	**Mutation Type**
Cushing's Disease	*USP8*	Inhibit epidermal growth factor receptor (EGFR) degradation and prolonged EGF signaling, resulting in increased activity in the proopiomelanocortin (POMC) promoter and transcription	Somatic GOF hotspot mutations
	MEN1	A putative tumor suppressor gene	Germline loss of function mutations/ deletions
	CDKN1B/p27Kip1	CDK inhibitor; inhibits corticotroph cell proliferation	Germline nonsense mutation, Under expression
	AIP	A tumor suppressor	Silence mutation, Missense mutation
	DICER1	Tumor suppressor gene, a highly conserved RNase III enzyme,	Frameshift mutation, Missense mutation
	Abnormal Protein Expression		
	Protein	**Function**	**Levels**
	Brg1	Chromatin remodeling; facilitates GR response	
	HDAC2	Chromatin remodeling	Decreased
	TR4	Transcriptional coregulator; stimulates POMC transcription and cell proliferation	Increased
	PTTG	Sister chromatid separation during metaphase; tumor progression	Increased
	EGFR	EGF receptor; proliferation, differentiation; stimulates ACTH synthesis	Increased

(Table 4) cont.....

	Gene Mutations		
Ectopic Acth Secretion	**Gene**	**Function**	**Mutation Type**
	RET	Oncogene	LOF mutations or Germline GOF mutations
	MEN1	A putative tumor suppressor gene	Germline LOF mutations/ deletions
Adrenal Cushing's Syndrome	**Bilateral Macronodular Adrenal Hyperplasia**		
	Gene Mutations		
	Gene	**Function**	**Mutation Type**
	ARMC5	A tumor suppressor	Germline and somatic LOF mutations
Adrenal Cushing's Syndrome	*ARMC5*	A tumor suppressor	Germline and somatic LOF mutations
	MEN1	A putative tumor suppressor gene	LOF mutations/deletion
	FH	Encodes an enzyme called fumarase which participates in Krebs cycle, which allows cells to use oxygen and generate energy.	LOF mutations
	GNAS1	Oncogene which encodes various proteins, including the α subunit of the stimulatory G protein (Gsα), extra-large αs and 55-kDa neuroendocrine secretory protein.	Mosaic GOF mutation
	PDE11A	Encodes phosphodiesterase11A4 which catalyzes the hydrolysis of cyclic adenosine monophosphate and cyclic guanosine monophosphate.	Germline LOF mutations
	PDE8B	Encodes a cyclic nucleotide phosphodiesterase (PDE) that catalyzes the hydrolysis of the second messenger cAMP.	Germline LOF mutation
	MC2R	Encodes adrenocorticotropic hormone (ACTH) receptor	Somatic mutations
	PRKACA	Encodes one of the catalytic subunits of protein kinase A which catalyze cAMP-dependent phosphorylation of proteins	Somatic GOF hotspot mutations, Germline amplification

(Table 4) cont.....

	Protein Expression		
	Protein	**Function**	**Levels**
	GPCR		
	POMC/ACTH	ACTH precursor	Increased
	PRKAR1A	Type 1 alpha subunit of an enzyme called protein kinase A which promotes cell growth and division (proliferation).	Increased
	Adrenal Adenoma		
	Gene Mutations		
	Gene	**Function**	**Mutation Type**
Adrenal Cushing's Syndrome	*PRKACA*	Encodes one of the catalytic subunits of protein kinase A which catalyze cAMP-dependent phosphorylation of proteins	Somatic GOF hotspot mutations,
	CTNNB1	Encodes a protein called beta-catenin which plays an important role in the Wnt signaling pathway, and in sticking cells together (cell adhesion) and in communication between cells.	Somatic LOF mutations
	GNAS1	Oncogene which encodes various proteins, including the α subunit of the stimulatory G protein (Gsα), extra-large αs and 55-kDa neuroendocrine secretory protein.	Somatic GOF mutations
	PRKAR1A	Encodes type 1 alpha subunit of an enzyme called protein kinase A which promotes cell growth and division (proliferation).	Germline LOF mutations/deletions
	Protein Expression		
	Protein	**Function**	**Levels**
	GPCR	G-protein coupled hormone receptors which can substitute for the normal function of ACTH or angiotensin-II.	Increased
	PRKAR1A	Type 1 alpha subunit of an enzyme called protein kinase A which promotes cell growth and division (proliferation).	Increased

(Table 4) cont.....

	Primary Pigmented Nodular Adrenocortical Disease		
	Gene Mutations		
	Gene	Function	Mutation Type
Adrenal Cushing's Syndrome	*PRKAR1A*	Encodes type 1 alpha subunit of an enzyme called protein kinase A which promotes cell growth and division (proliferation).	Germline LOF mutations/deletions,
	PDE11A	Encodes phosphodiesterase11A4 which catalyses the hydrolysis of cyclic adenosine monophosphate and cyclic guanosine monophosphate.	Germline LOF mutations
	PDE8B	Encodes a cyclic nucleotide phosphodiesterase (PDE) that catalyzes the hydrolysis of the second messenger cAMP.	Germline LOF mutation
	PRKACA	Encodes one of the catalytic subunits of protein kinase A which catalyze cAMP-dependent phosphorylation of proteins	Somatic GOF hotspot mutations or Germline amplification
	Protein Expression		
	Protein	Function	Levels
	PRKACA	The catalytic subunits of protein kinase A which catalyze cAMP-dependent phosphorylation of proteins	Increased

GOF: Gain of function; LOF: Loss of function;

Primary Aldosteronism

Hyperaldosteronism is an endocrine disorder that defined as a selective increase of mineralocorticoids caused by a disorder of the zona glomerulosa of the adrenal gland. Hyperaldosteronism may be primary or secondary [51].

In primary hyperaldosteronism, which is due to an abnormality within the adrenal gland, the initiating event is an autonomous increase in the secretion of aldosterone. Secondary hyperaldosteronism is initiated by activation of the renin-angiotensin system, which, in turn, increases the secretion of aldosterone. Thus, in secondary hyperaldosteronism, the increased production of aldosterone by the adrenal gland is due an external (extra-adrenal) stimulus.

Primary aldosteronism may be familial or sporadic; Familial forms 4 currently recognized subtypes (familial hyperaldosteronism [FH] types I–IV). The classification of sporadic PA is based on anatomic location of excess aldosterone: a) unilateral, caused by an aldosterone-producing adenoma (APA) and often treated surgically; and b) bilateral, caused by bilateral adrenal hyperplasia (BAH) and often treated medically with mineralocorticoid antagonist therapy [52].

FH-I was the first genetically defined form of human hypertension, while the genetic basis of FH-III and IV are known, but there is no information about the molecular basis of FH-II. The genetic defect leading to FH-I is a chimeric gene duplication resulting from unequal crossing over between the 11β-hydroxylase (*CYP11B1*) and aldosterone synthase genes (*CYP11B2*). a chimeric gene is created from the recombination of the ACTH responsive promoter region of the 11β-hydroxylase gene to coding sequences of the aldosterone synthase gene. Therefore, chimeric enzyme is regulated by ACTH and located ectopically in the zona fasciculata. Aldosterone synthase activity is thus colocalized with cortisol that can be metabolized further by the 18-hydroxylase and 18-oxidase activities of aldosterone synthase to overproduce the hybrid steroids 18-hydroxycortisol and 18-oxocortisol as is characteristic of this condition [52]. FH-III is caused by a germline heterozygous mutation in the *KCNJ5* gene (encoding the GIRK4 [G-protein–activated inward rectifier potassium channel 4]). The mutated K^+ channel GIRK4 (p.Thr158Ala) displayed a loss of selectivity for K^+ and an increase in Na^+ conductance that depolarizes the cell membrane. In zona glomerulosa cells, membrane depolarization causes the opening of voltage-dependent Ca^{2+} channels and Ca^{2+} influx, which activates Ca^{2+} signaling pathways and leads to an increase in aldosterone production. FH-IV is caused by a germline mutation in the *CACNA1H* gene that encodes the T-type (low voltage activated) Ca^{2+} channel Cav 3.2 (Cav 3.2 p.Met1549Val). Gain-of-function mutations in *CACNA1H* have been previously associated with epilepsy, seizures, and autism. Table **5** shows genetic and biochemical alterations of familial hyperaldosteronism types. Also, the known causative germline and somatic mutations associated with sporadic PA are summed in Table **6**.

Table 5. Clinical, genetic and biochemical data of patients with familial hyperaldosteronism (FH) [52 - 55].

	FH-I	FH-II	FH-III	FH-IV
Associated Gene	*CYP11B1/CYP11B2* hybrid gene	*CLCN2* mutations	*KCNJ5* mutations	*CACNA1H* mutations
Encoded protein	*CYP11B2*	CIC-2	GIRK4	Cav3.2

(Table 5) cont.....

	FH-I	FH-II	FH-III	FH-IV
Molecular mechanism	Chimeric fusion of *CYP11B1/CYP11B2* genes resulting in ACTH-dependent aldosterone synthesis in zona fasciculata	Unknown	Gain of function mutation of GIRK4 channel (*KCNJ5*) increases Na+ conductance, depolarizes cell, and opens voltage-gated calcium channels to increase aldosterone synthesis	*CACNA1H* encodes a voltage-gated calcium channel (CaV3.2) expressed in adrenal glomerulosa. Mutation drastically impaired channel inactivation and activation at more hyperpolarized potentials, producing increased intracellular Ca^{2+}, the signal for aldosterone production.
Inheritance	AD	AD	AD	AD
Male/Female ratio	1:1	1:1	1:1	Unknown
Hypertension	Normotensive to severely hypertensive	Normotensive to severely hypertensive	Severely hypertensive	Hypertensive
Biochemical findings	Normal to high aldosterone-to-renin ratio; Commonly normokalemia; High levels of 18-oxocortisol, 18-hydroxycortisol; Normal to markedly increased aldosterone levels	High aldosterone-to- renin ratio; Commonly hypokalemia; Normal to markedly increased aldosterone levels	High aldosterone-to-renin ratio; Commonly hypokalemia; High levels of 18-oxocortisol, 18-hydroxycortisol; Extremely high aldosterone levels	Elevated aldosterone levels despite low plasma renin activity, and abnormal adrenal steroid production.
Genetic testing	Germline sequencing	None	Germline sequencing of *KCNJ5*	Unknown
Treatment	Dexamethasone or mineralocorticoid receptor antagonist	Unilateral adrenalectomy or mineralocorticoid receptor antagonist	Bilateral adrenalectomy	Unknown

Table 6. The known causative germline and somatic mutations associated with sporadic PA [53].

Gene	Known Mutation Types	Protein	Molecular Mechanism
KCNJ5	Somatic and germline	The potassium ion channel Kir3.4	The mutations abolish the K^+ selectivity of the channel. which leads to higher Na^+ conductance and depolarization of the cell. Moreover, this depolarization results in the opening of the voltage-gated Ca^{2+} channels, which results in an influx of Ca^{2+} and increased aldosterone production.
ATP1A1	Somatic	The α1 subunit of Na^+/K^- ATPase (P-type ATPase)	The mutant protein displayed severely impaired ATPase activity, which indicates decreased Na^+ and K^+ binding. The mutant also showed considerably higher levels of membrane depolarization when expressed by an adrenal cell line, H295R. Membrane depolarization leads to opening of a voltage-gated ion channel, increased intracellular calcium, and subsequently enhanced production of aldosterone
ATP2B3	Germline, in-frame deletions	Plasma membrane calcium transporter, ATPase 3 (PMCA3)	The mutations potentially lead to the distortion of both Ca^{2+} binding regions.
CACNA1D	Somatic and *de novo* germline mutations	α1 subunit of L-type voltage calcium channel, Cav1.3	The mutant channels open early (lower potential) and have a sustained activation. Early activation at a lower depolarization leads to an increase in Ca^{2+} entry, which is associated with enhanced aldosterone production
CACNA1H	De novo germline, hot spot mutation	α1 subunit of the T-type voltage calcium channel, Cav3.2	Mutations delay the inactivation of the channel. Slower inactivation leads to prolonged opening of the channel, which results in higher Ca^{2+} influx.
CTNNB1	Somatic, germline	β-catenin	*CTNNB1* mutations relate to tumorigenesis rather than aldosterone production by activating Wnt/β-catenin signaling.
ARMC5	Somatic, germline	Armadillo-repeat-containing 5	Overexpression of mutant *ARMC5* was found to downregulate *CYP11B2*, encoding aldosterone synthase, expression.

CONCLUDING REMARKS

Hypertension is an important disease because of its high prevalence and mortality risk. Hence, it is one of the vital aims of researchers that to explain the mechanism of the disease and the causes contributing to the disease. Approximately 15% of hypertensive patients have secondary hypertension, namely hypertension develops in addition to an identifiable condition. The endocrine conditions causing secondary hypertension consist at least 15 endocrine disorders and the identification of genetic determinants has been most successful in these forms of hypertension. Moreover, the latest discoveries in genetic area of these diseases will provide an important basis for personalized therapy.

CONSENT FOR PUBLICATION

Not applicable.

CONFLICT OF INTEREST

The authors declare no conflict of interest, financial or otherwise.

ACKNOWLEDGEMENT

Declare none.

REFERENCES

[1]   Kearney PM, Whelton M, Reynolds K, Muntner P, Whelton PK, He J. Global burden of hypertension: analysis of worldwide data. Lancet 2005; 365(9455): 217-23.
        [http://dx.doi.org/10.1016/S0140-6736(05)17741-1] [PMID: 15652604]

[2]   Whelton PK, Carey RM, Aronow WS, *et al.* 2017 ACC/AHA/AAPA/ABC/ACPM/AGS/APhA/ASH/ ASPC/NMA/PCNA Guideline for the Prevention, Detection, Evaluation, and Management of High Blood Pressure in Adults: A Report of the American College of Cardiology/American Heart Association Task Force on Clinical Practice Guidelines. J Am Coll Cardiol 2018; 71(19): e127-248.
        [http://dx.doi.org/10.1016/j.jacc.2017.11.006] [PMID: 29146535]

[3]   Koch CA, Chrousos GP. Overview of Endocrine Hypertension http://www.ncbi.nlm.nih.gov/pubmed/ 259052142000.

[4]   Puar THK, Mok Y, Debajyoti R, Khoo J, How CH, Ng AK. Secondary hypertension in adults. Singapore Med J 2016; 57(5): 228-32.
        [http://dx.doi.org/10.11622/smedj.2016087] [PMID: 27211205]

[5]   Gupta-Malhotra M, Banker A, Shete S, *et al.* Essential hypertension *vs.* secondary hypertension among children. Am J Hypertens 2015; 28(1): 73-80.
        [http://dx.doi.org/10.1093/ajh/hpu083] [PMID: 24842390]

[6]   Koivuviita N. Secondary hypertension http://www.ebm-guidelines.com/go/ebm/ebm00075.html 2018.

[7]   Chapter 12. Secondary hypertension. Hypertens Res 2009; 32: 78-90.
        [http://dx.doi.org/10.1038/hr.2008.13]

[8]   Young WF, Calhoun DA, Lenders JWM, *et al.* Screening for endocrine hypertension: An endocrine society scientific statement. Endocr Rev 2017; 38: 103-22.
        [http://dx.doi.org/10.1210/er.2017-00054]

[9]   Thomas RM, Ruel E, Shantavasinkul PC, Corsino L. Endocrine hypertension: An overview on the current etiopathogenesis and management options. World J Hypertens 2015; 5(2): 14-27.
        [http://dx.doi.org/10.5494/wjh.v5.i2.14] [PMID: 26413481]

[10]   Pacak K, Tella SH. Pheochromocytoma and Paraganglioma http://www.ncbi.nlm.nih.gov/pubmed/ 29465938 2000.

[11]   DeLellis RA. Pathology and genetics of tumours of endocrine organs http://publications.iarc.fr/ Book-And-Report-Series/Who-Iarc-Classification-Of-Tumours/Pathology-And-Genetics-Of-Tumours-Of-Endocrine-Organs-2004 2004.

[12]   Backman S, Maharjan R, Falk-Delgado A, *et al.* Global DNA methylation analysis identifies two discrete clusters of pheochromocytoma with distinct genomic and genetic alterations. Sci Rep 2017; 7: 44943.
[http://dx.doi.org/10.1038/srep44943] [PMID: 28327598]

[13]   Zuber SM, Kantorovich V, Pacak K. Hypertension in pheochromocytoma: characteristics and treatment. Endocrinol Metab Clin North Am 2011; 40(2): 295-311, vii. [vii.].
[http://dx.doi.org/10.1016/j.ecl.2011.02.002] [PMID: 21565668]

[14]   2017 Guideline for the Prevention, Detection, Evaluation, and Management of High Blood Pressure in Adults American College of Cardiology https://wwwaccorg/~/media/Non-Clinical/Files-PDFs-Ex-el-MS-Word-etc/Guidelines/2017/Guidelines_Made_Simple_2017_HBPpdf

[15]   Cano Megías M, Rodriguez Puyol D, Fernández Rodríguez L, *et al.* pheochromocytoma-paraganglioma: Biochemical and genetic diagnosis. Nefrol (English Ed.) 2016; 36: 481–488.

[16]   Jochmanova I, Pacak K. Pheochromocytoma: The first metabolic endocrine cancer. Clin Cancer Res 2016; 22(20): 5001-11.
[http://dx.doi.org/10.1158/1078-0432.CCR-16-0606] [PMID: 27742786]

[17]   Korpershoek E, van Nederveen FH, Komminoth P, *et al.* Familial endocrine tumours: pheochromocytomas and extra-adrenal paragangliomas – an update. Diagn Histopathol 2017; 23: 335-45.
[http://dx.doi.org/10.1016/j.mpdhp.2017.06.001]

[18]   Amar L, Bertherat J, Baudin E, *et al.* Genetic testing in pheochromocytoma or functional paraganglioma. J Clin Oncol 2005; 23(34): 8812-8.
[http://dx.doi.org/10.1200/JCO.2005.03.1484] [PMID: 16314641]

[19]   Flynn A, Dwight T, Harris J, *et al.* Pheo-type: A diagnostic gene-expression assay for the classification of pheochromocytoma and paraganglioma. J Clin Endocrinol Metab 2016; 101(3): 1034-43.
[http://dx.doi.org/10.1210/jc.2015-3889] [PMID: 26796762]

[20]   Fishbein L, Leshchiner I, Walter V, *et al.* Comprehensive molecular characterization of pheochromocytoma and paraganglioma. Cancer Cell 2017; 31(2): 181-93.
[http://dx.doi.org/10.1016/j.ccell.2017.01.001] [PMID: 28162975]

[21]   Amorim-Pires D, Peixoto J, Lima J. Hypoxia pathway mutations in pheochromocytomas and paragangliomas. Cytogenet Genome Res 2016; 150(3-4): 227-41.
[http://dx.doi.org/10.1159/000457479] [PMID: 28231563]

[22]   Taïeb D, Pacak K. New insights into the nuclear imaging phenotypes of cluster 1 pheochromocytoma and paraganglioma. Trends Endocrinol Metab 2017; 28(11): 807-17.
[http://dx.doi.org/10.1016/j.tem.2017.08.001] [PMID: 28867159]

[23]   Wigerup C, Påhlman S, Bexell D. Therapeutic targeting of hypoxia and hypoxia-inducible factors in cancer. Pharmacol Ther 2016; 164: 152-69.
[http://dx.doi.org/10.1016/j.pharmthera.2016.04.009] [PMID: 27139518]

[24]   Crona J, Taïeb D, Pacak K. New perspectives on pheochromocytoma and paraganglioma: Toward a molecular classification. Endocr Rev 2017; 38(6): 489-515.
[http://dx.doi.org/10.1210/er.2017-00062] [PMID: 28938417]

[25]   Vicha A, Musil Z, Pacak K. Genetics of pheochromocytoma and paraganglioma syndromes: New

advances and future treatment options. Curr Opin Endocrinol Diabetes Obes 2013; 20(3): 186-91.
[http://dx.doi.org/10.1097/MED.0b013e32835fcc45] [PMID: 23481210]

[26]   Pillai S, Gopalan V, Smith RA, Lam AK. Updates on the genetics and the clinical impacts on phaeochromocytoma and paraganglioma in the new era. Crit Rev Oncol Hematol 2016; 100: 190-208.
[http://dx.doi.org/10.1016/j.critrevonc.2016.01.022] [PMID: 26839173]

[27]   Kantorovich V, King KS, Pacak K. SDH-related pheochromocytoma and paraganglioma. Best Pract Res Clin Endocrinol Metab 2010; 24(3): 415-24.
[http://dx.doi.org/10.1016/j.beem.2010.04.001] [PMID: 20833333]

[28]   Bardella C, Pollard PJ, Tomlinson I. SDH mutations in cancer. Biochim Biophys Acta 2011; 1807(11): 1432-43.
[http://dx.doi.org/10.1016/j.bbabio.2011.07.003] [PMID: 21771581]

[29]   LaGory EL, Giaccia AJ. The ever-expanding role of HIF in tumour and stromal biology. Nat Cell Biol 2016; 18(4): 356-65.
[http://dx.doi.org/10.1038/ncb3330] [PMID: 27027486]

[30]   Cruz JB, Fernandes LPS, Clara SA, *et al.* Molecular analysis of the Von Hippel-Lindau (VHL) gene in a family with non-syndromic pheochromocytoma: the importance of genetic testing. Arq Bras Endocrinol Metabol 2007; 51(9): 1463-7.
[http://dx.doi.org/10.1590/S0004-27302007000900008] [PMID: 18209888]

[31]   Jia D, Tang B, Shi Y, *et al.* A deletion mutation of the VHL gene associated with a patient with sporadic von Hippel-Lindau disease. J Clin Neurosci 2013; 20(6): 842-7.
[http://dx.doi.org/10.1016/j.jocn.2012.06.013] [PMID: 23632291]

[32]   Jochmanova I, Pacak K. Genomic landscape of pheochromocytoma and paraganglioma. Trends Cancer 2018; 4(1): 6-9.
[http://dx.doi.org/10.1016/j.trecan.2017.11.001] [PMID: 29413423]

[33]   El-Maouche D, Arlt W, Merke DP. Congenital adrenal hyperplasia. Lancet 2017; 390(10108): 2194-210.
[http://dx.doi.org/10.1016/S0140-6736(17)31431-9] [PMID: 28576284]

[34]   Société française d'endocrinologie. MG, Tardy V, Nicolino M, et al. Annales d'endocrinologie = Annals of endocrinology. Elsevier Masson. http://www.em-consulte.com/en/article/76394 2008, accessed 16 September 2018.

[35]   Huynh T, McGown I, Cowley D, *et al.* The clinical and biochemical spectrum of congenital adrenal hyperplasia secondary to 21-hydroxylase deficiency. Clin Biochem Rev 2009; 30(2): 75-86.
[PMID: 19565027]

[36]   Khattab A, Haider S, Kumar A, *et al.* Clinical, genetic, and structural basis of congenital adrenal hyperplasia due to 11β-hydroxylase deficiency. Proc Natl Acad Sci USA 2017; 114(10): E1933-40.
[http://dx.doi.org/10.1073/pnas.1621082114] [PMID: 28228528]

[37]   Krone N, Arlt W, Merke DP. Genetics of congenital adrenal hyperplasia. Best Pract Res Clin Endocrinol Metab 2009; 23(2): 181-92.
[http://dx.doi.org/10.1016/j.beem.2008.10.014] [PMID: 19500762]

[38]   New M, Yau M, Lekarev O, *et al.* Congenital Adrenal Hyperplasia. Endotext: South Dartmouth (MA): MDTextcom, Inc 2000. http://www.ncbi.nlm.nih.gov/pubmed/259051882000

[39]   Bakris GL, Sorrentino MJ. Hypertension: A companion to Braunwald's heart disease. Amsterdam: Elsevier Health Science 2017.

[40]   Melmed S, Polonsky K, Larsen PR, Kronenberg H. Williams textbook of endocrinology. Saunders Elsevier 2011.

[41]   Black HR. https://books.google.com.tr/books?id=ZEDm7j2dq70C&pg=PA86&lpg=PA86&dq=primary+cortisol+resistance&source=bl&ots=eBHsETOInt&sig=gbB0Zx3atLSOqZwOTno0u_9lq-

c&hl=tr&sa=X&ved=2ahUKEwiK8IGKxbHeAhWrlIsKHYymAok4HhDoATAKegQIBxAB#v=onepage&q=primary 2013.

[42]   Lacroix A, Feelders RA, Stratakis CA, Nieman LK. Cushing's syndrome. Lancet 2015; 386(9996): 913-27.
[http://dx.doi.org/10.1016/S0140-6736(14)61375-1] [PMID: 26004339]

[43]   Daniel E, Newell-Price J. Recent advances in understanding Cushing disease: resistance to glucocorticoid negative feedback and somatic USP8 mutations. F1000 Res 2017; 6: 613.
[http://dx.doi.org/10.12688/f1000research.10968.1] [PMID: 28529722]

[44]   Hernández-Ramírez LC, Stratakis CA. Genetics of Cushing's Syndrome. Endocrinol Metab Clin North Am 2018; 47(2): 275-97.
[http://dx.doi.org/10.1016/j.ecl.2018.02.007] [PMID: 29754632]

[45]   Hernández-Ramírez LC, Gam R, Valdés N, *et al.* Loss-of-function mutations in the *CABLES1* gene are a novel cause of Cushing's disease. Endocr Relat Cancer 2017; 24(8): 379-92.
[http://dx.doi.org/10.1530/ERC-17-0131] [PMID: 28533356]

[46]   Yau M, Haider S, Khattab A, *et al.* Clinical, genetic, and structural basis of apparent mineralocorticoid excess due to 11β-hydroxysteroid dehydrogenase type 2 deficiency. Proc Natl Acad Sci USA 2017; 114(52): E11248-56.
[http://dx.doi.org/10.1073/pnas.1716621115] [PMID: 29229831]

[47]   Ferrari P, Krozowski Z. Role of the 11β-hydroxysteroid dehydrogenase type 2 in blood pressure regulation. Kidney Int 2000; 57(4): 1374-81.
[http://dx.doi.org/10.1046/j.1523-1755.2000.00978.x] [PMID: 10760070]

[48]   Walker BR, Stewart PM, Edwards CRW. Enzyme modulation of access to corticosteroid receptors. Princ Med Biol 1997; 10: 297-310.
[http://dx.doi.org/10.1016/S1569-2582(97)80038-4]

[49]   Parthasarathy HK, MacDonald TM. Primary hyperaldosteronism and other forms of mineralocorticoid hypertension. Compr Hypertens 2007; pp. 809-25.
[http://dx.doi.org/10.1016/B978-0-323-03961-1.50070-2]

[50]   White PC. 11beta-hydroxysteroid dehydrogenase and its role in the syndrome of apparent mineralocorticoid excess. Am J Med Sci 2001; 322(6): 308-15.
[http://dx.doi.org/10.1097/00000441-200112000-00003] [PMID: 11780688]

[51]   Bertorini TE, Perez A. Neurologic complications of disorders of the adrenal glands. Handb Clin Neurol 2014; 120: 749-71.
[http://dx.doi.org/10.1016/B978-0-7020-4087-0.00050-4] [PMID: 24365350]

[52]   Vaidya A, Hamrahian AH, Auchus RJ. Genetics of primary aldosteronism. Endocr Pract 2015; 21(4): 400-5.
[http://dx.doi.org/10.4158/EP14512.RA] [PMID: 25667376]

[53]   Dutta RK, Söderkvist P, Gimm O. Genetics of primary hyperaldosteronism. Endocr Relat Cancer 2016; 23(10): R437-54.
[http://dx.doi.org/10.1530/ERC-16-0055] [PMID: 27485459]

[54]   Stowasser M, Pimenta E, Gordon RD. Familial or genetic primary aldosteronism and Gordon syndrome. Endocrinol Metab Clin North Am 2011; 40(2): 343-368, viii.
[http://dx.doi.org/10.1016/j.ecl.2011.01.007] [PMID: 21565671]

[55]   Aristizabal Prada ET, Castellano I, Sušnik E, *et al.* Comparative genomics and transcriptome profiling in primary aldosteronism. Int J Mol Sci 2018; 19(4): 1124.
[http://dx.doi.org/10.3390/ijms19041124] [PMID: 29642543]

CHAPTER 9

The Use of Calcium Channel Blockers and Risk of the Breast Cancer

Berrin Papila Kundaktepe[1] and **Hafize Uzun[2,*]**

[1] *Department of General Surgery, Cerrahpaşa Faculty of Medicine Istanbul, Turkey*

[2] *Department of Medical Biochemistry, Cerrahpaşa Faculty of Medicine, Istanbul University-Cerrahpasa, Istanbul, Turkey*

Abstract: Hypertension is one of the most common diseases responsible for death. There are five classes of medication for the treatment of hypertension, including those which have increasing prescription ratings year after year; angiotensin receptors blockers (ARBs) and calcium channel blockers (CCBs). Like all medications, CCBs were questioned about their long-term effects. Due to the important role of calcium (Ca^{2+}) in cell physiology and apoptosis, investigators started to follow up patients using CCBs for cancers, especially breast cancer. Theories were consistent about the blockade of cytoplasmic Ca^{2+} and failure of apoptosis. There have been a lot of studies (cohorts, case-control and observational studies) in this area. Studies with a small sample size and short-term follow-up reported that the use of CCBs increases the risk of cancer, whereas larger studies and meta-analyses were in favor of CCBs. In conclusion, CCBs are very important agents in hypertension, arrhythmia and angina treatment. In theory, they may seem to inhibit apoptosis and increase cancer growth but with the right consideration of patients' characteristics, time of use and age of the patient at the onset of the treatment, they are considered safe and efficient drugs unless studies with larger sample size and long-term follow-up claim opposite.

Keywords: Angiotensin receptors blockers, calcium channel blockers, breast cancer, apoptosis, hypertension, arrhythmia, angina treatment.

HYPERTENSION

Prevalence

Hypertension is a chronic and progressive disease which leads to two most common reasons of death (cardiovascular and cerebrovascular diseases) in the adult population. In 2010, a review estimated that 31 percent of the global popul-

* **Corresponding author at Hafize Uzun:** Department of Medical Biochemistry, Cerrahpaşa Faculty of Medicine, Istanbul University-Cerrahpasa, Istanbul, Turkey; Fax: +90 212 633 29 87; Tel: +90 212 414 30 56;
E-mail: huzun59@hotmail.com

Hafize Uzun & Pınar Atukeren (Eds.)

ation (1.39 billion people) suffers from hypertension [1]. Awareness of hypertension is not high as expected, thus only 48 percent of patients have been receiving medical treatment [2].

Treatment

There are five major classes of medication used in hypertension treatment. Each class can be prescribed according to characteristics of the patient and physician's choice. A study enrolling 772 patients in Switzerland revealed the intake of antihypertensive medications. According to the study, 42.8 percent of patients use diuretics, 51.7 percent use angiotensin receptor blockers (ARBs), 25.5 percent use angiotensin-converting enzyme inhibitors (ACEIs), 33 percent use beta-blockers (BBs) and 20.7 percent us calcium channel blockers (CCBs). The study suggested increasing intake of ARBs and CCBs [3]. Intake rats for antihypertensives are shown in Fig. (1).

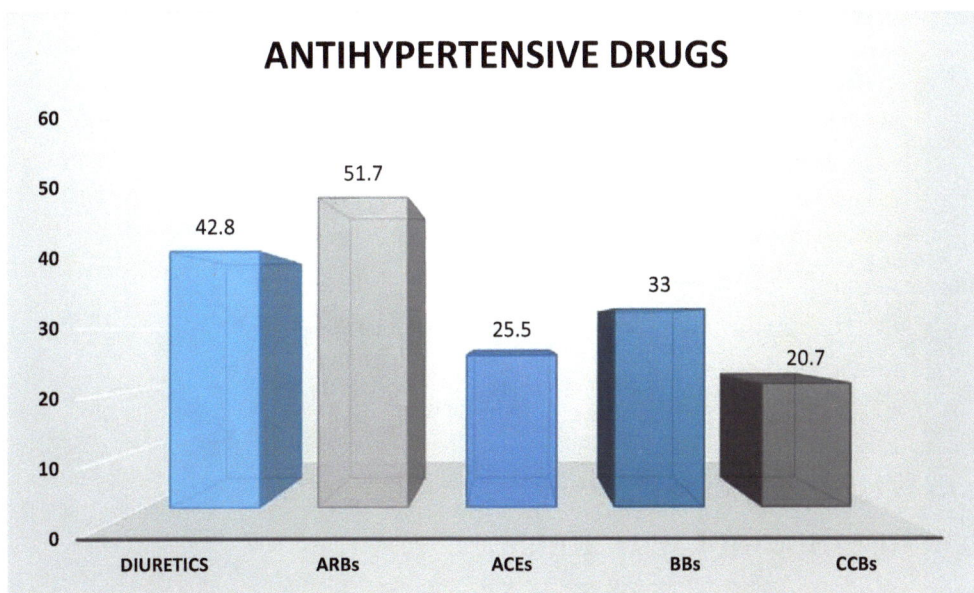

Fig. (1). Intake rates for antihypertensives.

As the prevalence of the disease and treatment rate increase, the burden of disease and complications also increase. There are several side effects of treatment options. Dehydration and electrolyte imbalances for diuretics, cough and some renal complications for ARBs and ACEIs, erectile dysfunction and fatigue for BBs, constipation and headache for CCBs are the examples of side effects. Most of those effects do not manifest with discontinuation of treatment.

TIMELINE OF ANTIHYPERTENSIVE TREATMENT

Relatively old medications such as diuretics and BBs are well-known for their long-term effects. Likewise, the other classes caused some question marks at the beginning and it seems that they still do.

In this chapter, we will discuss CCBs and their effects on breast cancer. Timeline of antihypertensive treatment are shown in Fig. (**2**).

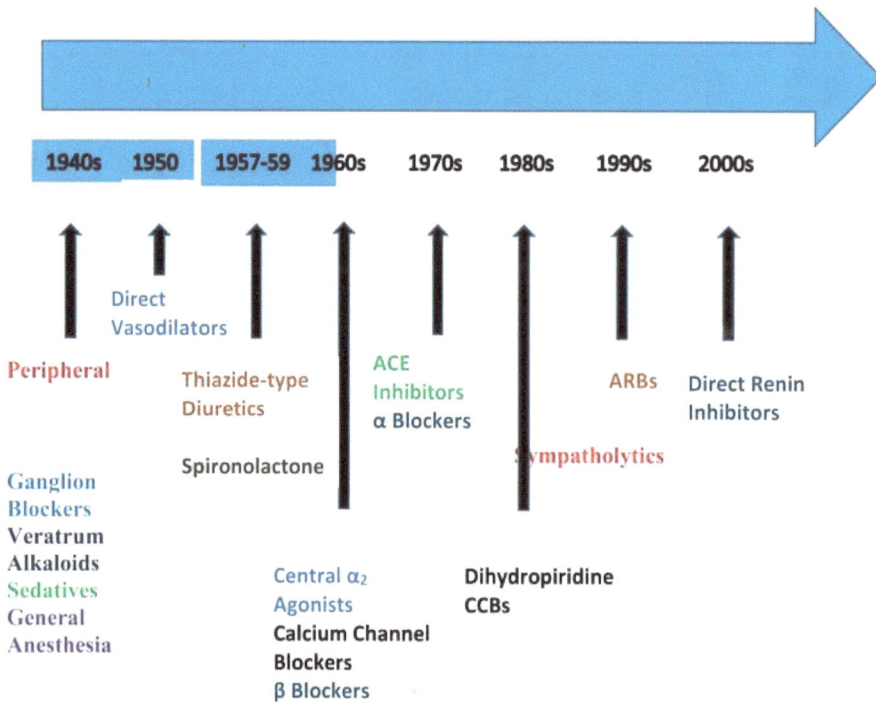

Fig. (2). Timeline of Antihypertensive Treatment.

CALCIUM CHANNEL BLOCKERS

Definition

CCBs are a group of medicine that block the entry of calcium to muscle cells of the heart and arteries. Calcium is crucial for conduction of electrical signal in muscle cells for contraction. Contraction provides blood pumping in the heart and constriction in arteries. The blockage of the entry of calcium into the cells initiates dilation of the arteries, which results in reduction of blood pressure. This eases the burden of the heart while pumping the blood. Also, with dilation, arteries carry more blood with a high level of oxygen to the heart.

Mechanism of Action

The entry of calcium into the smooth muscle cell is controlled by channels which are located on the cell membrane. Calcium channels have three types; voltage-gated, receptor-operated and leak channels. CCBs affect voltage-gated channels which divide into three subgroups; L-Type, T-Type and N-Type.

N-Type channels are common in neurons and nephrons. Calcium causes sympathetic activation and constriction on efferent arterioles. T-Type is common in neurons, nephrons and cardiac cells. Calcium causes an increase in the heart rate and also constriction of efferent arterioles. L-Type channels which are the main target of CCBs are common in smooth muscle cells, cardiac cells and neurons. When calcium reaches those channels, it causes vasoconstriction and increase of blood pressure. CCBs treatment areas and mechanisms of action are shown in Fig. (**3**) [4].

CCBs block depolarization and contraction of smooth muscle cells. Thus, CCBs cause negative chronotropic and ionotropic effects on the heart.

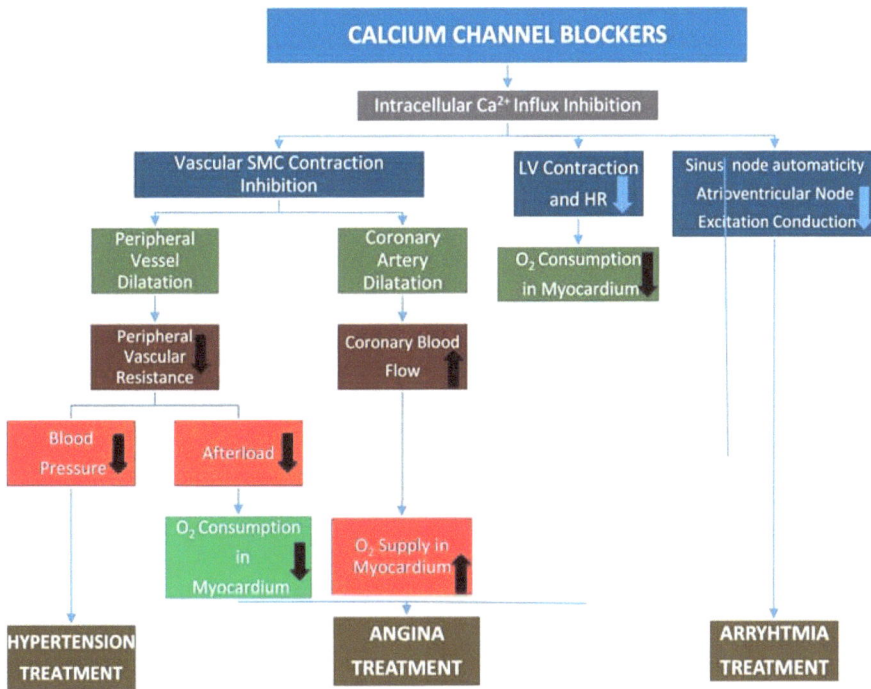

Fig. (3). CCBs Treatment Areas and Mechanisms of Action [4].
SMC: Smooth muscle cells; **LV:** left ventricular; **HR:** heart rate.

Classification

CCBs are divided into three subgroups: Phenylalkylamines (Verapamil); Benzothiazepines (Diltiazem) and Dihydropyridines (Nifedipine, Isradipine, Nicardipine, Felodipine, Amlodipine, Lacidipine, Lercanidipine, Benidipine, Manidipine, and Barnidipine). Classification of CCBs is shown in Fig. (**4**).

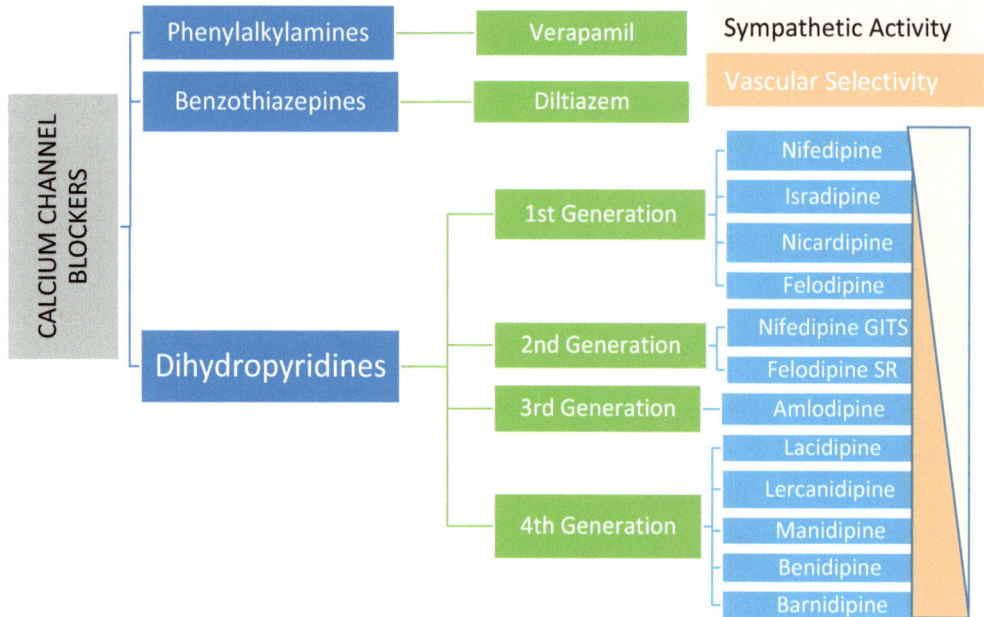

Fig. (4). Classification of CCBs.

Usage

CCBs are commonly used for hypertension, angina and arrhythmia treatment. They can be also used for pulmonary hypertension, Raynaud's phenomenon, cardiomyopathy and migraine.

Side Effects

CCBs can cause some side effects. Especially, dihydropyridines cause feet ankle edema, flushing and headache. Verapamil may cause hypotension, bradycardia and heart failure. All subgroups may cause drowsiness, constipation, increased appetite, gastroesophageal reflux and sexual dysfunction.

Contraindications of using CCBs are heart failure, severe aortic stenosis, bradycardia and complete atrioventricular (AV) block and acute coronary syndrome.

BREAST CANCER

Overview

Breast cancer is the most common (29%) malignancy and second common (%15) cause of cancer death in women.

Epidemiology

Gender (women), age (advanced age), race (Caucasian), geography (Japan, Thailand-the lowest incidence, and North America-the highest incidence) and socioeconomic status (directly proportional).

Survival

Due to the advances in screening and therapy, survival rates are increased in years. 8 years of survival chance is 90% for stage 1, 70% for stage 2 and 10% for stage 4.

Risk Factors

- *Genetical:* BRCA1, BRCA2, TP53, PTEN genes
- *Family History:* Relative risk of having a first-degree relative with breast cancer is 1.7.
- *Proliferative Breast Disease:* Ductal hyperplasia and sclerosing adenosis
- *Personal Cancer History:* Being diagnosed with breast cancer increases the risk of having breast cancer again.
- *Menstrual and Reproductive Factors:* Early onset of menarche and late onset of menopause increase, first full-term pregnancy before the age of 30 decreases the risk.
- *Radiation Exposure*
- *Exogenous Hormone Use*
- *Alcohol*
- *High-Fat Diet*
- *Obesity* [5].

Diagnosis

Physical exam (by physician and/or patient), mammogram, ultrasound, biopsy, MRI

Types

- Ductal Carcinoma in Situ (DCIS)

- Invasive Ductal Carcinoma (IDC) - most common (*Tubular, Medullary, Mucinous, Papillary, Cribriform*)
- Invasive Lobular Carcinoma (ILC)
- Inflammatory Breast Cancer
- Lobular Carcinoma in Situ (LCIS)
- Male Breast Cancer
- Paget's Disease
- Phyllodes Tumors
- Metastatic Tumors

Treatment Options

- Surgery (Lumpectomy, Mastectomy, Axillary lymph node dissection, Sentinel lymph node biopsy, Reconstructive surgery)
- Radiation Therapy
- Systemic Therapy
- Chemotherapy
- Hormonal Therapy
- Targeted Therapy

HYPOTHESIS ABOUT CCBS AND CANCER

Cancer is defined as abnormal and uncontrolled cell proliferation. Carcinogenesis damages DNA or alters enzymes which are necessary for DNA replication. In this situation, the cell has three options; malignant proliferation, apoptosis or postponement of replication until the damage is repaired [6].

Apoptosis is an effective mechanism to remove cells with genetic abnormalities; thus preventing cancer. Calcium plays a crucial role in the mechanism of apoptosis. Different decoding of Ca^{2+}-linked stimuli evoking cell activation or apoptosis is shown in Fig. (**5**).

Transmembrane calcium signals trigger cell differentiation and genetically programmed cell death (apoptosis), both important for inhibiting cancer growth [7 - 10]. Sustained rise of cytosolic ionized calcium leads cell to apoptosis. It is also involved in the activation of endonuclease enzyme which leads to DNA fragmentation [11].

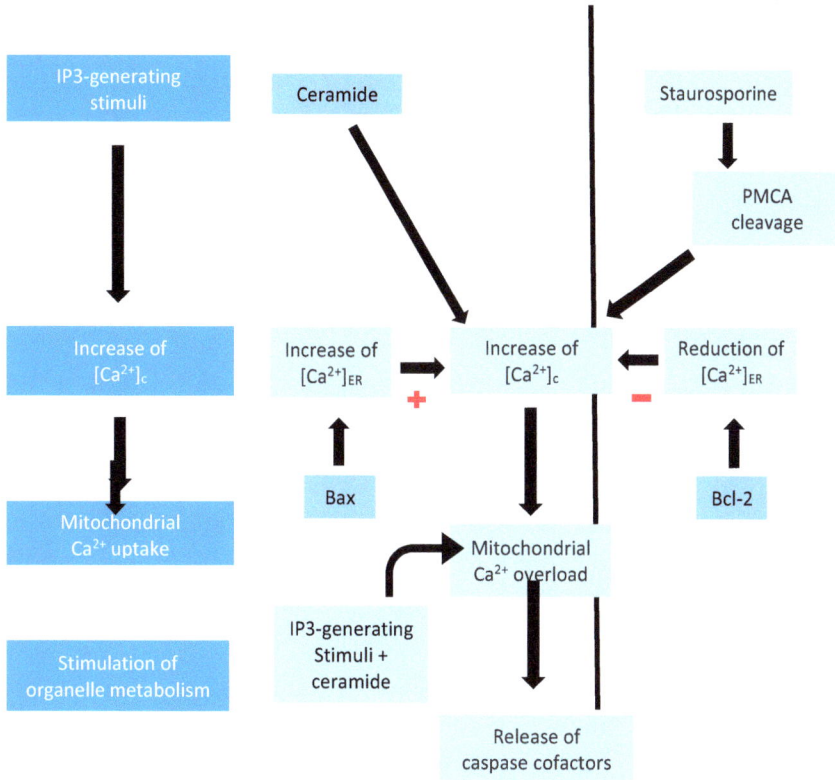

Fig. (5). Differential decoding of Ca^{2+}-linked stimuli evoking cell activation or apoptosis [12]. $[Ca^{2+}]_c$: Cytoplasmic calcium, $[Ca^{2+}]_{ER}$: Calcium in endoplasmic reticulum, PMCA: plasma membrane Ca^{2+} ATPase.

STUDIES AND CONTROVERSIAL RESULTS

In 1996, Pahor *et al.* [6] studied the relationship between CCBs and cancer. They enrolled 750 hypertensive individuals with the age greater than 71 and no cancer diagnosis formerly. Patients using CCBs and other antihypertensives were compared by means of the risk assessment of cancer development. In conclusion, CCBs have increased cancer risk. Most probably this study was the first study to draw attention to the relationship between CCBs and cancer.

In one of the earlier studies, which was conducted by Fitzpatrick *et al.* [13], 3.198 postmenopausal women aged greater than 65 years were enrolled. They compared patients taking CCBs to patients using other antihypertensive drugs. They conclude that breast cancer risk in patients using CCBs increased 2.6-fold and there was no association between other antihypertensives and breast cancer. The risk was highest in patients using estrogens with immediate release CCBs [13].

After Pahor's study [6], researchers started to suspect the relationship between

CCBs usage and cancer. Olsen *et al.* [14] conducted a study with 17.911 patients in a Danish county and revealed no association with CCBs use and any kind of cancer. After this study, a cohort study of 18.635 female nurses was conducted. This study also concluded that there is no significant cancer risk in patients using CCBs compared to the patients using other antihypertensives [15].

In the year 2013, Saltzman *et al.* [16] conducted a prospective cohort of 3.201 women equal to or greater than 65 years of age. Compared with women using no antihypertensives, CCBs users had a 1.6-fold increased risk of breast cancer. The risk was 2.4-fold increased with immediate-release CCBs.

A case-control study conducted in 2013 by Li *et al.* [17], enrolled post-menopausal 1907 patients diagnosed with breast cancer and 856 cancer-free controls between 55–74 years of age. The aim of the study was to evaluate all antihypertensive drug classes associated with breast cancer. None of the antihypertensives were found related to breast cancer in current, former or short-term use. CCBs use for 10 years or longer was found associated with breast cancer. The risk of short-acting CCBs was found to be higher. Also, the use of ACEs for 10 years or longer was found to be associated with reduced breast cancer risk [17].

Another meta-analysis published in 2014 conducted by Chen *et al.* [18] evaluated 11 studies (five cohorts, four case-control, and two nested case-control). These studies reported no evidence that CCBs use is associated with breast cancer. However, there may be a positive association between immediate-release CCBs use and risk of breast cancer.

A meta-analysis in 2014 conducted by Li *et al.* [19] including 17 studies (9 cohorts and 8 case-control) evaluated CCBs and breast cancer risk among 149,607 patients, among which 53,812 patients were using CCBs. The study revealed an increased risk of breast cancer in patients using CCBs.

A study on a cohort of 210,641 U.S. registered nurses followed up for 23-24 years by Devore *et al.* [20] was published in 2015. There was no significant increase in the risk of breast cancer in patients using CCBs.

In 2015, Grimaldi-Bensouda *et al.* [21] conducted a large population-based cohort study in the UK including patients using CCBs, patients using other antihypertensives and patients using no medications. In conclusion, no association was revealed between CCBs and the risk of breast cancer.

In 2016, Wilson *et al.* [22] enrolled 50,757 women patients aged between 35 and 74. They named this study as "The Sister Study" because patients with no breast cancer were allowed to include their sisters who were diagnosed with breast cancer. With this effect, genetic factors could also be evaluated. 3316 patients were currently using CCBs at study baseline. 1965 patients were diagnosed with breast cancer during the study at 10 years' follow-up. There was no significant difference in the risk of breast cancer between patients using CCBs and others who didn't receive CCBs in these 10 years.

In 2016, Fryzek *et al.* [23] studied breast cancer incidence among 49,950 women aged between 50-67 years in Denmark in order to determine if breast cancer risk is associated with any of the classes of antihypertensives. There has been no increase in the risk of breast cancer with antihypertensive drugs including CCBs.

A population-based cohort study was conducted by Azoulay *et al.* [24] in 2016, with 273,152 patients. There was no increased risk of breast cancer in patients using CCBs regardless of subtypes and duration of use.

A case-control study conducted by Gómez-Acebo *et al.* [25] with 1,736 breast cancer patients and 1,895 healthy controls in 2016. revealed that CCBs were associated with 72% increase in breast cancer risk in postmenopausal women. This risk was doubled in patients with a BMI greater than 25.

Ye *et al.* [26] conducted a large meta-analysis including 24 studies and 711,479 female patients followed up for 3-16 years and reported that long-term use of CCBs had a significant relationship with breast cancer [26].

Raebel *et al.* [27] wanted to figure out the controversy about CCBs and ACEs causing breast cancer in long-term use in 2017. They enrolled 109,752 women patients who have used the drugs for 1-12 years and were older than age 55. CCBs users (17.9%) and ACEs users (82.1%) were evaluated separately. In conclusion, long-term CCBs use didn't increase breast cancer risk, whereas long-term ACEs (2-12 years) use conferred a protective association against relatively short-term use (1-2 years), similar to Li *et al.*'s study in 2013 [17].

In 2017, Brasky *et al.* [28] enrolled 28.561 postmenopausal women from the Women's Health Initiative using antihypertensive drugs including CCBs. 1402 patients were diagnosed with breast cancer in 12 years of follow-up. The use of CCBs was not found to be associated with breast cancer.

Ni *et al.* [29] conducted a meta-analysis which included twenty-one observational studies with 3,116,266 patients in 2017. Studies with major antihypertensive classes (ARBs, ACEs, BBs and CCBs) were evaluated. Six retrospective and seven prospective studies were included in the analysis of breast cancer risk among CCBs users. Random effect pool analysis suggested no relationship between breast cancer and CCBs use. Subgroup analysis showed a positive association among retrospective studies but a negative association among prospective studies.

DISCUSSION

Calcium may play an important role in the regulation of human breast carcinoma cells. A Ca^{2+}/ Mg^{2+}-dependent endonuclease activation is a critical step of apoptosis in human breast tumors [13].

Blocking calcium entry to the cell may inhibit apoptosis which is a natural defensive mechanism against cancer growth. On the other hand, breast cancer is more related to inhibition of apoptosis mechanism than other cancers which can be explained with the contribution of hormones. Some studies suggested an increased risk of breast cancer in postmenopausal women which can be explained by apoptosis inhibition by CCBs and cell proliferation by estrogens. Gynecomastia in men was found to be associated with the use of CCBs, pertaining to a mechanism involving hormones [30, 31].

It has been proposed that CCBs also have different effects on apoptosis. A study suggested that low intracytoplasmic Ca^{2+} levels prevent cation-mediated charge neutralization of DNA and stimulate the apoptosis [32 - 34]. Antiapoptotic effect of CCBs does not always cause cancer growth. Some studies showed CCBs can present their antiapoptotic effect on noncancerous cells too which is beneficial as blocking the apoptotic destruction of pancreatic beta-cells [33, 34].

On the contrary to studies suggesting CCBs may cause cancer, verapamil can interfere with the function of the membrane-bound multi-drug resistance protein 1 (MDR1) protein and improve the efficacy of anti-cancer agents [34 - 37]. Another study suggested that CCBs can be used for the treatment of Ca^{2+}-dependent cancers like breast cancer by maintaining the normal calcium homeostasis. CCBs can reduce excessive cell Ca^{2+} levels linked to abnormal cell growth and dramatically inhibit tumor growth as compared to controls. As a result, they can be useful in the treatment of breast cancer [34, 38].

Antihypertensives are one of the most prescribed drug groups worldwide. CCBs are in the first-line treatment of hypertension and stable angina. In addition, they are the most preferred drugs with diuretics in combined hypertension treatment. Besides some mild side effects like headache and edema, they are well-tolerated drugs with a strong antihypertensive effect. Therefore, CCBs are indispensable in hypertension management.

As a result of studies conducted during the last three decades, CCBs could not be held responsible for causing breast cancer. There are contradictory results of studies. Ignoring the fact that every study has strengths and weaknesses, lots of medications can be held responsible for cancer propagation by their mechanism of action. Regarding CCBs, there were two points which attracted our attention. Firstly, most of these studies suggested that using CCBs over 10 years may be held responsible for cancer growth. Secondly, using CCBs at postmenopausal stage may increase cancer propagation with an additional risk of hormone replacement therapy. However, there are still no contraindications of using CCBs in these patients.

In conclusion, CCBs are commonly used drugs with their pros and cons. There is a need of independent studies with larger and various patient groups in the near future.

CONSENT FOR PUBLICATION

Not applicable.

CONFLICT OF INTEREST

The authors confirm that this chapter contents have no conflict of interest.

ACKNOWLEDGEMENTS

Declared none.

REFERENCES

[1] Mills KT, Bundy JD, Kelly TN, *et al.* Global disparities of hypertension prevalence and control: A systematic analysis of population-based studies from 90 countries. Circulation 2016; 134(6): 441-50.
[http://dx.doi.org/10.1161/CIRCULATIONAHA.115.018912] [PMID: 27502908]

[2] Melgarejo JD, Maestre GE, Thijs L, *et al.* Prevalence, treatment, and control rates of conventional and ambulatory hypertension across 10 populations in 3 continents. Hypertension 2017; 70(1): 50-8.
[http://dx.doi.org/10.1161/HYPERTENSIONAHA.117.09188] [PMID: 28483916]

[3] Christe V, Waeber G, Vollenweider P, Marques-Vidal P. Antihypertensive drug treatment changes in the general population: the CoLaus study. BMC Pharmacol Toxicol 2014; 15: 20.
[http://dx.doi.org/10.1186/2050-6511-15-20] [PMID: 24685255]

[4] Sueta D, Tabata N, Hokimoto S. Clinical roles of calcium channel blockers in ischemic heart diseases. Hypertens Res 2017; 40(5): 423-8.
[http://dx.doi.org/10.1038/hr.2016.183] [PMID: 28123178]

[5] Jardines L, Goyal S, Fisher P, Weitzel J, Royce M, Goldfarb SB. Breast Cancer Overview: Risk Factors, Screening, Genetic Testing, and Prevention. http://www.cancernetwork.com/cancer-management/breast-cancer-overview-risk-factors-screening-genetic-testing-and-prevention 2015.

[6] Koivuviita N. Secondary hypertension. 2018. http://www.ebm-guidelines.com/go/ebm/ebm00075.html

[7]   Whitfield JF. Calcium signals and cancer. Crit Rev Oncog 1992; 3(1-2): 55-90.
        [PMID: 1550862]

[8]   Carson DA, Ribeiro JM. Apoptosis and disease. Lancet 1993; 341(8855): 1251-4.
        [http://dx.doi.org/10.1016/0140-6736(93)91154-E] [PMID: 8098400]

[9]   Martin SJ, Green DR. Apoptosis and cancer: the failure of controls on cell death and cell survival. Crit
        Rev Oncol Hematol 1995; 18(2): 137-53.
        [http://dx.doi.org/10.1016/1040-8428(94)00124-C] [PMID: 7695828]

[10]   Trump BF, Berezesky IK. Calcium-mediated cell injury and cell death. FASEB J 1995; 9(2): 219-28.
        [http://dx.doi.org/10.1096/fasebj.9.2.7781924] [PMID: 7781924]

[11]   Nicotera P, Zhivotovsky B, Orrenius S. Nuclear calcium transport and the role of calcium in apoptosis.
        Cell Calcium 1994; 16(4): 279-88.
        [http://dx.doi.org/10.1016/0143-4160(94)90091-4] [PMID: 7820847]

[12]   Rizzuto R, Pinton P, Ferrari D, *et al.* Calcium and apoptosis: facts and hypotheses. Oncogene 2003;
        22(53): 8619-27.
        [http://dx.doi.org/10.1038/sj.onc.1207105] [PMID: 14634623]

[13]   Fitzpatrick AL, Daling JR, Furberg CD, Kronmal RA, Weissfeld JL. Use of calcium channel blockers
        and breast carcinoma risk in postmenopausal women. Cancer 1997; 80(8): 1438-47.
        [http://dx.doi.org/10.1002/(SICI)1097-0142(19971015)80:8<1438::AID-CNCR11>3.0.CO;2-6]
        [PMID: 9338468]

[14]   Olsen JH, Sørensen HT, Friis S, *et al.* Cancer risk in users of calcium channel blockers. Hypertension
        1997; 29(5): 1091-4.
        [http://dx.doi.org/10.1161/01.HYP.29.5.1091] [PMID: 9149671]

[15]   Michels KB, Rosner BA, Walker AM, *et al.* Calcium channel blockers, cancer incidence, and cancer
        mortality in a cohort of U.S. women: the nurses' health study. Cancer 1998; 83(9): 2003-7.
        [http://dx.doi.org/10.1002/(SICI)1097-0142(19981101)83:9<2003::AID-CNCR17>3.0.CO;2-3]
        [PMID: 9806660]

[16]   Saltzman BS, Weiss NS, Sieh W, *et al.* Use of antihypertensive medications and breast cancer risk.
        Cancer Causes Control 2013; 24(2): 365-71.
        [http://dx.doi.org/10.1007/s10552-012-0122-8] [PMID: 23224328]

[17]   Li CI, Daling JR, Tang MT, Haugen KL, Porter PL, Malone KE. Use of antihypertensive medications
        and breast cancer risk among women aged 55 to 74 years. JAMA Intern Med 2013; 173(17): 1629-37.
        [http://dx.doi.org/10.1001/jamainternmed.2013.9071] [PMID: 23921840]

[18]   Chen Q, Zhang Q, Zhong F, *et al.* Association between calcium channel blockers and breast cancer: a
        meta-analysis of observational studies. Pharmacoepidemiol Drug Saf 2014; 23(7): 711-8.
        [http://dx.doi.org/10.1002/pds.3645] [PMID: 24829113]

[19]   Li W, Shi Q, Wang W, Liu J, Li Q, Hou F. Calcium channel blockers and risk of breast cancer: a
        meta-analysis of 17 observational studies. PLoS One 2014; 9(9) e105801.
        [http://dx.doi.org/10.1371/journal.pone.0105801] [PMID: 25184210]

[20]   Devore EE, Kim S, Ramin CA, *et al.* Antihypertensive medication use and incident breast cancer in
        women. Breast Cancer Res Treat 2015; 150(1): 219-29.
        [http://dx.doi.org/10.1007/s10549-015-3311-9] [PMID: 25701121]

[21]   Grimaldi-Bensouda L, Klungel O, Kurz X, *et al.* Calcium channel blockers and cancer: a risk analysis
        using the UK Clinical Practice Research Datalink (CPRD). BMJ Open 2016; 6(1) e009147.
        [http://dx.doi.org/10.1136/bmjopen-2015-009147] [PMID: 26747033]

[22]   Wilson LE, D'Aloisio AA, Sandler DP, Taylor JA. Long-term use of calcium channel blocking drugs and breast cancer risk in a prospective cohort of US and Puerto Rican women. Breast Cancer Res 2016; 18(1): 61.
[http://dx.doi.org/10.1186/s13058-016-0720-6] [PMID: 27378129]

[23]   Fryzek JP, Poulsen AH, Lipworth L, *et al.* A cohort study of antihypertensive medication use and breast cancer among Danish women. Breast Cancer Res Treat 2006; 97(3): 231-6.
[http://dx.doi.org/10.1007/s10549-005-9091-x] [PMID: 16791484]

[24]   Azoulay L, Soldera S, Yin H, Bouganim N. Use of Calcium Channel Blockers and Risk of Breast Cancer: A Population-based Cohort Study. Epidemiology 2016; 27(4): 594-601.
[http://dx.doi.org/10.1097/EDE.0000000000000483] [PMID: 27031042]

[25]   Gómez-Acebo I, Dierssen-Sotos T, Palazuelos C, *et al.* The use of antihypertensive medication and the risk of breast cancer in a case-control study in a spanish population: The MCC-spain study. PLoS One 2016; 11(8) e0159672.
[http://dx.doi.org/10.1371/journal.pone.0159672] [PMID: 27508297]

[26]   Ye X, Du Q, Li H, Yu B, Zhai Q. Calcium channel blockers and risk of breast cancer: a meta-analysis. Int J Clin Exp Med 2016; 9(10): 20425-31.

[27]   Raebel MA, Zeng C, Cheetham TC, *et al.* Risk of breast cancer with long-term use of calcium channel blockers or angiotensin-converting enzyme inhibitors among older women. Am J Epidemiol 2017; 185(4): 264-73.
[http://dx.doi.org/10.1093/aje/kww217] [PMID: 28186527]

[28]   Brasky TM, Krok-Schoen JL, Liu J, *et al.* Use of calcium channel blockers and breast cancer risk in the women's health initiative. Cancer Epidemiol Biomarkers Prev 2017; 26(8): 1345-8.
[http://dx.doi.org/10.1158/1055-9965.EPI-17-0096] [PMID: 28765339]

[29]   Ni H, Rui Q, Zhu X, Yu Z, Gao R, Liu H. Antihypertensive drug use and breast cancer risk: a meta-analysis of observational studies. Oncotarget 2017; 8(37): 62545-60.
[http://dx.doi.org/10.18632/oncotarget.19117] [PMID: 28977968]

[30]   Tanner LA, Bosco LA. Gynecomastia associated with calcium channel blocker therapy. Arch Intern Med 1988; 148(2): 379-80.
[http://dx.doi.org/10.1001/archinte.1988.00380020123017] [PMID: 3341839]

[31]   Boyd IW. Adverse Drug Reactions Advisory Committee. Gynaecomastia in association with calcium antagonists. Med J Aust 1994; 161(5): 328.
[http://dx.doi.org/10.5694/j.1326-5377.1994.tb127457.x] [PMID: 7830672]

[32]   Whyte MK, Hardwick SJ, Meagher LC, Savill JS, Haslett C. Transient elevations of cytosolic free calcium retard subsequent apoptosis in neutrophils in vitro. J Clin Invest 1993; 92(1): 446-55.
[http://dx.doi.org/10.1172/JCI116587] [PMID: 8392090]

[33]   Juntti-Berggren L, Larsson O, Rorsman P, *et al.* Increased activity of L-type Ca2+ channels exposed to serum from patients with type I diabetes. Science 1993; 261(5117): 86-90.
[http://dx.doi.org/10.1126/science.7686306] [PMID: 7686306]

[34]   Mason RP. Calcium channel blockers, apoptosis and cancer: is there a biologic relationship? J Am Coll Cardiol 1999; 34(7): 1857-66.
[http://dx.doi.org/10.1016/S0735-1097(99)00447-7] [PMID: 10588195]

[35]   Hargrave RM, Davey MW, Davey RA, Kidman AD. Development of drug resistance is reduced with idarubicin relative to other anthracyclines. Anticancer Drugs 1995; 6(3): 432-7.
[http://dx.doi.org/10.1097/00001813-199506000-00011] [PMID: 7670142]

[36]   Chauffert B, Pelletier H, Corda C, *et al.* Potential usefulness of quinine to circumvent the anthracycline resistance in clinical practice. Br J Cancer 1990; 62(3): 395-7.
[http://dx.doi.org/10.1038/bjc.1990.305] [PMID: 2206948]

[37] Timcheva CV, Todorov DK. Does verapamil help overcome multidrug resistance in tumor cell lines and cancer patients? J Chemother 1996; 8(4): 295-9.
[http://dx.doi.org/10.1179/joc.1996.8.4.295] [PMID: 8873836]

[38] Taylor JM, Simpson RU. Inhibition of cancer cell growth by calcium channel antagonists in the athymic mouse. Cancer Res 1992; 52(9): 2413-8.
[PMID: 1533173]

CHAPTER 10

Neurogenic Hypertension

Gonul Simsek[*] and **Aykut Oruc**

Department of Physiology, Istanbul University-Cerrahpaşa, Cerrahpasa Faculty of Medicine Istanbul, Turkey

Abstract: In this section, we discuss the cardiovascular pathways of the central nervous system (CNS), neural regulation of circulation and patophysiologic mechanisms of neurogenic hypertension. The pathophysiologic mechanisms underlying the increased arterial pressure in neurogenic hypertension are not clear. It has been suggested that sympathetic overactivity is present in hypertensive patients. The role of sympathetic outflow in the pathogenesis of hypertension has been an issue of continuous interest recently. Why sympathetic activity rises in neurogenic hypertension is unclear. In this section, proposed causes of increased sympathetic tone in essential hypertension; especially the factors causing impaired baroreflex sensitivity (*i.e.* aldosterone and locally produced chemical factors such as prostacyclin, prostaglandins, nitric oxide (NO), reactive oxygen species (ROS) and platelet factors),direct effects of NO, ROS, angiotensin II, salt and proinflammatuar cytokines to CNS factors that play role on impaired sympathetic activity in aging and obesity processes (*i.e.* leptin, insulin, insulin resistance, adiponectin and ghrelin) are discussed.

Keywords: Adiponectin, Aging, Angiotensin II, Baroreceptor sensitivity, Blood pressure, Chemoreceptors, Dietary salt, Ghrelin, Inflammation, Insulin resistance, Insülin, Leptin, Neurogenic hypertension, Nitric oxide, Obesity, Oxidative stress, Prostacyclin, Prostaglandins, Sympathetic activity, Vasopressin.

Neurogenic hypertension can be defined as hypertension in patients in whom the sympathetic nervous system plays a dominant role as a driving force of their hypertension [1]. Neurogenic hypertension applies whether the true origin of the hypertension is neural, such as the primary underlying issue is in the brain or in afferent or efferent nerves, or the origin is nonneural but results in neurally mediated increase in ABP [2].

---

[*] **Corresponding author Gonul Simsek:** Department of Physiology, Istanbul University-Cerrahpaşa, Cerrahpasa Faculty of Medicine Istanbul, Turkey; Tel: +90 212 414 30 56; Fax: +90 212 633 29 87; E-mail: gdincsimsek@yahoo.com

Hafize Uzun & Pınar Atukeren (Eds.)

In order to better understand the mechanisms of neurogenic hypertension within this section, the cardiovascular pathways of the central nervous system (CNS) and neural regulation of circulation will be explained first.

CNS CARDIOVASCULAR PATHWAYS

Neurons can be defined as "cardiovascular neurons" if their stimulations or lesions cause response in circulatory system; or if changes in blood pressure or stimulation of arterial or cardiopulmonary baroreceptors cause a response in neurons [3].

As is known, parasympathetic and sympathetic nerve system innervates the heart. The parasympathetic fibers innervating the heart are tonically active, even while in resting. Acetylcholine (ACh) released from these fibers binds to muscarinic receptors of sinoatrial (SA) and atrioventricular nodes as well as to special conductive tissues. The induction of parasympathetic fibers causes the heart rate and the rate of transmission to slow down. Ventricular muscle has seldom innervation by parasympathetic nerve fibers, and the stimulation of these fibers has only a small negative inotropic effect on the heart. Some cardiac parasympathetic fibers end on sympathetic nerves and inhibit norepinephrine (NE) release from sympathetic nerve fibers. Therefore, in the presence of sympathetic nervous system activity, parasympathetic activation reduces cardiac contractility.

The sympathetic fibers of heart are also tonically active and release NE binding to the β1-adrenergic receptors in the SA node, the atrioventricular node in the special conductive tissues and the myocardium. The stimulation of these fibers leads to increased heart rate, conduction rate and contractility. Activity along the two divisions of the autonomic nervous system (ANS) changes in a reciprocal manner to cause changes in heart rate. For example, an increase in heart rate results in a simultaneous decrease in parasympathetic fiber stimulation and an increase in sympathetic nerve activity in the heart. However, the parasympathetic effect of controlling heart rate is overwhelming. Activation of parasympathetic system may slow down the heart rate even when the sympathetic system is maximally active. During submaximal sympathetic stimulation, activation of the vagus nerve may completely suppress the SA node and may cause the heart to stop. Contrary to controlling heart rate, the control of cardiac contractility is dominated by the sympathetic nervous system. The inotropic condition is only minimally affected by the vagal effect, and therefore myocardial contractility is modulated primarily by the activity level of sympathetic nerves innervating the ventricular muscle [4 - 6].

Sympathetic fibers innervate arteries and veins of all the major systemic organs except the brain. These fibers release NE binding to α1-adrenergic and β2-adrenergic receptors in blood vessels. However, systemic circulatory activation of sympathetic nerves causes vasoconstriction and so an increase in systemic vascular resistance (SVR), since arteries of all vascular beds outside the heart and brain contain more α1-adrenergic receptors than β2-adrenergic receptors. The circulating epinephrine, which is released from modified sympathetic nerve endings in the adrenal medulla binds to both α1-adrenergic and β2-adrenergic receptors in vascular and smooth muscle cells. However, the affinity of epinephrine for both β1 and β2 receptors is greater than the norepinephrine. Thus, at low circulating concentrations, the epinephrine essentially activates only β receptors, with a decrease in SVR, despite an increase in cardiac output (chronotropic and inotropic effects) [4, 6].

In addition to sympathetic vasoconstrictor innervations, resistance vessels in skeletal muscles of the limbs are also innervated by cholinergic vasodilator fibers **(sympathetic cholinergic vasodilator system).** These nerves are inactive at rest but can be activated during stress or exercise. Evidence for a sympathetic cholinergic vasodilator system in humans is lacking. It is more likely that vasodilation of skeletal muscle vasculature in response to activation of the sympathetic nervous system is due to the actions of epinephrine released from the adrenal medulla. Activation of β2-adrenoceptors on skeletal muscle blood vessels promotes vasodilation [5].

Even the arterioles and the other resistance vessels are most densely innervated, all blood vessels except capillaries and venules contain smooth muscle and receive motor nerve fibers from the sympathetic division of the autonomic nervous system. The fibers innervating the resistance vessels regulate tissue blood flow and arterial pressure. The fibers innervating the venous capacitance vessels vary the volume of blood "stored" in the veins. Venoconstriction is produced by stimuli that also activate the vasoconstrictor nerves to the arterioles. The resultant decrease in venous capacity increases venous return, shifting blood to the arterial side of the circulation [5].

The activity, or tone of sympathetic nerve, to blood vessels, the heart, and the adrenal medulla produces a background level of sympathetic vasoconstriction, cardiac stimulation, and adrenal epinephrine secretion in the body. All of these factors contribute to the maintenance of normal blood pressure. This tonic activity is generated by excitatory signals from the medulla oblongata [4].

AUTONOMIC OUTPUTS AND BULBOSPINAL CENTERS

The autonomic outputs include the parasympathetic cardiac vagal motoneurons, the sympathetic preganglionic motoneurons to the heart, to the various peripheral beds and to the adrenal medulla. The vagal motoneurons are located in the nucleus ambiguus and the dorsal vagal motor nucleus of the medulla and innervate the heart and coronary vessels (Fig. 1).

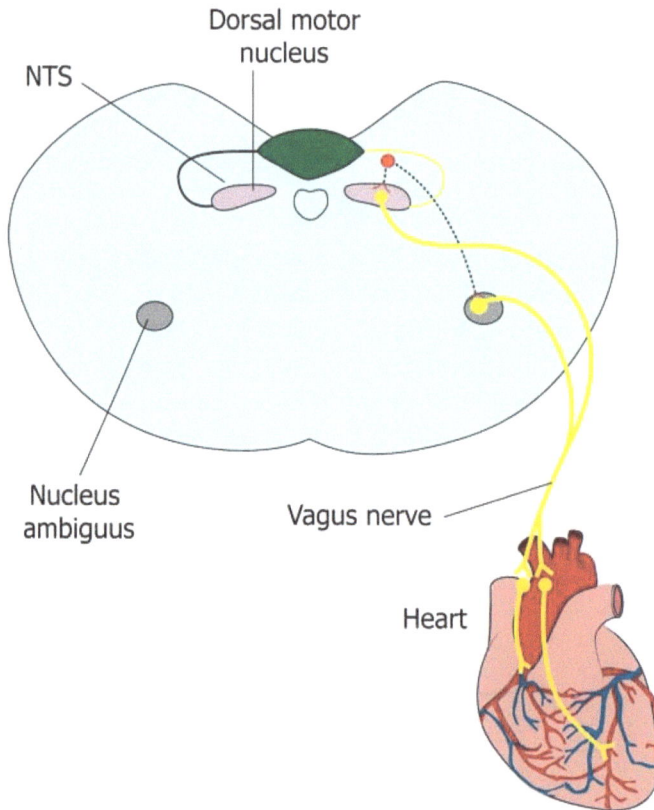

Fig. (1). Basic pathways controlling the heart rate by vagus nerves (Modified from Ganong's Review of Medical Physiology, 25th Ed [5]);
NTS: Nucleus Tractus Solitarius.

The sympathetic preganglionic motoneurons are located in the intermediol-ateralnucleus (IML) of the thoracolumbar segments of the spinal cord. Their axons project to the sympathetic ganglia and the postganglionic nerves innervate the heart and the resistance vessels of various regional beds. The cells of the adrenal medulla are innervated directly by preganglionic fibers from IML sympathetic motoneurons [3, 7] (Fig. 2).

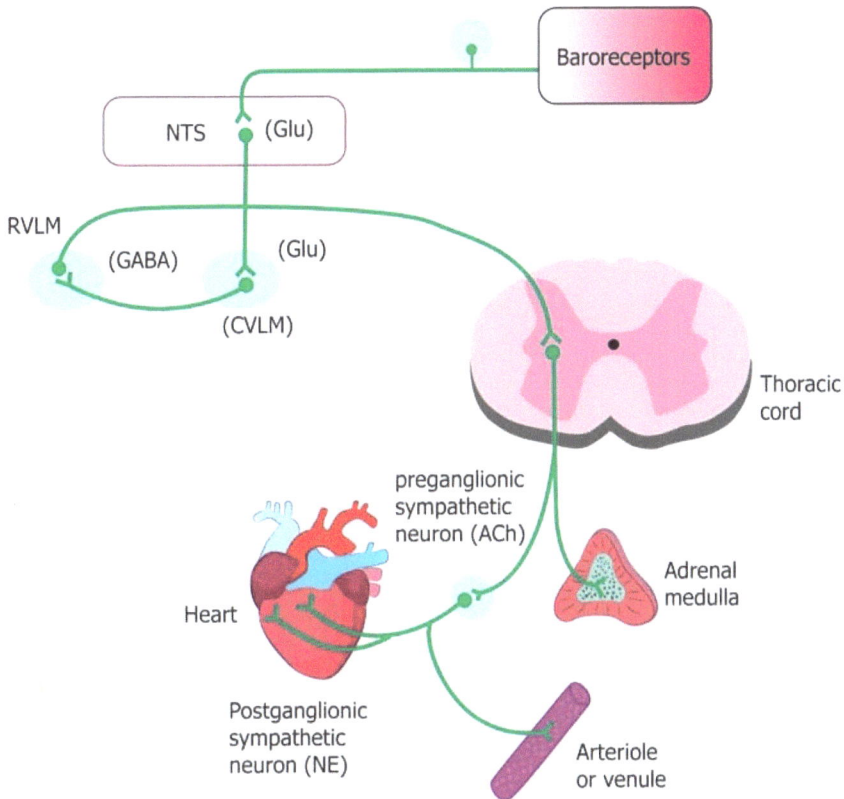

Fig. (2). Basic neural pathways involved in the control of blood pressure(Modified from Ganong's Review of Medical Physiology, 25th Ed [5])
NTS: Nucleus tractus solitarious, Glu: Glutamate, RVLM: Rostral ventrolateral medulla, CVLM: Caudal ventrolateral medulla, IML: Intermediolateral nucleus, ACh: Acetylcholine, NE: Norepinephrine.

Integrative activity takes place at all levels of the neuraxis, including the spinal motoneurons and the premotor neurons of the rostral ventrolateral medulla (RVLM) and caudalventrolateral medulla (CVLM), the rostral ventromedial medulla, the caudal raphe nuclei, the hypothalamic paraventricular nucleus (PVN) and other hypothalamic nuclei, the midbrain periaqueductalgray region, and others [3].

The RVLM neurons are an important source of normal resting sympathetic tone [8]. They receive afferent projections from many sources including projections from the arterial and cardiopulmonary baroreceptors, respiratory receptors, chemoreceptors and others (Table **1**). Their afferents synapse in the nucleus tractus solitarii (NTS), and their projections reach RVLM via the caudal ventrolateral medulla [3, 5]. The axons of RVLM neurons course dorsally and medially and then descend in the lateral column of the spinal cord to the thoracolumbar intermediolateral cell column [3, 5, 9] (Fig. **2**).

However, resting sympathetic tone also comes from sources above the pons, and from hypothalamic nuclei, various hindbrain and midbrain centers, and many regions from forebrain and cerebellum [3, 9] (Fig. **3**).

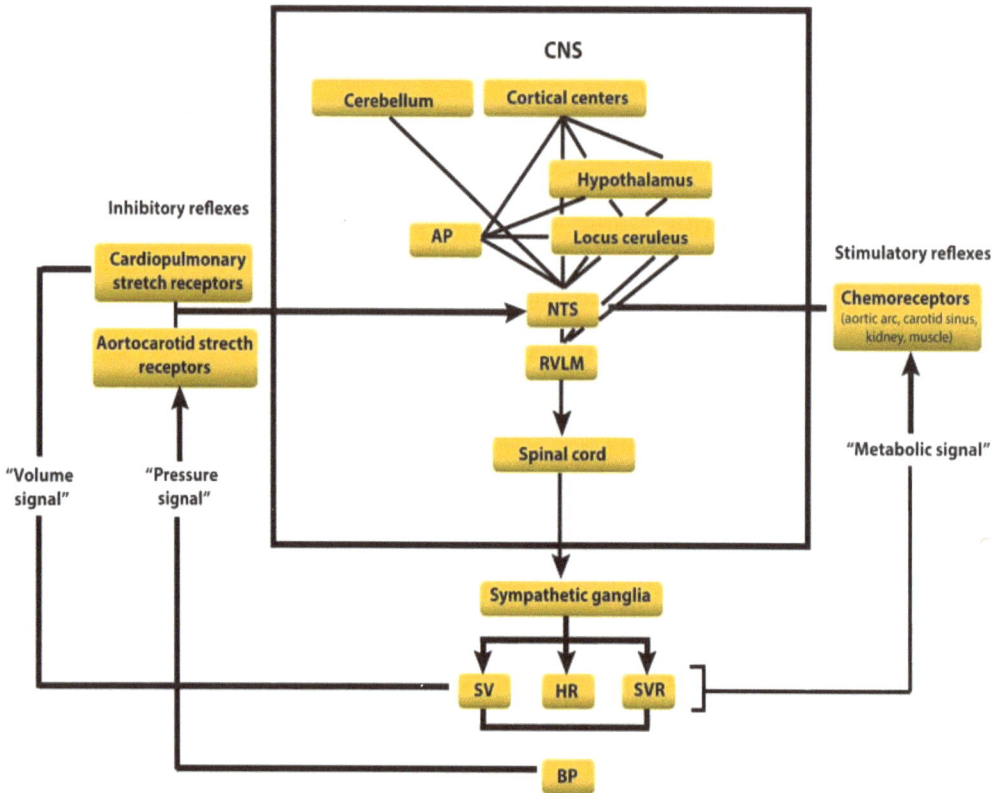

Fig. (**3**). **Sympathetic control by central nervous system** (Modified from Hypertension, Companion to Brenner & Rector's The Kidney, 2nd Ed. [10])
AP: Area Postrema, NTS: Nucleus Tractus Solitarius, RVLM: Rostral Ventrolateral Medulla, SV: Stroke Volume, HR: Heart Rate, SVR: Systemic Vascular Resistance, BP: Blood Pressure.

The most critical RVLM inputs comes from the adjacent NTS. Signals from the NTS inhibit RVLM sympathetic outflow and buffer acute blood pressure changes. The NTS integrates a variety of signals from stimulatory and inhibitory centers in the brain stem, basal ganglia, and cortex, including the circumventricular organs (CVOs). The NTS is also controlled by the signals from the CVOs, which do not have a blood brain barrier. For example, the CVOs are sensitive to circulation angiotensin II (AgII), which suppresses the inhibitory effect of the NTS, resulting in an increase in RVLM dependent sympathetic nerve system (SNS) outflow [11 - 13]. The sympathoexcitatory effect of AgII will be discussed under the

''Patophysiologic Mechanisms of Neurogenic Hypertension'' topic.

The cell bodies of cardiac preganglionic parasympathetic neurons are located in the nucleus ambiguus. The activity of these neurons is affected by reflex inputs and inputs from respiratory neurons [4, 5].

Neurons in NTS project to cardiac preganglionic parasympathetic neurons primarily in the nucleus ambiguus and excite them. Some cardiac preganglionic parasympathetic neurons are also located in the dorsal motor nucleus of the vagus (Fig. **1**) [5, 14]. Many factors determine the activity of RVLM neurons. They primarily include fibers from arterial baroreceptors, also fibers from other parts of the nervous system and from the carotid and aortic chemoreceptors. In addition, some stimuli act directly on RVLM neurons to increase their firing rate. There are descending tracts to the vasomotor area from the cerebral cortex, especially the limbic cortex, that relays in the hypothalamus. These fibers are responsible for the increased blood pressure and heart rate triggered by emotions such as stress, sexual excitement, and anger.

Inflation of the lungs causes vasodilation and a decreased blood pressure. This response is mediated via vagal afferents from the lungs that inhibit RVLM and sympathetic nerve activities. Pain usually causes a rise in blood pressure via afferent impulses converging in the RVLM. On the other hand, prolonged severe pain may cause vasodilation and fainting [4, 5] (Table **1**).

Table 1. Factors Affecting the Activity of RVLM (Adapted from Ganong's Review of Medical Physiology, 25ᵗʰ Ed [5]). RVLM: Rostral Ventrolateral Medulla.

Factors Affecting the Activity of RVLM
Direct Stimulation
CO_2
Hypoxia
Excitatory Signals
Cortex via Hypothalamus
Mesencephalic Periaquaductal Gray Matter
Pain
Somatic Afferents (Somatosympathetic Reflex)
Carotid and Aortic Chemoreceptors
Skeletal Muscle Chemoreceptors
Renal Chemoreceptors and Mechanoreceptors
Brainstem Reticular Formation

(Table 1) cont.....

Inhibitory Signals
Cortex via Hypothalamus
Caudal Ventrolateral Medulla
Caudal Medullary Raphe Nuclei
Lung Inflation
Carotid, Aortic and Cardiopulmonary Baroreceptors
Prolonged Severe Pain

REFLEX MECHANISMS MAINTAINING BLOOD PRESSURE REGULATION

By far the best known of the nervous mechanisms for arterial pressure control is the baroreceptor reflex. Basically, this reflex is initiated by stretch receptors located at specific points in the walls of several large systemic arteries, called baroreceptors (high-pressure receptors). A rise in arterial pressure stretches the baroreceptors and causes an excitation transmitting to the central nervous system. "Feedback" signals are then sent back through the autonomic nervous system to the circulation to reduce arterial pressure to the normal level. Mechanoreceptors in the atria, ventricles, and pulmonary vessels primarily sense pressure changes due to changes in blood volume. Therefore, these receptors are called as volume-receptors, low-pressure baroreceptors, or cardiopulmonary baroreceptors. The carotid and aortic bodies located in the areas of the carotid sinus, and aortic arch play an important role on the control of ABP [4 - 6].

Circulatory Reflex Initiated By The Baroreceptors

Baroreceptors are nerve endings which are located in the walls of the arteries; they are stimulated when stretched. A few baroreceptors are located in the wall of almost every large artery of the thoracic and neck regions; but, they are extremely abundant in the wall of each internal carotid artery slightly above the carotid bifurcation, an area known as the carotid sinus, and the wall of the aortic arch [6, 14].

The baroreceptors are stimulated by distension of the structures in which they are located. Their afferent fibers pass via the glossopharyngeal and vagus nerves to the medulla. Most of them end in the NTS, and they secrete the excitatory transmitter glutamate. Excitatory projections that secretes glutamate extend from the NTS to CVLM, where they stimulate γ-aminobutyric acid (GABA)-secreting inhibitory neurons that project to the RVLM (Fig. **2**). Excitatory projections also extend from the NTS to the vagal motor neurons in the nucleus ambiguus and dorsal motor nucleus. Thus, increased baroreceptor discharge inhibits the tonic discharge of sympathetic nerves and excites the vagal innervation of the heart. These neural changes produce vasodilation, venodilation, hypotension, bradycardia, and a decrease in cardiac output [5]. In chronic hypertension, the baroreceptor reflex mechanism is *"reset"* to higher levels of blood pressure. Little is known about how and why this occurs, but this resetting occurs rapidly in experimental animals [5].

An important property of the baroreceptor reflex is adapting during a period of 1 to 2 days to the prevailing mean ABP. When the mean ABP is suddenly raised, baroreceptor firing increases. If arterial pressure is held at the higher level, baroreceptor firing declines during the next few seconds. Firing rate then continues to decline more slowly until it returns to the original firing rate over the next 1 to 2 days. Consequently, if the mean ABP is maintained at an elevated level, the tendency for the baroreceptors to initiate a decrease in blood pressure quickly disappears. This is an example of receptor adaptation. A "resetting" of the reflex in the CNS occurs as well [4].

"Resetting" of the baroreceptors may attenuate their potency as a control system for correcting disturbances that tend to change arterial pressure for longer than a few days. It has been suggested that the baroreceptors do not completely reset and may therefore contribute to long-term blood pressure regulation, especially by affecting sympathetic nerve activity of the kidneys. For example, with prolonged increases in ABP, the baroreceptor reflexes may mediate decreases in renal sympathetic nerve activity that promote increased excretion of sodium and water by the kidneys. This situation decreases blood volume, which helps to restore ABP toward normal [5].

Blood pressure initially rises following a bilateral section of baroreceptor nerves or bilateral lesions of the NTS. However, after a period of time, even the mean AVP returns to near control levels, there become large fluctuations in blood pressure during the day [5].

Supramedullary responses can override the baroreceptor reflex. For example, the fight-or-flight response increases the heart rate despite a simultaneous rise in ABP. In such circumstances, the neurons connecting the hypothalamus to medullary areas suppress the baroreceptor reflex and allow the corticohypothalamic response to predominate [4].

This override occurs acutely in situations where the activity of the sympathetic nervous system is increased by excitement. When the neural excitement persists for a long time, it enters the chronic phase due to sympathetic activity [4].

A long-term change in blood pressure resulting from loss of baroreceptor reflex control is called **neurogenic hypertension** [5].

Cardiopulmonary Baroreceptors (Low-Pressure Receptors)

Atria, ventriculi and the pulmonary arteries have in their walls stretch receptors called low pressure receptors. These low-pressure receptors play an important role, especially in minimizing arterial pressure changes in response to changes in blood volume [6].

Even the low-pressure receptors in the pulmonary artery and in the atria cannot detect the systemic arterial pressure, they do detect simultaneous increases in pressure in the low pressure areas of the circulation caused by increase in volume. They elicit reflexes parallel to the baroreceptor reflexes to make the total reflex system more potent for control of ABP [6].

These receptors initiate reflex responses of the ANS that alter ABP. The central terminals for these receptors are located in NTS in the medulla oblongata. Neurons from the NTS project to the RVLM and nucleus ambiguus, where they influence the firing of sympathetic and parasympathetic nerves [4].

Stretch of the atria also causes significant reflex dilation of the afferent arterioles in the kidneys. And still other signals are transmitted simultaneously from the atria to the hypothalamus to decrease secretion of vasopressin (VP). The decreased afferent arteriolar resistance in the kidneys causes the glomerular capillary pressure to rise, with resultant increase in filtration of fluid into the kidney tubules. The reduction of VP decreases the reabsorption of water from the tubules. Combination of these two effects— increase in glomerular filtration and decrease in reabsorption of the fluid—increases fluid loss by the kidneys and reduces an increased blood volume back toward normal [6]. Also, decreased stretch of the cardiopulmonary baroreceptors activates the renin angiotensin aldosterone system [4].

Sensory receptors located near the endocardial surfaces of the ventricles initiate reflex effects similar to those elicited by the arterial baroreceptors. Excitation of these endocardial receptors reduces the heart rate and peripheral resistance. These left ventricular stretch receptors may play a role in the maintenance of vagal tone that keeps the heart rate low at rest. Other sensory receptors have been identified in the epicardial regions of the ventricles. Although all these ventricular receptors are excited by various mechanical and chemical stimuli, their exact physiological functions remain unclear [5, 14].

Relationship between altered sensitivity of cardiopulmonary baroreflexes and increased SNS will be explained below.

Control of Arterial Pressure by Chemoreceptors

The carotid and aortic bodies are specialized structures located in the areas of the carotid sinus and aortic arch that sense changes in blood O_2, CO_2, and pH. These structures are known as chemoreceptors. Peripheral chemoreceptors send impulses to the NTS and exhibit increased firing rate when, either the PO_2 or pH of the arterial blood is low, the PCO_2 of arterial blood is increased, the flow through the bodies is low or stopped, or a chemical is given that blocks oxidative metabolism in the chemoreceptor cells. There are also central medullary chemoreceptors that increase their firing rate primarily in response to elevated arterial PCO_2, which causes a decrease in brain pH. The increased firing of both peripheral and central chemoreceptors via the NTS and RVLM leads to a significant elevation in ABP.

The chemoreceptor reflex is important in the cardiovascular response to severe hypotension [4].

Each carotid or aortic body is supplied with an abundant blood flow through a small nutrient artery, so that the chemoreceptors always monitor arterial blood. When the ABP falls below a critical level, the chemoreceptors become stimulated because diminished blood flow causes decreased oxygen as well as excess buildup of carbon dioxide and hydrogen ions that are not removed by the slowly flowing blood [6].

The chemoreceptor reflex, however, does not respond to a change in blood pressure itself until mean arterial pressure decreases to about 80 mm Hg. Therefore, this reflex is not involved in maintenance of normal blood pressure on a moment-to-moment basis, but rather serves as a secondary emergency reflex if blood pressure continues to fall in spite of activation of the baroreceptor reflex [4, 6]. It has been suggested that the overactivity of carotid body can contribute to neurogenic hypertension. This issue will be discussed below.

Pulmonary Stretch Receptors

Inflation of the lungs causes vasodilation and a decrease in blood pressure. This response is mediated via vagal afferents from the lungs that inhibit RVLM and sympathetic nerve activities [5].

PATOPHYSIOLOGIC   MECHANISMS   OF   NEUROGENIC HYPERTENSION

The hypothesis that essential hypertension may include in its multifactorial aetiology an abnormality in the autonomic modulation of blood pressure homeostasis, for example a sympathetic activation coupled with a parasympathetic inhibition, has been investigated for a long time, both in experimental animals and in humans. The results of these studies have led to the so-called 'neurogenic hypothesis of hypertension', which emphasizes the potential pathophysiological relevance of the sympathetic and parasympathetic neural abnormalities seen in patients with essential hypertension [15].

The pathophysiologic mechanisms underlying the increased ABP in neurogenic hypertension are not clear. The role of sympathetic outflow in the pathogenesis of hypertension has been an issue of continuous interest recently. It has been suggested that sympathetic overactivity is present in hypertensive patients [16].

In a rat model of neurogenic hypertension there is a significant increase in sympathetic activity and vascular resistance even in neonatal and juvenile rats [17, 18]. Additionally, sympathectomy in young spontaneous hypertensive (SH) rats prevents the increase in ABP and vascular hypertrophy [19, 20]. The neural origin of high blood pressure was also supported by an experimental approach based on the manipulation of cardiovascular reflexogenic areas or of neural pathways involved in cardiovascular homeostasis [15, 21].

Surgical denervation of sino-aortic baroreceptors or lesioning of the central relay station of the baroreflex, NTS, was followed by an increase in ABP immediately [15, 21]. The development of hypertension can be prevented or delayed by chemical sympathectomy or by denervating the kidneys in a animal model study [22].

Why sympathetic activity rises in neurogenic hypertension is unclear [23]. The factors that stimulate sympathetic tone in human essential hypertension remains hypotheses [1].

Proposed causes of increased sympathetic tone in essential hypertension is given in Table **2** and will be explained in detail below.

It still remains considerable uncertainty as to whether the stimulus for increased sympathetic tone in patients with neurogenic hypertension originates mainly in the kidneys or in the central nervous system [15, 24, 25]. The origin of increased sympathetic tone likely differs among patients with different phenotypes of neurogenic hypertension. Therefore, for example, in patients with chronic kidney disease or resistant hypertension, increased sympathetic tone might result from renal injury. The renal nerves likely play a role in neurogenic hypertension, but its role is incompletely understood. On the other hand, in patients with labile forms of hypertension, a central nervous system origin appears more likely [1].

Table 2. Proposed causes of increased sympathetic tone in essential hypertension (Adapted from 'Samuel J. Mann - "Neurogenic hypertension: pathophysiology, diagnosis and management" [1]).

Impaired Baroreceptor Reflexes
Carotid Body Overactivity
Augmented Central Respiratory–Sympathetic Coupling
Vascular Compression of the Medulla
Aging
Psychological Factors
Nitric Oxide
Reactive Oxygen Species
Angiotensin II
Dietary Salt and Vasopressin
Obesity
a. Leptin
b. Insulin resistance
c. Adiponectin
d. Ghrelin
e. Insulin
f. Oxidative Stress
Proinflammatory Cytokines
Genetic Factors

There is also uncertainty as if sympathetic effects on ABP in patients with neurogenic hypertension are due mainly to effects on renal function or to direct effects on systemic hemodynamics. It is suggested that the main effects of the SNS in driving sustained hypertension derive from its effects on renal function, whereas sympathetic effects on systemic hemodynamics, for example, cardiac output and SVR, are responsible mainly for transient blood pressure elevation [1].

Proposed Causes of İncreased Sympathetic Tone in Essential Hypertension

Impaired Baroreceptor Reflexes

Impairment of the baroreflex function, called as baroreflex failure syndrome, has been demonstrated in patients with lesions in the afferent portion of the baroreflex, caused by physical damage to the glossopharyngeal and vagus nerves or other anatomical structures. These patients have striking, paroxysmal increases in ABP [26]. However, other than in these selected groups of patients with obvious lesions in the afferent baroreceptors, the role of baroreflex abnormalities in neurogenic hypertension is not clear, and clarity is also lacking as to whether it is a cause of hypertension or a consequence of hypertension and arterial stiffening [1].

Baroreceptor activity is modulated by several mechanisms under physiological conditions and in pathological conditions. These mechanisms may involve changes in the mechanical properties of the vascular wall of the carotid sinuses and aortic arch, actions on a new class of mechanosensitive ion channel that blunts or enhances the magnitude of depolarization evoked by mechanical stimulation of the endings, and/or by actions on voltage-dependent Na^+ and K^+ channels at the spike initiating zone (SIZ) that alter the threshold for action potential discharge and the frequency of afferent activity. Modulation of voltage-dependent channels at the SIZ by changes in membrane potential, action potential discharge, and paracrine factors released from nearby cells is an important mechanism contributing to changes in baroreceptor activity during acute hypertension and in pathological situations related with endothelial dysfunction, platelet activation and oxidative stress [27].

Circulating hormones and locally produced chemical factors have been shown to modulate baroreceptor activity [27].

Chronically infusion of aldosterone decreases the sensitivity of baroreceptor afferents. Administration of ouabain restores baroreceptor sensitivity in aldosterone-infused dogs, suggesting that the inhibitory effect is mediated by increased Na+ pump activity [28].

Inhibitors of Na^+ pump (*e.g.* oubain and low K^+) significantly attenuate post excitatory depression and baroreceptor resetting and blunting [29, 30].

The predominant prostanoid produced in large arteries is prostacyclin. Increased blood flow (shear stress) and pulsatile pressure stimulate prostacyclin release from endothelium. Prostacyclin is a vasodilator and a powerful inhibitor of platelet aggregation [31].

Injection of prostacyclin into the isolated carotid sinus increases baroreceptor sensitivity without altering the carotid pressure-diameter relation, suggesting a direct action on baroreceptors [32, 33]. Inhibitors of prostanoid production such as indomethacin decrease baroreceptor activity, suggesting a role of endogenous prostacyclin in activation of baroreceptors [32, 33] Decreased production of prostacyclin in atherosclerosis and chronic hypertension may contribute to decreased baroreceptor sensitivity in these pathologic states [33].

Prostaglandins are prostanoids formed from the conversion of arachidonic acid by the cyclooxygenase (COX) enzyme [34]. Consistent with these findings, administration of pharmacological substances reducing prostanoid synthesis into the isolated carotid sinus impairs both afferent baroreceptor and efferent baroreflex responses [35].

Thus systemic modulation of prostanoid levels may be hypothesized to increase baroreflex sensitivity (BRS) through a facilitory influence on arterial baroreceptors or decrease BRS through impairment in baroreceptor responsiveness mediated by cardiac-related afferents [36].

Monahan KD and Ray AC suggest that reductions in prostanoid levels in animals with hypertension results with impaired baroreflex function [35]. They hypothesized that it is possible that NSAID ingestion could mimic the effects of cardiovascular disease by impairing baroreflex function secondary to reducing endogenous prostanoid levels. But they reported that acute pharmacological antagonism of the COX enzyme does not impair BRS (cardiovagal or sympathetic) or augment pressor reactivity in healthy young adults [36].

Nitric oxide (NO) is an potent vasodilator released from vascular endothelial cells in response to shear stress and various chemical factors [37, 38].

When NO is injected into the isolated carotid sinus, there occured a decrease in baroreceptor sensitivity independently of its vasodilator action [35].

Subsequent studies have demonstrated that NO is produced by various cells including certain types of neurons [38].The neuronal isoform of NO synthase (nNOS) has been demonstrated in vagal afferent fibers [40], in baroreceptor nerves innervating the carotid sinus [41].

Li Z *et al.* indicated that NO and NO-related species inhibit the Na^+ current (INa) of baroreceptor neurons. Their results all suggest that NO and NO-related species modulate baroreceptor INa and activity by a cGMP-independent mechanism [37].

A recent study also demonstrated that NO donors injected into the isolated carotid sinus of rabbits decrease the action potential frequency of baroreceptor fibers [33].

It has been demonstrated that gene transfer of the endothelial isoform of NOS to carotid sinus adventitia of rabbits resets the baroreceptor pressure-activity curve to higher pressures [42].

On the other hand, Bock JM *et al.* recently illustrated that inorganic nitrate supplementation attenuates peripheral chemoreflex sensitivity but does not improve cardiovagal baroreflex sensitivity in older adults [43].

There are studies showing that factors secreted from platelets can effect BRS. It has been suggested that platelet activation in carotid sinuses with carotid sinus pressure maintained constant rapidly increases the activity of type II baroreceptors that tend to profound hypotension [44, 45]. The rapid platelet-induced inhibition of sympathetic activity and hypotension is mediated by platelet-derived serotonin acting on 5-HT3, and to a lesser extent 5-HT2 receptors on the type II baroreceptors [44].

On the other hand, Alper RH demonstrated that the serotonin reuptake inhibitor fluoxetine did not effect baroreceptor sensitivity [46].

Tomiya Yasumasu *et al.* assessed whether BRS is influenced by risk factors of cardiovascular disease. Their study showed that increased platelet count may result in increased platelet activity and indicated that BRS is inversely related to platelet count in the elderly population. The precise mechanism of this correlation is unknown, but platelet factors released from platelet aggregates can potentially influence vascular function and modify BRS [47].

Reactive oxygen species (ROS) produced in various pathological conditions including ischemia/reperfusion, atherosclerosis, diabetes, and aging contribute to dysfunction of multiple organ systems. The carotid sinuses are particularly susceptible to development of atherosclerotic lesions. It has been suggested that ROS generated close to the nerve endings contribute to baroreflex dysfunction in atherosclerosis and that gene transfer of antioxidant enzymes to carotid sinus can restore reflex sensitivity [39].

Li Z *et al.* suggest that in atherosclerotic rabbits, oxygen-derived free radicals contribute to baroreceptor dysfunction. Therefore they treated the carotid sinus with the superoxide dismutase (SOD) and catalase that are ROS scavengers for 10–15 minutes, and they indicated a significantly increase in baroreceptor activity of atherosclerotic rabbits but no change in normal healthy rabbits [48]. Gene transfer of SOD and catalase to carotid sinus adventitia enhances the pressor reflex due to carotid artery occlusion in apoE knockout mice with atherosclerosis but does not influence the reflex in normal control C57BL/6 mice [49].

Nightingale AK *et al.* showed that acute intravenous infusion of vitamin C partially restores BRS in patients with chronic heart failure. There was no improvement in BRS in chronic heart failure patients given chronic oral vitamin C. Thus acute intravenous, but not chronic oral, vitamin C improved BRS in patients with chronic heart failure. There was no effect of intravenous vitamin C in healthy subjects. This results suggest that the mechanisms of vitamin C are either by free radical scavenging or due to central effects [50].

It has been suggested that an implantation of a surgical device which elicits chronic stimulation of the carotid baroreflex may be a suitable approach to targeting the sympathetic nervous system in resistant hypertension [51].

Carotid Body Overactivity

Peripheral chemoreceptors located in carotid body may play an important role in development of cardiovascular diseases, including neurogenic hypertension [23, 52, 53]. Peripheral chemoreceptor reflex sensitivity has been shown to be significantly enhanced in both patients with neurogenic hypertension and SH rats [23, 54]. Regarding this, Moraes DA *et al.* have hypothesized that chronic activation of carotid body chemoreceptors can cause long-term synaptic plasticity within brainstem sympatho-excitatory networks, by increasing the respiratory synaptic inputs to RVLM pre-sympathetic neurones. They suggested that carotid body overactivity induces respiratory neurone channelopathy contributing to neurogenic hypertension [23]. Moraes DJ *et al.* supported that the notion of targeting the carotid body as a potential novel therapeutic approach for reducing sympathetic vasomotor tone in neurogenic hypertension [55].

Augmented Central Respiratory–Sympathetic Coupling

Respiratory modulation of autonomic neural activity, with consequent phasic alteration of cardiac and vascular function, has been observed in many species including humans and is considered an index of cardiovascular health. Functional links between the brainstem circuitry generating the respiratory rhythm and neurons are responsible for generate sympathetic and parasympathetic activity to the cardiovascular system. Respiratory-sympathetic coupling is a result of feedback from peripheral baroreceptors, as venous return varies with intrathoracic pressure, and also a result of the inhibitory influence of activation of pulmonary stretch receptors on the sympathetic activity. Recent observations suggest that altered central respiratory coupling may play a role in the development of hypertension and in the maintenance of elevated levels of sympathetic vasomotor activity in disease. The mechanism(s) driving this enhanced coupling remain uncertain [17].

Vascular Compression of the Medulla

Compression of the RVLM by an abnormally located artery is regarded as one possible cause of arterial hypertension. Although, increased sympathetic activity in patients with RVLM compression may lead to arterial hypertension, Solar *et al.* could not observed increased sympathetic activity in patients with neurovascular compression of RVLM [56]. On the other hand, Sasaki S *et al.* supported that the operative decompression of the RVLM could lower BP *via* restoration of sympathetic nerve activities and the renin-angiotensin system [57].

Aging

Aging increases SNS activity [58]. This increase may be resulted from, the increased peripheral chemoreflex sensitivity and reduction of BRS. This situation collectively increases the risk of cardiovascular disease [43].

Baroreflex control of the heart rate is impaired in hypertensive subjects and decreases with age. The decrease in BRS is often described as decreased distension of the pressure-sensing arterial wall segments. However, alterations in the sensing and processing of neural signals may be involved as well [59].

As mentioned above, increased ROS may attenuate BRS. Aging increases ROS production [60].This condition may be the reason of the increased SNS activity on elderly people. Furthermore, it is reported that ROS in CNS can induce SNS activity. This will be mentioned below.

Long-standing hypertension causes chronic arterial baroreflex blunting. Baroreflex blunting is associated with conditions such as aging, chronic hypertension, in all of which there may be increased arterial stiffness and reduced arterial mechanoreceptor distensibility [3, 61 - 63].

Altered sensitivity of cardiopulmonary reflexes may also play a significant role in chronic increases in SNS activity with aging and hypertension. Hajduczok *et al.* demonstrated that the age-related increases in SNS activity may be resulted from impaired cardiopulmonary baroreflexes [58].

When cardiac filling is reduced equally, borderline hypertensives exhibit augmented muscle sympathetic activation compared with normotensives [64 - 67].

Psychological Factors

It has been usually suggested that there may be a link between hypertension and psychological factors [1, 68]. Acute laboratory-based stress tasks (*i.e.* mental arithmetic) have been shown to evoke increases in sympathetic vasoconstrictor tone and ABP [69]. A greater reactivity to such acute stressors has been suggested to be prognostic for the future development of hypertension [51, 70, 71]. Transient and moment-to-moment increases in blood pressure in response to emotional and physical stressors are mediated by the instant systemic hemodynamic effects of sympathetic activation. These immediate increases in ABP are likely independent of sympathetic stimulation effects on renal function [1].

It has been suggested that the emotional factors may not play a role in more sustained ABP elevation. Chronic stress or chronic emotional distress, such as anger and anxiety does not result with sustained hypertension, or stress reduction does not provide a sustained effect in the management of chronic hypertension [69, 72 - 75]. Emotional factors play a potential role in less-sustained forms of hypertension, such as labile or paroxysmal hypertension [76].

In labile hypertension, patients experience intermittent, sometimes substantial, increases in ABP. The blood pressure usually falls spontaneously without intervention [77, 78]. It has been suggested that there are no recognized criteria for diagnosing or treating labile hypertension, and as yet there is no consensus on to the long-term benefit of treatment. However, in patients with paroxysmal hypertension experience a sudden increase in ABP and can continue for minutes, hours, or even days [68, 72]. There are treatments that can attenuate or eliminate paroxysms in most patients and enable most to resume a normal life [79, 80].

It has been suggested that stress reduction methods may have beneficial effects by lowering SNA and blood pressure [81]. Thus this is clearly an area worthy of further investigation [51].

Nitric Oxide

As mentioned above, it is suggested that NO can attenuate the BRS. However, it is suggested that central NO can decrease SNA. All NOS isoforms are expressed in the central nervous system and animal and human studies suggest that NO is a key signalling molecule involving the sympathetic outflow from the brainstem [82]. Systemic infusion of a competitive NOS inhibitor in healthy humans causes sympathetic activation and marked elevations in ABP [83, 84]. Additionally, an increase of an endogenous NOS inhibitor may raise SNA. Plasma concentrations of an endogenous NOS inhibitor, asymmetric dimethlarginine (ADMA) has been shown to be strongly associated with plasma concentrations of noradrenaline [85]. It is unclear the contribution of excessive ADMA to central SNA increases in essential hypertension [51].

In a study we conducted, we found that plasma eNOS and total NO levels were lower in hypertensive patients compared to normotensives, and in white-coat hypertensive patients, no significant difference was observed compared to normotensives [86].

Reactive Oxygen Species

It has been mentioned above that ROS can increase SNA by attenuating BRS. It is reported that ROS levels are elevated in patients with hypertension, and vascular oxidative stress can play a role in the pathogenesis of essential hypertension [87]. In a study, we found that both white coat hypertensives and hypertensive subjects had significantly higher levels of malondialdehyde (MDA), an oxidative stress indicator, than the normotensives. With respect to an HDL-associated esterase paraoxonase (PON1), the HT and WCH groups had significantly lower levels than the normotensive group. MDA correlated positively with both systolic and diastolic blood pressures, while PON1 correlated with both of them negatively [88]. However, it has been suggested that increases in ROS within the CNS may scavenge NO, and also directly activate or sensitise sympathetic neurones [89]. Reducing ROS may not only provide a decrease in central sympathetic drive but would also cause an improvement of endothelial function by reducing NO. The therapeutic approaches targeting of ROS may be an suitable strategy to reduce vasomotor tone and ABP [51].

Angotensin II

Toney GM *et al.* suggest that angiotensin II (AgII) plays an important role in the developement of neurogenic hypertension. Especially the brain renin–angiotensin system contributes to neurogenic hypertension instead of circulating AgII [90]. Animal studies show that sympathetic outflow is increased when renin–angiotensin system (RAS) is stimulated and results with noradrenaline release from adrenergic nerve terminals and amplifying adrenergic receptor responsiveness [13, 91 - 94].

AgII is a neuropeptide that has plenty actions on the brain. The distribution of its AT1 receptor in the CNS coincides with several cerebral regions known to regulate cardiovascular and body fluid homeostasis [95, 96]. It is likely that an intrinsic brain RAS exists [97]. Neither renin nor Ag peptides pass readily from the blood into the brain interstitium [98]. Therefore, it is necessary to distinguish those cerebral regions that are separated by the blood–brain barrier from the environment of the systemic circulation, from those few regions—the CVOs, that lack the blood–brain barrier and are influenced directly by the peripheral RAS [12]. The CVOs is responsive to circulating AgII. Circulating AgII suppresses the inhibitory effect of the NTS, and this increases SNS outflow from RVLM [11 - 13]. Blood Ag II interacts with the brain through AT1 receptors located on neurons in these CVOs and these neurons may project to many other brain regions behind the blood–brain barrier [11, 12].

Angiotensin-converting enzyme (ACE) inhibitors reduce sympathetic outflow in addition to antagonizing the RAS [99].

Angiotensinogen is synthesised in most regions of the brain, especially in medulla, hypothalamus [100, 101]. This synthesis occurs mostly in glial cells [101].

Renin is present in the CNS with a low concentration and its spatial relationship to centrally synthesised angiotensinogen is not yet clear [13, 102].

In the brain, very high concentrations of ACE is located in the circumventricular organs such as the subfornical organ, OVLT, area postrema and median eminence [103]. In these CVOs, ACE locally converts AgI came from peripheral circulation to AgII. AgII binds to angiotensin receptors within these regions. ACE has been also identified in other brain regions *i.e.* caudate nucleus, putamen, substantia nigra pars reticularis, NTS, dorsal motor nucleus, median preoptic nucleus by binding studies or immunohistochemistry in rat, human, rabbit, sheep, monkey [104 - 106]. This ACE may generate AgII locally in the brain [107].

AT1 receptor binding are especially occurs on neurons in the lamina terminalis, hypothalamic paraventricular nucleus and the NTS [95]. Within the lamina terminalis; the subfornical organ and organum vasculosum lamina terminalis (OVLT) exposed to circulating angiotensins contain AT1 receptors [108].

Neurons in the subfornical organ, OVLT and median preoptic nucleus that express AT1 receptor mRNA, have polysynaptic connections to peripheral organs such as the kidney via renal sympathetic nerves [109]. However, Osborn JW and Foss JD suggested that AgII does not increase renal sympathetic nerve activity [110]. AT1 receptors also exists in neurons of the hindbrain region that have important roles in cardiovascular regulation, ie. in the NTS, the RVLM and CVLM, and the midline raphe [96, 97]. In the NTS, a considerable proportion of these receptors may exist presynaptically on vagal afferent terminals [111, 112]. This may suggest that the parasympathetic effect, which would ocur from afferent signals from baroreceptors, may be suppressed by AgII. An angiotensinergic neural pathway from parvocellular neurons of the hypothalamic PVN may drive pre-motor neurons in RVLM to increase sympathetic activity and ABP [13]. AT1 receptors can be seen in parts of the limbic system *i.e.* amygdala, bed nucleus of the stria terminalis and cingulate cortex additionally. Other regions that express the AT1 receptor are the hippocampus, the olfactory bulb, the piriform cortex [95, 96]. AT1 receptors may be up or down regulated in specific regions of the brain depending on the physiological state such as dehydration, sodium or chloride depletion, hypertension and stress [113 - 117].

Immunohistochemical and neuropharmacological studies suggest that angiotensinergic neural pathways release AgII as a neurotransmitter or neuromodulator in the several brain regions [13]. AgII may increase arterial pressure at these brain sites. Micro-injection of AgII into the lateral or third ventricle, hypothalamic PVN, several forebrain regions, RVLM, NTS, the area postrema and subfornical organ increases ABP [118 - 124].

Centrally administered AT1 receptor antagonists inhibit sympathetic activity and reduce ABP in certain physiological or pathophysiological conditions [13].

Dietary Salt and Vasopressin

Excess dietary salt intake is a major contributing factor to the pathogenesis of hypertension and affect the regulation of SNA and ABP [2]. Specialized neurons located in the organum vasculosum of the lamina terminalis or subfornical organ (SFO) detect changes in extracellular NaCl levels or osmolality [125, 126]. Direct stimulation of organum vasculosum of the lamina terminalis neurons with injection of hypertonic NaCl increases lumbar SNA, adrenal SNA, and ABP with a dependency of concentration [127]. Importantly, inhibition of organum vasculosum of the lamina terminalis neurons largely attenuates sympathoexcitatory responses to central infusion of hypertonic NaCl [127]. Central hypernatremia increases glutamatergic activation of bulbospinal neurons in the RVLM to increase SNA [128]. Blockade of excitatory amino receptors or angiotensin type I receptors in the RVLM reduces ABP in Dahl salt–sensitive rats fed a high salt diet [129, 130].

Dietary salt intake also alters the excitability of hypothalamic vasopressin (VP) neurons to exaggerate VP secretion or regulate SNA through local release within the hypothalamic PVN [131]. Blockade of V1a receptors in the PVN decreases lumbar SNA and ABP after chronic salt loading [132]. Stocker *et al.* suggested that dietary salt may adversely affect the gain of sympathetic regulatory networks and future experiments are needed to identify the mechanism(s) by which this occurs [2].

Obesity

Studies show gaining weight is strongly associated with hypertension [133]. Obesity is linked with increased sympathetic tone [134, 135]. In one study, combined alpha and beta blockade were shown to be more effective in obese than in non-obese hypertensives [136].

In obesity-related hypertension elevations in muscle SNA, and renal noradrenaline spillover have been identified [137]. Although the underlying mechanisms remain to be fully elucidated impairments in arterial baroreflex function, alterations in central neural pathways, activation of the renin-angiotensin-aldosterone system, sleep disordered breathing, genetic factors and elevations in circulating concentrations of insulin and leptin have all been implicated [138].

Intracerebroventricular infusion of leptin or insulin receptor antagonists decrease ABP in high-fat-fed rabbits [139]. Leptin, but not insulin, receptor blockade reduces renal SNA [140]. Moreover, deletion of leptin receptors on specific hypothalamic neurons using transgenic mice also prevents leptin-induced hypertension [140, 141]. The sympathoexcitatory actions of leptin and insulin are mediated by activation of melanocortin but inhibition of neuropeptide Y pathways. The central actions of leptin and insulin largely originate in the arcuate nucleus that contains proopiomelanocortin and neuropeptide Y neurons [140, 142, 143]. Leptin and insulin act through the melanocortin pathway as pharmacological blockade of central melanocortin receptors or deletion of melanocortin-4 receptors attenuates these acute and chronic sympathoexcitatory effects [144 - 147]. A parallel neuropeptide Y pathway also contributes to leptin- and insulin-induced sympathoexcitation. Blockade of neuropeptide Y receptors in the hypothalamic PVN raises SNA and ABP, and injection of neuropeptide Y to hypothalamic PVN suppresses the sympathoexcitatory response to insulin [25, 148]. Future studies are needed to address the contribution of neuropeptide Y to obesity related hypertension [1].

It has been suggested that there is a relationship between obesity and insulin resistance [149]. Insulin sentizing drugs, such as metformin, have been found to decrease SNS activity and ABP [150]. Given the diabetic actions of catecholamines, it is likely that increased SNS activity itself causes insulin resistance [151]. However, it is unclear whether insulin resistance is a cause, or a consequence, of increased sympathetic tone [140, 142, 143].

It has been suggested that impaired adiponectin secretion promotes insulin resistance [152]. Total and HMW adiponectin oligomers are inversely correlated to BMI [153]. Low adiponectin levels are linked to SNS activation, although their role in SNS regulation is unclear [154]. In a study, we found that adiponectin levels were low in patients with metabolic syndrome and that there was a negative correlation between adiponectin levels and systolic blood pressure [155]. Importantly, weight loss following caloric restriction alone or in combination with exercise training has been associated with reductions in muscle SNA and heart rate variability indicating cardiac SNA, in obese individuals [156 - 158].

Ghrelin levels are low in obesity and even lower in morbidly obeses. This shows that ghrelin is a consequence rather than a cause of overeating [159, 160]. Guarino *et al.* suggested that decreased ghrelin levels may be the other cause of increased SNA in obesity [161]. Beyond its established role in appetite regulation, ghrelin has beneficial effects on ABP and cardiovascular function, possibly modulating ANS activity [161, 162]. In experimental animals, it has been observed that intracerebral infusion of ghrelin may reduce ABP; however, it is unclear if this effect was observed by modulation of sympathetic traffic or not [163, 164]. Lambert *et al.* investigated the effects of supraphysiological doses of intravenous ghrelin in lean and obese individuals. They showed that ghrelin did not influence SNS activity controlling calf vascular tone in resting; however, ghrelin infusion blunted ABP and muscle sympathetic nerve activity responses to acute mental stress after short-term ghrelin infusion either in lean or obese individuals [165].

On the other hand, obesity and the aging increase oxidative stress [166]. In a study, we found increased oxidative stress in morbidly obese patients. Our findings indicated that in morbid obesity, weight loss after surgery had positive effects on oxidative stress and antioxidant activity [167].

We also mentioned above that ROS may reduce BRS and in CNS, ROS may amplify SNS activity directly [39, 89]. Thus, increased ROS in obesity may attenuate BRS and/or directly activate or sensitise sympathetic neurones.

The sympathetic nervous system plays a major role in some types of chronic hypertension, with activation of the renal sympathetic nerves. Excess weight gain and obesity often lead to sympathetic nerve activation resulting in the stimulation of the renal sympathetic nerves, impairing pressure-natriuresis in the kidney and causing chronic hypertension [6].

Proinflammatory Cytokines

Shi *et al.* suggested that inflammation may play a key role in developement of hypertension and cardiovascular disorders. However, the role of inflammatory processes in neurogenic hypertension is still unclear [168]. Peripheral immune events and inflammation elevate SNA and contribute to neurally mediated hypertension. Intravenous or intrainternal carotid artery injection of proinflammatory cytokines such as TNF-α (tumor necrosis factor-α) or IL-1β (interleukin-1β) increases renal SNA, heart rate, and ABP, and lesion of the SFO attenuates these responses [169]. Microinjection of either TNF-α or IL-1β into the SFO increases renal SNA and ABP. SFO pretreatment with either an angiotensin-converting enzyme inhibitor or angiotensin receptor blocker attenuates these responses [170]. Furthermore, injection of TNF-α or IL-1β into the SFO increases expression of inflammatory signaling pathways in PVN and these signaling pathways in the PVN can increase ABP [170 - 172]. According to these findings, Stocker *et al.* suggest that proinflammatory cytokines act in the SFO via renin–angiotensin system to activate a downstream pathway to the PVN and elevate SNA and ABP [2].

Shi *et al.* indicated that angiotensin II-induced hypertension involves activation of microglia, and increases in proinflammatory cytokines in the PVN [168].

Targeted deletion of brain microglia reduces ABP in both angiotensin II–induced and L-NAME (*N*-nitroarginine methyl ester)-induced hypertension [173].

PTX3 blood levels are low in normal conditions rapidly increase in plasma during inflammation (*i.e.*, sepsis, endotoxin shock, and other inflammatory conditions) so that it acts like a acute phase protein [174]. In a study we conducted on diabetic patients, we determined that plasma PTX-3 levels, an important indicator of inflammation, are significantly related to systolic blood pressure [175].

It has been suggested that proinflammatory molecules, such as junctional adhesion molecule 1 (JAM-1) are highly expressed in the NTS of an animal model of human essential hypertension, the spontaneously hypertensive rat (SHR), compared with normotensive rats (Wistar–Kyoto, WKY) [176]. The functional role for JAM-1 in the NTS was tested by adenovirus-mediated overexpression in adult normotensive (15-week-old) WKY rats *in vivo*. Seven days after adenovirus-mediated JAM-1 expression, blood pressure was increased significantly [177]. These data indicate a novel prohypertensive property for JAM-1 [176]. Waki H *et al.* suggested that JAM-1 and leukotriene B4 12-hydroxydehydrogenase (LTB4) may, in part, contribute to the leukocyte accumulation in NTS microvessels of the SHR [176]. They also suggested a novel hypothetical mechanisms involving specific inflammatory responses that affect neuronal function in the nucleus tractus NTS and may contribute to neurogenic hypertension in the spontaneously hypertensive SHR: Some proinflammatory molecules, such as JAM-1 and LTB4, are abnormally expressed in the NTS of SHR in neonatal period before hypertension has manifested. During development, this abnormal condition may induce leukocyte accumulation in capillaries that may obstruct blood flow and result in highly localized hypoxia. They have also hypothesized that local disturbance of blood supply in the dorsomedial region of the medulla oblongata, including NTS regions, evokes neurogenic hypertension to ensure adequate brain blood flow [176].

Waki *et al.* also suggested that the mRNA of some proinflammatory factors, such as JAM-1 and enzymes regulating expression levels of LTB4, are abnormally expressed in the NTS of SHR. This may be due to a genetic predisposition of the SHR [176]. However, recent evidence suggests that the brainstem of the SHR is hypoperfused [178]. Hypoperfusion and oxygen starvation are known to trigger an inflammatory state within the microvasculature [179]. Thus, Waki H *et al.* suggested that inflamation may occur within the brainstem of the SHR [176].

Additionally, AgII, a major peptide associated with cardiovascular disease and known to be upregulated in the SHR, could also trigger the proinflammatory state in the NTS [180]. Waki H et al suggested that a combination of hypoperfusion and raised AgII could have a facilitatory effect on inflammation [176].

High circulating AgII directly activates AT1-R at the CVO and/or PVN. The resultant signals cause microglial activation, increased ROS and cytokine production in the PVN. AgII activity causes nicotinamide adenine dinucleotide phosphate-mediated increase in oxidative stress in autonomic nuclei within the medulla oblongata (for example, RVLM). Increased oxidative stress and cytokine concentration at the PVN and RVLM augment sympathetic neuronal activity. The upregulation of AT1-R on cerebral blood vessels due to elevated circulating AgII levels will facilitate sympathetic neural outflow. The associated local oxidative stress, inflammation and upregulation of JAM promote leukocyte adhesion within the brain microvasculature. The subsequently increased cerebral vascular tone could impair perfusion, cause local tissue hypoxia and evoke reflex sympathoexcitation [181].

Genetic Factors

Genetic factors are also being investigated [182 - 186].

Hereditary spontaneous hypertension was detected in different rat species and at least one dog species. In these rat species, Okamoto is the most studied type of spontaneous hypertensive rats. There is evidence that the sympathetic nervous system is more active in the early stages of hypertension formation in these rats than in normal rats [6].

Genome-wide linked studies focusing on hypertension have clarified many candidate genes with very small effect in population studies. More recent studies are investigating the role of micro RNA and epigenetic mechanisms, although their role in neurogenic hypertension is not yet known [2].

NEUROPLASTICITY IN HYPERTENSION

As that can be understanded, there are many factors that can cause neurogenic hypertension. However, the interaction among these and other factors is likely much more complex. Recent studies suggest a previous exposure to one stimulus may sensitize the response to a subsequent hypertensive stimulus. Essential hypertension is a complex disease that likely originates from a constellation of contributing factors summated over time. Rather than a single stimulus or challenge, hypertension may result from the integration of previous challenges or experiences with current environmental factors but temporally separated. These previous experiences or exposures impact how the brain responds to subsequent stimuli [2].Subsequent studies show that angiotensin II−induced hypertension is exacerbated by pre-exposure with aldosterone, high-fat diet, leptin, and TNF-α [187 - 189].

CONCLUDING REMARKS

In many patients, hypertension may be due to neurogenic origin. Therefore, it is important to distinguish neurogenic hypertension from non-neurogenic hypertension. It has been suggested that sympathetic overactivity appears to be present before the hypertensive phenotype and its early antagonism should be considered a potential preventative measure before end organ damage becomes irreversible and hypertension becomes drug resistant [16, 18, 181, 190]. This implies that SNA should be measured in patients first presenting hypertensive trends and targeted to arrest the inevitable pathological cascade and ultimate disease progression [181].

Future studies about additional factor that impairing sympathetic tone directly or indirectly, and therapeutic strategies targeting neurogenic hypertension will make important contributions to treatment.

Lifestyle modification including exercise training, diet therapy, weight loss, stress reduction may play an important role on reducing excessive central sympathetic activation.

CONSENT FOR PUBLICATION

Not applicable.

CONFLICT OF INTEREST

The authors declare no conflict of interest, financial or otherwise.

ACKNOWLEDGEMENTS

Declare none.

REFERENCES

[1]   Mann SJ. Neurogenic hypertension: pathophysiology, diagnosis and management. Clin Auton Res 2018; 28(4): 363-74.
[http://dx.doi.org/10.1007/s10286-018-0541-z] [PMID: 29974290]

[2]   Stocker SD, Kinsman BJ, Sved AF. Recent advances in neurogenic hypertension: dietary salt, obesity, and inflammation. Hypertension 2017; 70: 474-8.
[http://dx.doi.org/10.1161/HYPERTENSIONAHA.117.08936] [PMID: 28739972]

[3]   Korner PI. CNS cardiovascular pathways: Role of fast and slow transmitters. In: Korner PI, Ed. Essential Hypertension and Its Causes: Neural and Non-Neural Mechanisms. USA: Oxford University Press 2007; pp. 207-40.

[4]   Bell DR. Control mechanisms in circulatory function. In: Rhoades RA, Bell DR, Eds. Medical Physiology - Principles for Clinical Medicine. 4th Ed. Baltimore: Lippincott Williams & Wilkins, a Wolters Kluwer business 2013; pp. 311-7.

[5]   Barrett KE, Barman SM, Boitano S, Brooks. HL, Eds. Cardiovascular regulatory mechanisms. Ganong's Review of Medical Physiology. 25th Ed. New York: McGraw-Hill Education 2016; pp. 585-99.

[6]   Hall JE. Nervous regulation of the circulation, and rapid control of arterial pressure. In: Guyton AC, Hall JE, Eds. Textbook of Medical Physiology. 13th Ed. Philadelphia: Elsevier 2016; pp. 204-15.

[7]   Petras JM, Cummings JF. Autonomic neurons in the spinal cord of the Rhesus monkey: a correlation of the findings of cytoarchitectonics and sympathectomy with fiber degeneration following dorsal rhizotomy. J Comp Neurol 1972; 146(2): 189-218.
[http://dx.doi.org/10.1002/cne.901460205] [PMID: 4627467]

[8]   Dampney RA. Functional organization of central pathways regulating the cardiovascular system. Physiol Rev 1994; 74(2): 323-64.
[http://dx.doi.org/10.1152/physrev.1994.74.2.323] [PMID: 8171117]

[9]   Spyer KM. Central nervous mechanisms responsible for cardio-respiratory homeostasis. Adv Exp Med Biol 1995; 381: 73-9.
[http://dx.doi.org/10.1007/978-1-4615-1895-2_8] [PMID: 8867825]

[10] Izzo JL Jr. The sympathetic nervous system in acute and chronic blood pressure elevation.Hypertension : A Companionto Brenner & Rector's The Kidney. 2nd Edition. Philedelphia: Elsevier Mosby 2015; pp. 60-9.
[http://dx.doi.org/10.1016/B978-0-7216-0258-5.50096-X]

[11] Giles ME, Fernley RT, Nakamura Y, *et al.* Characterization of a specific antibody to the rat angiotensin II AT1 receptor. J Histochem Cytochem 1999; 47(4): 507-16.
[http://dx.doi.org/10.1177/002215549904700409] [PMID: 10082752]

[12] McKinley MJ, McAllen RM, Mendelsohn FAO, *et al.* Circumventricular organs: Neuroendocrine interfaces between the brain and the hemal milieu. Front Neuroendocrinol 1990; 11: 91-127.

[13] McKinley MJ, Albiston AL, Allen AM, *et al.* The brain renin-angiotensin system: location and physiological roles. Int J Biochem Cell Biol 2003; 35(6): 901-18.
[http://dx.doi.org/10.1016/S1357-2725(02)00306-0] [PMID: 12676175]

[14] Pappano JA. Regulation of the Heart and Vasculature. In: Koeppen BM, Stanton BA, Eds. Berne & Levy Physiology. Philadelphia: Elsevier Mosby 2010; pp. 370-93.

[15] Grassi G, Seravalle G, Quarti-Trevano F. The 'neuroadrenergic hypothesis' in hypertension: current

evidence. Exp Physiol 2010; 95(5): 581-6.
[http://dx.doi.org/10.1113/expphysiol.2009.047381] [PMID: 20008032]

[16]   Grassi G. Role of the sympathetic nervous system in human hypertension. J Hypertens 1998; 16(12 Pt 2): 1979-87.
[http://dx.doi.org/10.1097/00004872-199816121-00019] [PMID: 9886886]

[17]   Simms AE, Paton JFR, Allen AM, Pickering AE. Is augmented central respiratory-sympathetic coupling involved in the generation of hypertension? Respir Physiol Neurobiol 2010; 174(1-2): 89-97.
[http://dx.doi.org/10.1016/j.resp.2010.07.010] [PMID: 20674806]

[18]   Simms AE, Paton JF, Pickering AE, Allen AM. Amplified respiratory-sympathetic coupling in the spontaneously hypertensive rat: does it contribute to hypertension? J Physiol 2009; 587(3): 597-610.
[http://dx.doi.org/10.1113/jphysiol.2008.165902] [PMID: 19064613]

[19]   Korner P, Bobik A, Oddie C, Friberg P. Sympathoadrenal system is critical for structural changes in genetic hypertension. Hypertension 1993; 22(2): 243-52.
[http://dx.doi.org/10.1161/01.HYP.22.2.243] [PMID: 8340160]

[20]   Zicha J, Kunes J. Ontogenetic aspects of hypertension development: analysis in the rat. Physiol Rev 1999; 79(4): 1227-82.
[http://dx.doi.org/10.1152/physrev.1999.79.4.1227] [PMID: 10508234]

[21]   Korner PI. Whole-Organism Baroreflexes.Essential Hypertension and its Causes. New York: Oxford University Press 2007; pp. 241-84.

[22]   Winternitz SR, Katholi RE, Oparil S. Role of the renal sympathetic nerves in the development and maintenance of hypertension in the spontaneously hypertensive rat. J Clin Invest 1980; 66(5): 971-8.
[http://dx.doi.org/10.1172/JCI109966] [PMID: 7000828]

[23]   Moraes DJ, Machado BH, Paton JFR. Carotid body overactivity induces respiratory neurone channelopathy contributing to neurogenic hypertension. J Physiol 2015; 593(14): 3055-63.
[http://dx.doi.org/10.1113/JP270423] [PMID: 25900825]

[24]   Larsen R, Thorp A, Schlaich M. Regulation of the sympathetic nervous system by the kidney. Curr Opin Nephrol Hypertens 2014; 23(1): 61-8.
[http://dx.doi.org/10.1097/01.mnh.0000437610.65287.db] [PMID: 24275767]

[25]   Hering D, Schlaich M. The role of central nervous system mechanisms in resistant hypertension. Curr Hypertens Rep 2015; 17(8): 58.
[http://dx.doi.org/10.1007/s11906-015-0570-0] [PMID: 26070453]

[26]   Grassi G, Seravalle G, Brambilla G, *et al.* Marked sympathetic activation and baroreflex dysfunction in true resistant hypertension. Int J Cardiol 2014; 177(3): 1020-5.
[http://dx.doi.org/10.1016/j.ijcard.2014.09.138] [PMID: 25449517]

[27]   Chapleau MW, Li Z, Meyrelles SS, Ma X, Abboud FM. Mechanisms determining sensitivity of baroreceptor afferents in health and disease. Ann N Y Acad Sci 2001; 940: 1-19.
[http://dx.doi.org/10.1111/j.1749-6632.2001.tb03662.x] [PMID: 11458669]

[28]   Wang W. Chronic administration of aldosterone depresses baroreceptor reflex function in the dog. Hypertension 1994; 24(5): 571-5.
[http://dx.doi.org/10.1161/01.HYP.24.5.571] [PMID: 7960015]

[29]   Heesch CM, Abboud FM, Thames MD. Acute resetting of carotid sinus baroreceptors. II. Possible involvement of electrogenic Na+ pump. Am J Physiol 1984; 247(5 Pt 2): H833-9.
[PMID: 6093597]

[30]   Saum WR, Brown AM, Tuley FH. An electrogenic sodium pump and baroreceptor function in normotensive and spontaneously hypertensive rats. Circ Res 1976; 39(4): 497-505.
[http://dx.doi.org/10.1161/01.RES.39.4.497] [PMID: 963833]

[31]   Mombouli JV, Vanhoutte PM. Endothelial dysfunction: from physiology to therapy. J Mol Cell

Cardiol 1999; 31(1): 61-74.
[http://dx.doi.org/10.1006/jmcc.1998.0844] [PMID: 10072716]

[32]   Chen HI, Chapleau MW, McDowell TS, Abboud FM. Prostaglandins contribute to activation of baroreceptors in rabbits. Possible paracrine influence of endothelium. Circ Res 1990; 67(6): 1394-404.
[http://dx.doi.org/10.1161/01.RES.67.6.1394] [PMID: 2245501]

[33]   Matsuda T, Bates JN, Lewis SJ, Abboud FM, Chapleau MW. Modulation of baroreceptor activity by nitric oxide and S-nitrosocysteine. Circ Res 1995; 76(3): 426-33.
[http://dx.doi.org/10.1161/01.RES.76.3.426] [PMID: 7859388]

[34]   Smith WL, Marnett LJ, DeWitt DL. Prostaglandin and thromboxane biosynthesis. Pharmacol Ther 1991; 49(3): 153-79.
[http://dx.doi.org/10.1016/0163-7258(91)90054-P] [PMID: 1905023]

[35]   Xie PL, Chapleau MW, McDowell TS, Hajduczok G, Abboud FM. Mechanism of decreased baroreceptor activity in chronic hypertensive rabbits. Role of endogenous prostanoids. J Clin Invest 1990; 86(2): 625-30.
[http://dx.doi.org/10.1172/JCI114754] [PMID: 2117025]

[36]   Monahan KD, Ray CA. Cyclooxygenase inhibition and baroreflex sensitivity in humans. Am J Physiol Heart Circ Physiol 2005; 288(2): H737-43.
[http://dx.doi.org/10.1152/ajpheart.00357.2004] [PMID: 15486039]

[37]   Li Z, Chapleau MW, Bates JN, Bielefeldt K, Lee HC, Abboud FM. Nitric oxide as an autocrine regulator of sodium currents in baroreceptor neurons. Neuron 1998; 20(5): 1039-49.
[http://dx.doi.org/10.1016/S0896-6273(00)80484-5] [PMID: 9620707]

[38]   Moncada S, Higgs EA. Endogenous nitric oxide: physiology, pathology and clinical relevance. Eur J Clin Invest 1991; 21(4): 361-74.
[http://dx.doi.org/10.1111/j.1365-2362.1991.tb01383.x] [PMID: 1718757]

[39]   Chapleau MW, Li Z, Meyrelles SS, Ma X, Abboud FM. Mechanisms determining sensitivity of baroreceptor afferents in health and disease. Ann N Y Acad Sci 2001; 940: 1-19.
[http://dx.doi.org/10.1111/j.1749-6632.2001.tb03662.x] [PMID: 11458669]

[40]   Dun NJ, Dun SL, Chiba T, Förstermann U. Nitric oxide synthase-immunoreactive vagal afferent fibers in rat superior cervical ganglia. Neuroscience 1995; 65(1): 231-9.
[http://dx.doi.org/10.1016/0306-4522(94)00455-E] [PMID: 7538645]

[41]   Tanaka K, Chiba T. Nitric oxide synthase containing neurons in the carotid body and sinus of the guinea pig. Microsc Res Tech 1994; 29(2): 90-3.
[http://dx.doi.org/10.1002/jemt.1070290205] [PMID: 7529074]

[42]   Meyrelles SS, Mao HZ, Sharma RV, Chapleau MW. Baroreceptor resetting and vessel remodeling after gene transfer of nitric oxide synthase to carotidsinus (abstr.). FASEB J. 1998; 12(5)PtII: A687.

[43]   Bock JM, Ueda K, Schneider AC, *et al.* Inorganic nitrate supplementation attenuates peripheral chemoreflex sensitivity but does not improve cardiovagal baroreflex sensitivity in older adults. Am J Physiol Heart Circ Physiol 2018; 314(1): H45-51.
[http://dx.doi.org/10.1152/ajpheart.00389.2017] [PMID: 28971842]

[44]   Mao HZ, Li Z, Chapleau MW. Platelet activation in carotid sinuses triggers reflex sympathoinhibition and hypotension. Hypertension 1996; 27(3 Pt 2): 584-90.
[http://dx.doi.org/10.1161/01.HYP.27.3.584] [PMID: 8613208]

[45]   Chapleau MW, Su X, Li Z. Platelets aggregating in carotid-sinus selectively modulate activity of baroreceptor fiber types. FASEB J 1995; 9(3): A7.

[46]   Alper RH. Effects of the selective serotonin reuptake inhibitor fluoxetine on baroreceptor reflex sensitivity and body weight in young and old rats. J Gerontol 1992; 47(4): B130-6.
[http://dx.doi.org/10.1093/geronj/47.4.B130] [PMID: 1624689]

[47]   Yasumasu T, Takahara K, Sadayasu T, *et al.* Influence of coronary artery disease risk factors on baroreflex sensitivity in the elderly. Clin Auton Res 2003; 13(5): 330-6.
[http://dx.doi.org/10.1007/s10286-003-0108-4] [PMID: 14564655]

[48]   Li Z, Mao HZ, Abboud FM, Chapleau MW. Oxygen-derived free radicals contribute to baroreceptor dysfunction in atherosclerotic rabbits. Circ Res 1996; 79(4): 802-11.
[http://dx.doi.org/10.1161/01.RES.79.4.802] [PMID: 8831504]

[49]   Impaired carotid occlusion reflex in apoE deficient mice and its reversal by gene transfer to carotid sinus (abstr.). J Hypertens 2012; 18 (Suppl. 4): S202.

[50]   Nightingale AK, Blackman DJ, Field R, *et al.* Role of nitric oxide and oxidative stress in baroreceptor dysfunction in patients with chronic heart failure. Clin Sci (Lond) 2003; 104(5): 529-35.
[http://dx.doi.org/10.1042/CS20020334] [PMID: 12549975]

[51]   Fisher JP, Fadel PJ. Therapeutic strategies for targeting excessive central sympathetic activation in human hypertension. Exp Physiol 2010; 95(5): 572-80.
[http://dx.doi.org/10.1113/expphysiol.2009.047332] [PMID: 20304932]

[52]   Abdala AP, McBryde FD, Marina N, *et al.* Hypertension is critically dependent on the carotid body input in the spontaneously hypertensive rat. J Physiol 2012; 590(17): 4269-77.
[http://dx.doi.org/10.1113/jphysiol.2012.237800] [PMID: 22687617]

[53]   Paton JF, Ratcliffe L, Hering D, Wolf J, Sobotka PA, Narkiewicz K. Revelations about carotid body function through its pathological role in resistant hypertension. Curr Hypertens Rep 2013; 15(4): 273-80.
[http://dx.doi.org/10.1007/s11906-013-0366-z] [PMID: 23828147]

[54]   Siński M, Lewandowski J, Przybylski J, *et al.* Tonic activity of carotid body chemoreceptors contributes to the increased sympathetic drive in essential hypertension. Hypertens Res 2012; 35(5): 487-91.
[http://dx.doi.org/10.1038/hr.2011.209] [PMID: 22158114]

[55]   Moraes DJ, Machado BH, Paton JF. Carotid body induced post-inspiratory neuron channelopathy for neurogenic hypertension. FASEB J 2014; 28 (1 Suppl.): 872.9.

[56]   Solar M, Ceral J, Zizka J, Eliás P. Neurovascular compression: sympathetic activity in severe arterial hypertension. Physiol Res 2009; 58(6): 913-6.
[PMID: 19093731]

[57]   Sasaki S, Tanda S, Hatta T, *et al.* Neurovascular decompression of the rostral ventrolateral medulla decreases blood pressure and sympathetic nerve activity in patients with refractory hypertension. J Clin Hypertens (Greenwich) 2011; 13(11): 818-20.
[http://dx.doi.org/10.1111/j.1751-7176.2011.00522.x] [PMID: 22051426]

[58]   Hajduczok G, Chapleau MW, Abboud FM. Increase in sympathetic activity with age. II. Role of impairment of cardiopulmonary baroreflexes. Am J Physiol 1991; 260(4 Pt 2): H1121-7.
[PMID: 2012218]

[59]   Kornet L, Hoeks AP, Janssen BJ, Houben AJ, De Leeuw PW, Reneman RS. Neural activity of the cardiac baroreflex decreases with age in normotensive and hypertensive subjects. J Hypertens 2005; 23(4): 815-23.
[http://dx.doi.org/10.1097/01.hjh.0000163151.50825.e2] [PMID: 15775787]

[60]   Zhang B, Bailey WM, McVicar AL, Gensel JC. Age increases reactive oxygen species production in macrophages and potentiates oxidative damage after spinal cord injury. Neurobiol Aging 2016; 47: 157-67.
[http://dx.doi.org/10.1016/j.neurobiolaging.2016.07.029] [PMID: 27596335]

[61]   Goldstein DS. Arterial baroreflex sensitivity, plasma catecholamines, and pressor responsiveness in essential hypertension. Circulation 1983; 68(2): 234-40.
[http://dx.doi.org/10.1161/01.CIR.68.2.234] [PMID: 6407776]

[62]   Gribbin B, Pickering TG, Sleight P, Peto R. Effect of age and high blood pressure on baroreflex sensitivity in man. Circ Res 1971; 29(4): 424-31.
       [http://dx.doi.org/10.1161/01.RES.29.4.424] [PMID: 5110922]

[63]   Randall OS, Esler MD, Bulloch EG, *et al.* Relationship of age and blood pressure to baroreflex sensitivity and arterial compliance in man. Clin Sci Mol Med Suppl 1976; 3: 357s-60s.
       [http://dx.doi.org/10.1042/cs051357s] [PMID: 1071645]

[64]   Westheim A, Os I, Kjeldsen SE, Fønstelien E, Eide IK. Renal haemodynamic and sympathetic responses to head-up tilt in essential hypertension. Scand J Clin Lab Invest 1990; 50(8): 815-22.
       [http://dx.doi.org/10.3109/00365519009104947] [PMID: 2084819]

[65]   Simon AC, Safar ME, Weiss YA, London GM, Milliez PL. Baroreflex sensitivity and cardiopulmonary blood volume in normotensive and hypertensive patients. Br Heart J 1977; 39(7): 799-805.
       [http://dx.doi.org/10.1136/hrt.39.7.799] [PMID: 884030]

[66]   Mark AL, Kerber RE. Augmentation of cardiopulmonary baroreflex control of forearm vascular resistance in borderline hypertension. Hypertension 1982; 4(1): 39-46.
       [http://dx.doi.org/10.1161/01.HYP.4.1.39] [PMID: 7061127]

[67]   Rea RF, Hamdan M. Baroreflex control of muscle sympathetic nerve activity in borderline hypertension. Circulation 1990; 13(11): 818-20.
       [http://dx.doi.org/10.1161/01.CIR.82.3.856]

[68]   Mann SJ. The mind/body link in essential hypertension: time for a new paradigm. Altern Ther Health Med 2000; 6(2): 39-45.
       [PMID: 10710802]

[69]   Wallin BG, Esler M, Dorward P, *et al.* Simultaneous measurements of cardiac noradrenaline spillover and sympathetic outflow to skeletal muscle in humans. J Physiol 1992; 453: 45-58.
       [http://dx.doi.org/10.1113/jphysiol.1992.sp019217] [PMID: 1464839]

[70]   Chida Y, Steptoe A. Greater cardiovascular responses to laboratory mental stress are associated with poor subsequent cardiovascular risk status: a meta-analysis of prospective evidence. Hypertension 2010; 55(4): 1026-32.
       [http://dx.doi.org/10.1161/HYPERTENSIONAHA.109.146621] [PMID: 20194301]

[71]   Flaa A, Eide IK, Kjeldsen SE, Rostrup M. Sympathoadrenal stress reactivity is a predictor of future blood pressure: an 18-year follow-up study. Hypertension 2008; 52(2): 336-41.
       [http://dx.doi.org/10.1161/HYPERTENSIONAHA.108.111625] [PMID: 18574074]

[72]   Jorgensen RS, Johnson BT, Kolodziej ME, Schreer GE. Elevated blood pressure and personality: a meta-analytic review. Psychol Bull 1996; 120(2): 293-320.
       [http://dx.doi.org/10.1037/0033-2909.120.2.293] [PMID: 8831299]

[73]   Suls J, Wan CK, Costa PT Jr. Relationship of trait anger to resting blood pressure: a meta-analysis. Health Psychol 1995; 14(5): 444-56.
       [http://dx.doi.org/10.1037/0278-6133.14.5.444] [PMID: 7498116]

[74]   Mann AH. The psychological aspects of essential hypertension. J Psychosom Res 1986; 30(5): 527-41.
       [http://dx.doi.org/10.1016/0022-3999(86)90025-5] [PMID: 3772835]

[75]   Hunyor SN, Henderson RJ. The role of stress management in blood pressure control: why the promissory note has failed to deliver. J Hypertens 1996; 14(4): 413-8.
       [http://dx.doi.org/10.1097/00004872-199604000-00001] [PMID: 8761888]

[76]   Mann SJ, James GD. Defensiveness and essential hypertension. J Psychosom Res 1998; 45(2): 139-48.
       [http://dx.doi.org/10.1016/S0022-3999(97)00293-6] [PMID: 9753386]

[77]   Mann SJ. The clinical spectrum of labile hypertension: a management dilemma. J Clin Hypertens (Greenwich) 2009; 11(9): 491-7.

[http://dx.doi.org/10.1111/j.1751-7176.2009.00155.x] [PMID: 19751461]

[78]   Mann SJ. Labile and paroxysmal hypertension: common clinical dilemmas in need of treatment studies. Curr Cardiol Rep 2015; 17(11): 99.
[http://dx.doi.org/10.1007/s11886-015-0646-0] [PMID: 26370555]

[79]   Mann SJ. Severe paroxysmal hypertension (pseudopheochromocytoma). Curr Hypertens Rep 2008; 10(1): 12-8.
[http://dx.doi.org/10.1007/s11906-008-0005-2] [PMID: 18367021]

[80]   Vaclavik J, Krenkova A, Kocianova E, *et al.* 7B.04: Effect of sertraline in paroxysmal hypertension. J Hypertens 2015; 33 (Suppl. 1).e93
[http://dx.doi.org/10.1097/01.hjh.0000467601.49032.62]

[81]   Rozanski A, Blumenthal JA, Kaplan J. Impact of psychological factors on the pathogenesis of cardiovascular disease and implications for therapy. Circulation 1999; 99(16): 2192-217.
[http://dx.doi.org/10.1161/01.CIR.99.16.2192] [PMID: 10217662]

[82]   Thomas GD, Zhang W, Victor RG. Nitric oxide deficiency as a cause of clinical hypertension: promising new drug targets for refractory hypertension. JAMA 2001; 285(16): 2055-7.
[http://dx.doi.org/10.1001/jama.285.16.2055] [PMID: 11311074]

[83]   Lepori M, Sartori C, Trueb L, Owlya R, Nicod P, Scherrer U. Haemodynamic and sympathetic effects of inhibition of nitric oxide synthase by systemic infusion of N(G)-monomethyl-L-arginine into humans are dose dependent. J Hypertens 1998; 16(4): 519-23.
[http://dx.doi.org/10.1097/00004872-199816040-00013] [PMID: 9797197]

[84]   Young CN, Fisher JP, Gallagher KM, *et al.* Inhibition of nitric oxide synthase evokes central sympatho-excitation in healthy humans. J Physiol 2009; 587(Pt 20): 4977-86.
[http://dx.doi.org/10.1113/jphysiol.2009.177204] [PMID: 19723781]

[85]   Mallamaci F, Tripepi G, Maas R, Malatino L, Böger R, Zoccali C. Analysis of the relationship between norepinephrine and asymmetric dimethyl arginine levels among patients with end-stage renal disease. J Am Soc Nephrol 2004; 15(2): 435-41.
[http://dx.doi.org/10.1097/01.ASN.0000106717.58091.F6] [PMID: 14747391]

[86]   Yavuzer S, Yavuzer H, Cengiz M, *et al.* Endothelial damage in white coat hypertension: role of lectin-like oxidized low-density lipoprotein-1. J Hum Hypertens 2015; 29(2): 92-8.
[http://dx.doi.org/10.1038/jhh.2014.55] [PMID: 25007999]

[87]   Rodrigo R, Guichard C, Charles R. Clinical pharmacology and therapeutic use of antioxidant vitamins. Fundam Clin Pharmacol 2007; 21(2): 111-27.
[http://dx.doi.org/10.1111/j.1472-8206.2006.00466.x] [PMID: 17391284]

[88]   Uzun H, Karter Y, Aydin S, *et al.* Oxidative stress in white coat hypertension; role of paraoxonase. J Hum Hypertens 2004; 18(7): 523-8.
[http://dx.doi.org/10.1038/sj.jhh.1001697] [PMID: 14985779]

[89]   Peterson JR, Sharma RV, Davisson RL. Reactive oxygen species in the neuropathogenesis of hypertension. Curr Hypertens Rep 2006; 8(3): 232-41.
[http://dx.doi.org/10.1007/s11906-006-0056-1] [PMID: 17147922]

[90]   Toney GM, Pedrino GR, Fink GD, Osborn JW. Does enhanced respiratory-sympathetic coupling contribute to peripheral neural mechanisms of angiotensin II-salt hypertension? Exp Physiol 2010; 95(5): 587-94.
[http://dx.doi.org/10.1113/expphysiol.2009.047399] [PMID: 20228120]

[91]   Johns EJ, Kopp UC, DiBona GF. Neural control of renal function. Compr Physiol 2011; 1(2): 731-67.
[PMID: 23737201]

[92]   Saxena PR. Interaction between the renin-angiotensin-aldosterone and sympathetic nervous systems. J Cardiovasc Pharmacol 1992; 19 (Suppl. 6): S80-8.
[http://dx.doi.org/10.1097/00005344-199219006-00013] [PMID: 1382170]

[93]   Mancia G, Saino A. Interactions between the sympathetic nervous system and renin angiotensin system.Hypertension: pathophysiology, diagnosis, and management. 2nd ed. New York: Raven Press 1995; pp. 399-407.

[94]   Ball SG. The sympathetic nervous system and converting enzyme inhibition. J Cardiovasc Pharmacol 1989; 13 (Suppl. 3): S17-21.
[http://dx.doi.org/10.1097/00005344-198900133-00005] [PMID: 2474095]

[95]   Allen AM, Oldfield BJ, Giles ME, *et al.* Localization of angiotensin receptors in the nervous system.Handbook of Chemical Neuroanatomy. 2000; Vol. 16: pp. 79-124.

[96]   Lenkei Z, Palkovits M, Corvol P, Llorens-Cortès C. Expression of angiotensin type-1 (AT1) and type-2 (AT2) receptor mRNAs in the adult rat brain: a functional neuroanatomical review. Front Neuroendocrinol 1997; 18(4): 383-439.
[http://dx.doi.org/10.1006/frne.1997.0155] [PMID: 9344632]

[97]   Bader M, Ganten D. It's renin in the brain: transgenic animals elucidate the brain renin angiotensin system. Circ Res 2002; 90(1): 8-10.
[http://dx.doi.org/10.1161/res.90.1.8] [PMID: 11786510]

[98]   Fei DTW, Abrahams SF, Coghlan JP, *et al.* Angiotensin II in CSF of sheep. Clin Exp Pharmacol Physiol 1982; 9: 564-5.

[99]   Grassi G, Turri C, Dell'Oro R, Stella ML, Bolla GB, Mancia G. Effect of chronic angiotensin converting enzyme inhibition on sympathetic nerve traffic and baroreflex control of the circulation in essential hypertension. J Hypertens 1998; 16(12 Pt 1): 1789-96.
[http://dx.doi.org/10.1097/00004872-199816120-00012] [PMID: 9869013]

[100]   Lynch KR, Hawelu-Johnson CL, Guyenet PG. Localization of brain angiotensinogen mRNA by hybridization histochemistry. Brain Res 1987; 388(2): 149-58.
[http://dx.doi.org/10.1016/0169-328X(87)90008-8] [PMID: 3476177]

[101]   Stornetta RL, Hawelu-Johnson CL, Guyenet PG, Lynch KR. Astrocytes synthesize angiotensinogen in brain. Science 1988; 242(4884): 1444-6.
[http://dx.doi.org/10.1126/science.3201232] [PMID: 3201232]

[102]   Dzau VJ, Ingelfinger J, Pratt RE, Ellison KE. Identification of renin and angiotensinogen messenger RNA sequences in mouse and rat brains. Hypertension 1986; 8(6): 544-8.
[http://dx.doi.org/10.1161/01.HYP.8.6.544] [PMID: 3519452]

[103]   Saavedra JM, Chevillard C. Angiotensin-converting enzyme is present in the subfornical organ and other circumventricular organs of the rat. Neurosci Lett 1982; 29(2): 123-7.
[http://dx.doi.org/10.1016/0304-3940(82)90340-8] [PMID: 6283434]

[104]   Chai SY, McKenzie JS, McKinley MJ, Mendelsohn FAO. Angiotensin converting enzyme in the human basal forebrain and midbrain visualized by *in vitro* autoradiography. J Comp Neurol 1990; 291(2): 179-94.
[http://dx.doi.org/10.1002/cne.902910203] [PMID: 2153714]

[105]   Chai SY, McKinley MJ, Mendelsohn FAO. Distribution of angiotensin converting enzyme in sheep hypothalamus and medulla oblongata visualized by in vitro autoradiography. Clin Exp Hypertens A 1987; 9(2-3): 449-60.
[http://dx.doi.org/10.3109/10641968709164212] [PMID: 3038409]

[106]   Chai SY, McKinley MJ, Paxinos G, Mendelsohn FAO. Angiotensin converting enzyme in the monkey (Macaca fascicularis) brain visualized by in vitro autoradiography. Neuroscience 1991; 42(2): 483-95.
[http://dx.doi.org/10.1016/0306-4522(91)90391-Z] [PMID: 1654536]

[107]   Rogerson FM, Schlawe I, Paxinos G, Chai SY, McKinley MJ, Mendelsohn FA. Localization of angiotensin converting enzyme by in vitro autoradiography in the rabbit brain. J Chem Neuroanat 1995; 8(4): 227-43.
[http://dx.doi.org/10.1016/0891-0618(95)00049-D] [PMID: 7669270]

[108] Allen AM, Chai SY, Clevers J, McKinley MJ, Paxinos G, Mendelsohn FA. Localization and characterization of angiotensin II receptor binding and angiotensin converting enzyme in the human medulla oblongata. J Comp Neurol 1988; 269(2): 249-64.
[http://dx.doi.org/10.1002/cne.902690209] [PMID: 2833536]

[109] Giles ME, Sly DJ, McKinley MJ, Oldfield BJ. Neurons in the lamina terminalis which project polysynaptically to the kidney express angiotensin AT1A receptor. Brain Res 2001; 898(1): 9-12.
[http://dx.doi.org/10.1016/S0006-8993(01)02113-8] [PMID: 11292444]

[110] Osborn JW, Foss JD. Renal nerves and long-term control of arterial pressure. Compr Physiol 2017; 7(2): 263-320.
[http://dx.doi.org/10.1002/cphy.c150047] [PMID: 28333375]

[111] Diz DI, Barnes KL, Ferrario CM. Contribution of the vagus nerve to angiotensin II binding sites in the canine medulla. Brain Res Bull 1986; 17(4): 497-505.
[http://dx.doi.org/10.1016/0361-9230(86)90217-0] [PMID: 3779450]

[112] Lewis SJ, Allen AM, Verberne AJ, Figdor R, Jarrott B, Mendelsohn FA. Angiotensin II receptor binding in the rat nucleus tractus solitarii is reduced after unilateral nodose ganglionectomy or vagotomy. Eur J Pharmacol 1986; 125(2): 305-7.
[http://dx.doi.org/10.1016/0014-2999(86)90043-9] [PMID: 3017730]

[113] Barth SW, Gerstberger R. Differential regulation of angiotensinogen and AT1A receptor mRNA within the rat subfornical organ during dehydration. Brain Res Mol Brain Res 1999; 64(2): 151-64.
[http://dx.doi.org/10.1016/S0169-328X(98)00308-8] [PMID: 9931478]

[114] Charron G, Laforest S, Gagnon C, Drolet G, Mouginot D. Acute sodium deficit triggers plasticity of the brain angiotensin type 1 receptors. FASEB J 2002; 16(6): 610-2.
[http://dx.doi.org/10.1096/fj.01-0531fje] [PMID: 11919170]

[115] Saavedra JM, Correa FM, Kurihara M, Shigematsu K. Increased number of angiotensin II receptors in the subfornical organ of spontaneously hypertensive rats. J Hypertens Suppl 1986; 4(5) (Suppl. 4): S27-30.
[PMID: 3471907]

[116] Sandberg K, Ji H, Catt KJ. Regulation of angiotensin II receptors in rat brain during dietary sodium changes. Hypertension 1994; 23(1) (Suppl.): I137-41.
[http://dx.doi.org/10.1161/01.HYP.23.1_Suppl.I137] [PMID: 7506698]

[117] Ray PE, Castrén E, Ruley EJ, Saavedra JM. Different effects of sodium or chloride depletion on angiotensin II receptors in rats. Am J Physiol 1990; 258(4 Pt 2): R1008-15.
[PMID: 2331021]

[118] Allen AM, Dampney RA, Mendelsohn FAO. Angiotensin receptor binding and pressor effects in cat subretrofacial nucleus. Am J Physiol 1988; 255(5 Pt 2): H1011-7.
[PMID: 2903678]

[119] Andreatta SH, Averill DB, Santos RA, Ferrario CM. The ventrolateral medulla. A new site of action of the renin-angiotensin system. Hypertension 1988; 11(2 Pt 2): I163-6.
[http://dx.doi.org/10.1161/01.HYP.11.2_Pt_2.I163] [PMID: 2831146]

[120] Averill DB, Diz DI, Barnes KL, Ferrario CM. Pressor responses of angiotensin II microinjected into the dorsomedial medulla of the dog. Brain Res 1987; 414(2): 294-300.
[http://dx.doi.org/10.1016/0006-8993(87)90009-6] [PMID: 3620933]

[121] Jensen LL, Harding JW, Wright JW. Role of paraventricular nucleus in control of blood pressure and drinking in rats. Am J Physiol 1992; 262(6 Pt 2): F1068-75.
[PMID: 1621811]

[122] Severs WB, Daniels-Severs AE. Effects of angiotensin on the central nervous system. Pharmacol Rev 1973; 25(3): 415-49.
[PMID: 4356083]

[123] Simpson JB. The circumventricular organs and the central actions of angiotensin. Neuroendocrinology 1981; 32(4): 248-56.
[http://dx.doi.org/10.1159/000123167] [PMID: 7012657]

[124] Thornton SN, Nicolaidis S. Blood pressure effects of iontophoretically applied bioactive hormones in the anterior forebrain of the rat. Am J Physiol 1993; 265(4 Pt 2): R826-33.
[PMID: 8238453]

[125] Bourque CW. Central mechanisms of osmosensation and systemic osmoregulation. Nat Rev Neurosci 2008; 9(7): 519-31.
[http://dx.doi.org/10.1038/nrn2400] [PMID: 18509340]

[126] Kinsman BJ, Nation HN, Stocker SD. Hypothalamic signaling in body fluid homeostasis and hypertension. Curr Hypertens Rep 2017; 19(6): 50.
[http://dx.doi.org/10.1007/s11906-017-0749-7] [PMID: 28528375]

[127] Kinsman BJ, Simmonds SS, Browning KN, Stocker SD. Organum vasculosum of the lamina terminalis detects NaCl to elevate sympathetic nerve activity and blood pressure. Hypertension 2017; 69(1): 163-70.
[http://dx.doi.org/10.1161/HYPERTENSIONAHA.116.08372] [PMID: 27895193]

[128] Stocker SD, Lang SM, Simmonds SS, Wenner MM, Farquhar WB. Cerebrospinal fluid hypernatremia elevates sympathetic nerve activity and blood pressure via the rostral ventrolateral medulla. Hypertension 2015; 66(6): 1184-90.
[http://dx.doi.org/10.1161/HYPERTENSIONAHA.115.05936] [PMID: 26416846]

[129] Ito S, Hiratsuka M, Komatsu K, Tsukamoto K, Kanmatsuse K, Sved AF. Ventrolateral medulla AT1 receptors support arterial pressure in Dahl salt-sensitive rats. Hypertension 2003; 41(3 Pt 2): 744-50.
[http://dx.doi.org/10.1161/01.HYP.0000052944.54349.7B] [PMID: 12623990]

[130] Ito S, Komatsu K, Tsukamoto K, Sved AF. Tonic excitatory input to the rostral ventrolateral medulla in Dahl salt-sensitive rats. Hypertension 2001; 37(2 Pt 2): 687-91.
[http://dx.doi.org/10.1161/01.HYP.37.2.687] [PMID: 11230357]

[131] Son SJ, Filosa JA, Potapenko ES, *et al.* Dendritic peptide release mediates interpopulation crosstalk between neurosecretory and preautonomic networks. Neuron 2013; 78(6): 1036-49.
[http://dx.doi.org/10.1016/j.neuron.2013.04.025] [PMID: 23791197]

[132] Ribeiro N, Panizza HdoN, Santos KM, Ferreira-Neto HC, Antunes VR. Salt-induced sympathoexcitation involves vasopressin V1a receptor activation in the paraventricular nucleus of the hypothalamus. Am J Physiol Regul Integr Comp Physiol 2015; 309(11): R1369-79.
[http://dx.doi.org/10.1152/ajpregu.00312.2015] [PMID: 26354848]

[133] Brown CD, Higgins M, Donato KA, *et al.* Body mass index and the prevalence of hypertension and dyslipidemia. Obes Res 2000; 8(9): 605-19.
[http://dx.doi.org/10.1038/oby.2000.79] [PMID: 11225709]

[134] Hall JE, da Silva AA, do Carmo JM, *et al.* Obesity-induced hypertension: role of sympathetic nervous system, leptin, and melanocortins. J Biol Chem 2010; 285(23): 17271-6.
[http://dx.doi.org/10.1074/jbc.R110.113175] [PMID: 20348094]

[135] DeMarco VG, Aroor AR, Sowers JR. The pathophysiology of hypertension in patients with obesity. Nat Rev Endocrinol 2014; 10(6): 364-76.
[http://dx.doi.org/10.1038/nrendo.2014.44] [PMID: 24732974]

[136] Wofford MR, Anderson DC Jr, Brown CA, Jones DW, Miller ME, Hall JE. Antihypertensive effect of alpha- and beta-adrenergic blockade in obese and lean hypertensive subjects. Am J Hypertens 2001; 14(7 Pt 1): 694-8.
[http://dx.doi.org/10.1016/S0895-7061(01)01293-6] [PMID: 11465655]

[137] Rumantir MS, Vaz M, Jennings GL, *et al.* Neural mechanisms in human obesity-related hypertension. J Hypertens 1999; 17(8): 1125-33.

[http://dx.doi.org/10.1097/00004872-199917080-00012] [PMID: 10466468]

[138] Davy KP, Orr JS. Sympathetic nervous system behavior in human obesity. Neurosci Biobehav Rev 2009; 33(2): 116-24.
[http://dx.doi.org/10.1016/j.neubiorev.2008.05.024] [PMID: 18602694]

[139] Anderson EA, Hoffman RP, Balon TW, Sinkey CA, Mark AL. Hyperinsulinemia produces both sympathetic neural activation and vasodilation in normal humans. J Clin Invest 1991; 87(6): 2246-52.
[http://dx.doi.org/10.1172/JCI115260] [PMID: 2040704]

[140] Reaven GM, Lithell H, Landsberg L. Hypertension and associated metabolic abnormalities--the role of insulin resistance and the sympathoadrenal system. N Engl J Med 1996; 334(6): 374-81.
[http://dx.doi.org/10.1056/NEJM199602083340607] [PMID: 8538710]

[141] Jamerson KA, Julius S, Gudbrandsson T, Andersson O, Brant DO. Reflex sympathetic activation induces acute insulin resistance in the human forearm. Hypertension 1993; 21(5): 618-23.
[http://dx.doi.org/10.1161/01.HYP.21.5.618] [PMID: 8491496]

[142] Masuo K, Mikami H, Ogihara T, Tuck ML. Sympathetic nerve hyperactivity precedes hyperinsulinemia and blood pressure elevation in a young, nonobese Japanese population. Am J Hypertens 1997; 10(1): 77-83.
[http://dx.doi.org/10.1016/S0895-7061(96)00303-2] [PMID: 9008251]

[143] Anderson EA, Mark AL. The vasodilator action of insulin. Implications for the insulin hypothesis of hypertension. Hypertension 1993; 21(2): 136-41.
[http://dx.doi.org/10.1161/01.HYP.21.2.136] [PMID: 8428776]

[144] Wenzel UO, Bode M, Kurts C, Ehmke H. Salt, inflammation, IL-17 and hypertension. Br J Pharmacol 2018.
[PMID: 29767465]

[145] Marques FZ, Morris BJ. Neurogenic hypertension: revelations from genome-wide gene expression profiling. Curr Hypertens Rep 2012; 14(6): 485-91.
[http://dx.doi.org/10.1007/s11906-012-0282-7] [PMID: 22639016]

[146] Jia H, Sharma P, Hopper R, Dickerson C, Lloyd DD, Brown MJ. Beta2-adrenoceptor gene polymorphisms and blood pressure variations in East Anglian Caucasians. J Hypertens 2000; 18(6): 687-93.
[http://dx.doi.org/10.1097/00004872-200018060-00005] [PMID: 10872552]

[147] Bray MS, Krushkal J, Li L, *et al.* Positional genomic analysis identifies the beta(2)-adrenergic receptor gene as a susceptibility locus for human hypertension. Circulation 2000; 101(25): 2877-82.
[http://dx.doi.org/10.1161/01.CIR.101.25.2877] [PMID: 10869257]

[148] Ziakas A, Gossios T, Doumas M, Karali K, Megarisiotou A, Stiliadis I. The pathophysiological basis of renal nerve ablation for the treatment of hypertension. Curr Vasc Pharmacol 2014; 12(1): 23-9.
[http://dx.doi.org/10.2174/157016111113119990145] [PMID: 23905601]

[149] Preis SR, Massaro JM, Robins SJ, *et al.* Abdominal subcutaneous and visceral adipose tissue and insulin resistance in the Framingham heart study. Obesity (Silver Spring) 2010; 18(11): 2191-8.
[http://dx.doi.org/10.1038/oby.2010.59] [PMID: 20339361]

[150] Petersen JS, DiBona GF. Acute sympathoinhibitory actions of metformin in spontaneously hypertensive rats. Hypertension 1996; 27(3 Pt 2): 619-25.
[http://dx.doi.org/10.1161/01.HYP.27.3.619] [PMID: 8613213]

[151] Izzo JL Jr, Swislocki ALM. Workshop III-Insulin resistance: is it truly the link? Am J Med 1991; 90 (2A): 26S-31S.
[http://dx.doi.org/10.1016/0002-9343(91)90033-T] [PMID: 1994712]

[152] Leal VdeO, Mafra D. Adipokines in obesity. Clin Chim Acta 2013; 419: 87-94.
[http://dx.doi.org/10.1016/j.cca.2013.02.003] [PMID: 23422739]

[153] De Rosa A, Monaco ML, Capasso M, *et al.* Adiponectin oligomers as potential indicators of adipose tissue improvement in obese subjects. Eur J Endocrinol 2013; 169(1): 37-43.
[http://dx.doi.org/10.1530/EJE-12-1039] [PMID: 23612446]

[154] Smith MM, Minson CT. Obesity and adipokines: effects on sympathetic overactivity. J Physiol 2012; 590(8): 1787-801.
[http://dx.doi.org/10.1113/jphysiol.2011.221036] [PMID: 22351630]

[155] Tabak O, Simsek G, Erdenen F, *et al.* The relationship between circulating irisin, retinol binding protein-4, adiponectin and inflammatory mediators in patients with metabolic syndrome. Arch Endocrinol Metab 2017; 61(6): 515-23.
[http://dx.doi.org/10.1590/2359-3997000000289] [PMID: 28977161]

[156] Trombetta IC, Batalha LT, Rondon MU, *et al.* Weight loss improves neurovascular and muscle metaboreflex control in obesity. Am J Physiol Heart Circ Physiol 2003; 285(3): H974-82.
[http://dx.doi.org/10.1152/ajpheart.01090.2002] [PMID: 12714324]

[157] Straznicky NE, Lambert EA, Lambert GW, Masuo K, Esler MD, Nestel PJ. Effects of dietary weight loss on sympathetic activity and cardiac risk factors associated with the metabolic syndrome. J Clin Endocrinol Metab 2005; 90(11): 5998-6005.
[http://dx.doi.org/10.1210/jc.2005-0961] [PMID: 16091482]

[158] Ashida T, Ono C, Sugiyama T. Effects of short-term hypocaloric diet on sympatho-vagal interaction assessed by spectral analysis of heart rate and blood pressure variability during stress tests in obese hypertensive patients. Hypertens Res 2007; 30(12): 1199-203.
[http://dx.doi.org/10.1291/hypres.30.1199] [PMID: 18344625]

[159] Shiiya T, Nakazato M, Mizuta M, *et al.* Plasma ghrelin levels in lean and obese humans and the effect of glucose on ghrelin secretion. J Clin Endocrinol Metab 2002; 87: 240-4.
[http://dx.doi.org/10.1210/jcem.87.1.8129]

[160] Geliebter A, Gluck ME, Hashim SA. Plasma ghrelin concentrations are lower in binge-eating disorder. J Nutri 2005; 135: 1326-30.
[http://dx.doi.org/10.1093/jn/135.5.1326]

[161] Guarino D, Nannipieri M, Iervasi G, Taddei S, Bruno RM. The role of the autonomic nervous system in the pathophysiology of obesity. Front Physiol 2017; 8: 665.
[http://dx.doi.org/10.3389/fphys.2017.00665] [PMID: 28966594]

[162] Virdis A, Lerman LO, Regoli F, Ghiadoni L, Lerman A, Taddei S. Human ghrelin: a gastric hormone with cardiovascular properties. Curr Pharm Des 2016; 22(1): 52-8.
[http://dx.doi.org/10.2174/1381612822666151119144458] [PMID: 26581223]

[163] Matsumura K, Tsuchihashi T, Fujii K, Abe I, Iida M. Central ghrelin modulates sympathetic activity in conscious rabbits. Hypertension 2002; 40(5): 694-9.
[http://dx.doi.org/10.1161/01.HYP.0000035395.51441.10] [PMID: 12411464]

[164] Prior LJ, Davern PJ, Burke SL, Lim K, Armitage JA, Head GA. Exposure to a high-fat diet during development alters leptin and ghrelin sensitivity and elevates renal sympathetic nerve activity and arterial pressure in rabbits. Hypertension 2014; 63(2): 338-45.
[http://dx.doi.org/10.1161/HYPERTENSIONAHA.113.02498] [PMID: 24191287]

[165] Lambert E, Lambert G, Ika-Sari C, *et al.* Ghrelin modulates sympathetic nervous system activity and stress response in lean and overweight men. Hypertension 2011; 58(1): 43-50.
[http://dx.doi.org/10.1161/HYPERTENSIONAHA.111.171025] [PMID: 21502567]

[166] Tavano-Colaizzi L, López-Teros M, Pérez-Lizaur AB, Martínez-Castro N, Isoard-Acosta F, Hernández-Guerrero C. The consumption of antioxidants protects against cognitive and physical disabilities in aged with obesity. Nutr Hosp 2018; 35(4): 811-9.
[PMID: 30070868]

[167] Uzun H, Zengin K, Taskin M, Aydin S, Simsek G, Dariyerli N. Changes in leptin, plasminogen

activator factor and oxidative stress in morbidly obese patients following open and laparoscopic Swedish adjustable gastric banding. Obes Surg 2004; 14(5): 659-65.
[http://dx.doi.org/10.1381/096089204323093453] [PMID: 15186635]

[168] Shi P, Diez-Freire C, Jun JY, *et al.* Brain microglial cytokines in neurogenic hypertension. Hypertension 2010; 56(2): 297-303.
[http://dx.doi.org/10.1161/HYPERTENSIONAHA.110.150409] [PMID: 20547972]

[169] Wei SG, Zhang ZH, Beltz TG, Yu Y, Johnson AK, Felder RB. Subfornical organ mediates sympathetic and hemodynamic responses to blood-borne proinflammatory cytokines. Hypertension 2013; 62(1): 118-25.
[http://dx.doi.org/10.1161/HYPERTENSIONAHA.113.01404] [PMID: 23670302]

[170] Wei SG, Yu Y, Zhang ZH, Felder RB. Proinflammatory cytokines upregulate sympathoexcitatory mechanisms in the subfornical organ of the rat. Hypertension 2015; 65(5): 1126-33.
[http://dx.doi.org/10.1161/HYPERTENSIONAHA.114.05112] [PMID: 25776070]

[171] Bardgett ME, Holbein WW, Herrera-Rosales M, Toney GM. Ang II-salt hypertension depends on neuronal activity in the hypothalamic paraventricular nucleus but not on local actions of tumor necrosis factor-α. Hypertension. 2014; 63: 527-534. 113.02429.

[172] Sriramula S, Cardinale JP, Francis J. Inhibition of TNF in the brain reverses alterations in RAS components and attenuates angiotensin II-induced hypertension. PLoS One 2013; 8(5)e63847.
[http://dx.doi.org/10.1371/journal.pone.0063847] [PMID: 23691105]

[173] Shen XZ, Li Y, Li L, *et al.* Microglia participate in neurogenic regulation of hypertension. Hypertension 2015; 66(2): 309-16.
[http://dx.doi.org/10.1161/HYPERTENSIONAHA.115.05333] [PMID: 26056339]

[174] Bottazzi B, Garlanda C, Cotena A, *et al.* The long pentraxin PTX3 as a prototypic humoral pattern recognition receptor: interplay with cellular innate immunity. Immunol Rev 2009; 227(1): 9-18.
[http://dx.doi.org/10.1111/j.1600-065X.2008.00719.x] [PMID: 19120471]

[175] Erdenen F, Güngel H, Altunoğlu E, *et al.* Association of Plasma Pentraxin-3 Levels with Retinopathy and Systemic Factors in Diabetic Patients. Metab Syndr Relat Disord 2018; 16(7): 358-65.
[http://dx.doi.org/10.1089/met.2018.0023] [PMID: 30036122]

[176] Waki H, Gouraud SS, Maeda M, Paton JF. Evidence of specific inflammatory condition in nucleus tractus solitarii of spontaneously hypertensive rats. Exp Physiol 2010; 95(5): 595-600.
[http://dx.doi.org/10.1113/expphysiol.2009.047324] [PMID: 19923159]

[177] Waki H, Liu B, Miyake M, *et al.* Junctional adhesion molecule-1 is upregulated in spontaneously hypertensive rats: evidence for a prohypertensive role within the brain stem. Hypertension 2007; 49(6): 1321-7.
[http://dx.doi.org/10.1161/HYPERTENSIONAHA.106.085589] [PMID: 17420334]

[178] Paton JF, Dickinson CJ, Mitchell G. Harvey Cushing and the regulation of blood pressure in giraffe, rat and man: introducing 'Cushing's mechanism'. Exp Physiol 2009; 94(1): 11-7.
[http://dx.doi.org/10.1113/expphysiol.2008.043455] [PMID: 18820004]

[179] Skurk T, Mack I, Kempf K, Kolb H, Hauner H, Herder C. Expression and secretion of RANTES (CCL5) in human adipocytes in response to immunological stimuli and hypoxia. Horm Metab Res 2009; 41(3): 183-9.
[http://dx.doi.org/10.1055/s-0028-1093345] [PMID: 18956302]

[180] Mateo T, Abu Nabah YN, Abu Taha M, *et al.* Angiotensin II-induced mononuclear leukocyte interactions with arteriolar and venular endothelium are mediated by the release of different CC chemokines. J Immunol 2006; 176(9): 5577-86.
[http://dx.doi.org/10.4049/jimmunol.176.9.5577] [PMID: 16622027]

[181] Fisher JP, Paton JF. The sympathetic nervous system and blood pressure in humans: implications for hypertension. J Hum Hypertens 2012; 26(8): 463-75.

[http://dx.doi.org/10.1038/jhh.2011.66] [PMID: 21734720]

[182] Rahmouni K, Haynes WG, Morgan DA, Mark AL. Role of melanocortin-4 receptors in mediating renal sympathoactivation to leptin and insulin. J Neurosci 2003; 23(14): 5998-6004.
[http://dx.doi.org/10.1523/JNEUROSCI.23-14-05998.2003] [PMID: 12853417]

[183] Tallam LS, da Silva AA, Hall JE. Melanocortin-4 receptor mediates chronic cardiovascular and metabolic actions of leptin. Hypertension 2006; 48(1): 58-64.
[http://dx.doi.org/10.1161/01.HYP.0000227966.36744.d9] [PMID: 16754792]

[184] Ward KR, Bardgett JF, Wolfgang L, Stocker SD. Sympathetic response to insulin is mediated by melanocortin 3/4 receptors in the hypothalamic paraventricular nucleus. Hypertension 2011; 57(3): 435-41.
[http://dx.doi.org/10.1161/HYPERTENSIONAHA.110.160671] [PMID: 21263116]

[185] do Carmo JM, da Silva AA, Ebaady SE, *et al.* Shp2 signaling in POMC neurons is important for leptin's actions on blood pressure, energy balance, and glucose regulation. Am J Physiol Regul Integr Comp Physiol 2014; 307(12): R1438-47.
[http://dx.doi.org/10.1152/ajpregu.00131.2014] [PMID: 25339680]

[186] Dubinion JH, do Carmo JM, Adi A, Hamza S, da Silva AA, Hall JE. Role of proopiomelanocortin neuron Stat3 in regulating arterial pressure and mediating the chronic effects of leptin. Hypertension 2013; 61(5): 1066-74.
[http://dx.doi.org/10.1161/HYPERTENSIONAHA.111.00020] [PMID: 23529161]

[187] Xue B, Zhang Z, Roncari CF, Guo F, Johnson AK. Aldosterone acting through the central nervous system sensitizes angiotensin II-induced hypertension. Hypertension 2012; 60(4): 1023-30.
[http://dx.doi.org/10.1161/HYPERTENSIONAHA.112.196576] [PMID: 22949534]

[188] Xue B, Thunhorst RL, Yu Y, *et al.* Central renin-angiotensin system activation and inflammation induced by high-fat diet sensitize angiotensin II-elicited hypertension. Hypertension 2016; 67(1): 163-70.
[http://dx.doi.org/10.1161/HYPERTENSIONAHA.115.06263] [PMID: 26573717]

[189] Xue B, Yu Y, Zhang Z, *et al.* Leptin mediates high-fat diet sensitization of angiotensin II-elicited hypertension by upregulating the brain renin-angiotensin system and inflammation. Hypertension 2016; 67(5): 970-6.
[http://dx.doi.org/10.1161/HYPERTENSIONAHA.115.06736] [PMID: 27021010]

[190] Smith PA, Graham LN, Mackintosh AF, Stoker JB, Mary DA. Relationship between central sympathetic activity and stages of human hypertension. Am J Hypertens 2004; 17(3): 217-22.
[http://dx.doi.org/10.1016/j.amjhyper.2003.10.010] [PMID: 15001194]

CHAPTER 11

The Link Between Obesity and Hypertension Through Molecular Mechanisms

Dildar Konukoglu[*]

Department of Biochemistry, Istanbul University-Cerrahpasa, Cerrahpasa Faculty of Medicine, Istanbul, Turkey

Abstract: People with a body mass index of 30 kg/m² or more are considered obese. Obesity is a complex common health problem. It may be the result of several causes and contributing factors and increases the risk of developing a large number of diseases *via* several mechanisms. Dysregulation of appetite control, endocrine mediators secreted from fat tissue, insulin resistance (IR), elevated oxidative and inflammatory stress, and genetic factors are associated with obesity. There are several factors in obesity related to hypertension, such as increased activity of the renin-angiotensin system (RAS), elevated oxidative stress, and endothelial dysfunction. This is a review of link between obesity and hypertension through molecular mechanisms.

Keywords: Endothelial Dysfunction, Hypertension, Inflammation, Insulin Resistance, Obesity.

INTRODUCTION

Obesity is defined as a condition of excess body fat and is associated with an imbalance between calories consumed and calories expended. It is among the most important health problems and is related to increased morbidity and mortality in all over the world. The worldwide prevalence of obesity became more than doubled between 1980 and 2014. Recent World Health Organization global estimates indicated that in 2014, more than 1.9 billion adults aged 18 years and older were overweight. Of these, more than 600 million adults were obese [1 - 3].

Obesity-related health consequences include respiratory problems, musculo-skeletal disorders (like osteoarthritis), skin problems, infertility, type 2 diabetes mellitus, gallbladder disease, cardiovascular disorders (such as hypertension and stroke), and cancers (such as endometrial, breast, and colon cancer) [4, 5]. It has been suggested that severe obesity is associated with a 12-fold increase in morta-

---

[*] **Corresponding author Dildar Konukoglu:** Department of Biochemistry, Istanbul University-Cerrahpasa, Cerrahpasa, Faculty of Medicine, Istanbul, Turkey; Tel:+904143000-21320; E-mail: dkonuk@yahoo.com

Hafize Uzun & Pınar Atukeren (Eds.)

lity when compared with lean individuals [6]. The association of obesity and hypertension has been well established.

Classification of Obesity

To assess obesity, the use of the body mass index (BMI) is commonly recommended (Table 1). BMI is calculated as weight (kg) divided by height in meters squared (m²). Individuals are classified as overweight (BMI=25.0-29.9 kg/m²), class I obese (BMI=30.0-34.9 kg/m²), class II obese (BMI=35.0-39.9 kg/m²), and class III or morbidly obese (BMI>40kg/m²). The ideal BMI is 18.5-24.9 kg/m². Lower BMI cut-off points are applied for some ethnic groups [1, 2, 7, 8]. In children, risk-based, fixed BMI values are not used. The most widely used values are based on age and sex-specific 85th and 95th percentiles for each year of age from 6 to 19 years [9 - 11].

BMI is highly correlated with the fat mass of the body. The accumulation of intra-abdominal fat (also as defined as central obesity or visceral, android, apple-shaped or upper body obesity), which is evaluated by waist circumference, is related to high risks for metabolic and cardiovascular diseases. Therefore, waist circumference should be also used in combination with BMI to examine health risks in both overweight and class I obese patients with a BMI of 30.0-34.9 kg/m² [2]. Waist circumference is measured in the horizontal plane midway between the superior iliac crest and the lower margin of the last rib. The cut-off levels for waist circumference are 94 cm in men and 80 cm in women. The risk of cardiovascular disease, in particular, increases with a waist circumference greater than the cut-off [11, 12].

Table 1. Classification of obesity and health risks [1, 2].

Body Mass Index (kg/m²)	Obesity Degree	Health Risk
<18.5	Underweight	Low
18.5-24.9	Normal/healthy	Average
25.0-29.9	Overweight/pre-obese	Low risk
30.0-34.9	Class I	Elevated risk
35.0-39.9	Class II	High risk
>40	Class III/ morbidly obese	Very high risk
Waist circumference in men <94 cm 94 -102 cm >102 cm	**Waist circumference in women** <80 cm 80-88 cm >88 cm	Low risk High risk Very high risk

Pathogenesis of Obesity

Obesity is a complex and multifactorial health problem. At the simplest level, obesity is a disorder of chronic energy imbalance. Energy balance is the relationship between energy intake and energy expenditure, which are both measured in calories. A positive energy imbalance correlates to increased body weight. The most characteristic feature of obesity is an increased adipose triglyceride content. As a result of long-term overeating, both the adipocyte volume and the adipocyte count increase in the adipose tissue. Therefore, it has been suggested that obesity develops through the combination of increased adipocyte size (hypertrophy) and number (hyperplasia). Complex interactions occur between the regulation of energy balance and fat stores. Biological (including genetic and epigenetic), behavioral, social, and environmental factors (including chronic stress) are involved in the pathogenesis of obesity. The degree of energy control is achieved through endocrine and neural mechanisms [13 - 15].

Adipose tissue not only has a storage function, it also plays an active role in the regulation of the metabolism and body weight, and has endocrine functions. Obesity can also cause changes in hormone levels, as excessive and low levels of hormones can lead to obesity [15 - 18]. Some drugs, such as anticonvulsants, selective serotonin reuptake inhibitors, antipsychotics, corticosteroids, oral contraceptives, and hypoglycemic medications have also been associated with weight gain or obesity [19]. Several mechanisms (inflammation, oxidative stress. or genetic) and many of molecules or hormones (adipokines and insulin) are involved in the pathogenesis of both obesity and obesity-related disorders.

Dysregulation of Appetite Control

Appetite is controlled by the hypothalamus, specifically, the melanocortin system, the arcuate nucleus (ARC) and the melanocortin receptors. The system contains both orexigenic (feeding-stimulating peptides) and anorexigenic neuropeptides (feeding-suppressing peptides). Agouti gene-related protein (AgRP) and neuropeptide Y (NPY) are the primary orexigenic peptides, pro-opiomelanocortin (POMC) and cocaine-amphetamine-regulated transcript (CART) are the primary anorexigenic peptides. There is feedback regulation between feeding and energy balance. Signals from fat tissues act on the melanocortin system to produce reciprocal activation or inhibition. In the hypothalamus, the paraventricular, ventromedial, and lateral nucleus express receptors for adipokines, which are secreted from adipose tissue. In the lateral hypothalamus, there are neurons that both stimulate and inhibit food intake (Fig. **1**). An imbalance between orexigenic and anorexigenic stimulants is related to weight loss or gain [20 - 22].

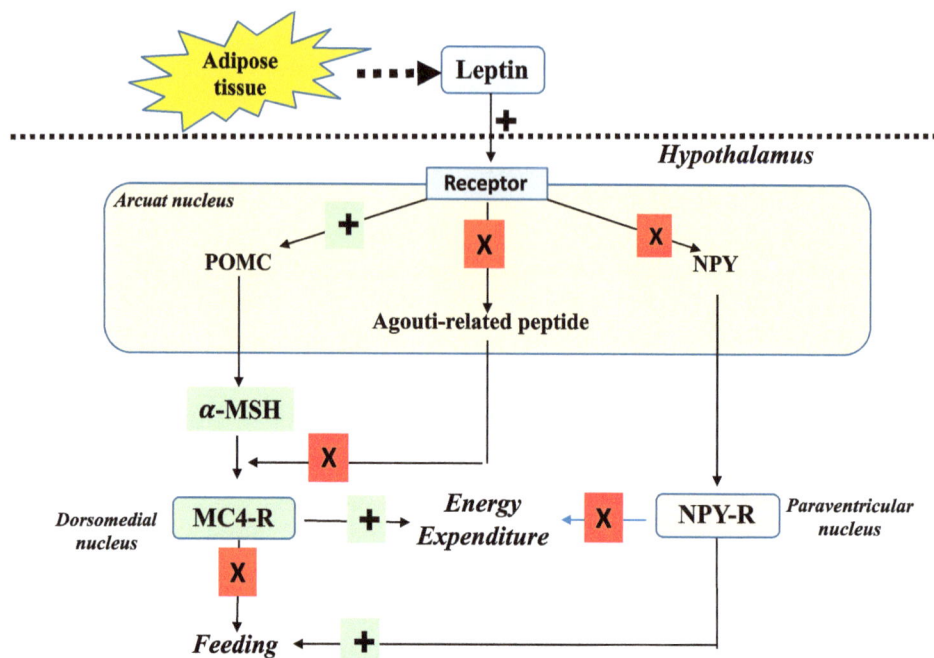

Fig. (1). Effects of leptin on feeding and energy expenditure. AGRP, agouti-related peptide; MCH, melano-cyte concentrating hormone; MC4-R, MSH receptors; MSH, melanocyte-stimulating hormone; NPY, neuropeptide Y; POMC, proopiomelanocortin.

Obesity and Adipokines

Adipokines are mediators secreted from fat tissue that demonstrates both endocrine activity and important roles in the development of obesity and IR (Table **2**). Leptin and adiponectin secreted from fat tissue are 2 basic adipokines [15].

Leptin has a role in energy homeostasis, appetite suppression, and modulation of immune and inflammatory processes. Leptin receptors are expressed in the ARC and the dorsomedial hypothalamus. Elevated anorexigenic POMC expression is related to the serum leptin level and is associated with an increase in anorexigenic POMC expression and a decrease in orexigenic NPY and AgRP. Leptin controls appetite *via* the phosphoinositol-3 kinase and AMP-activated protein kinase (AMPK) signaling pathways. The blockade of AMPK reverses the effect of leptin. Leptin inhibits NPY/AGRP neurons by decreasing AMPK activity, and thereby activates the melanocortin 4 receptor (MC4R) in the paraventricular nucleus of the hypothalamus (PVH) [20, 21]. Activated MC4R further decreases AMPK activity, which can lead to leptin-induced anorexia. Increased visceral adiposity causes hyperleptinemia and hyperinsulinemia, which are poorly regulated by the brain, perpetuating increased caloric intake. Leptin also induces the production of nitric oxide (NO) and several pro-inflammatory cytokines, such as tumor necrosis factor-alpha (TNF-a) and interleukin 6 (IL-6) in monocytes and macrophages [23 - 25].

Adiponectin is a collagen-like plasma protein that regulates several metabolic processes and is important in the control of glucose and fatty acid metabolism. Adiponectin has insulin-sensitizing, anti-atherogenic, and anti-inflammatory properties *via* AMPK and the p38 mitogen-activated protein kinase (MAPK) pathway in skeletal muscle tissue and the vascular endothelium. AdipoR1 and AdipoR2 are membrane receptors for adiponectin. The adaptor protein, phosphotyrosine interaction, PH domain, and leucine zipper-containing protein APPL1 interact directly with adiponectin receptors. APPL1 is necessary to exert the anti-inflammatory and cytoprotective effects of adiponectin on endothelial cells. Overexpression of APPL1 increases adiponectin signaling [26, 27]. Adiponectin also increases the expression and activity of peroxisome proliferator-activated receptors (PPARs), which decrease muscle lipids and improve insulin sensitivity [28]. It has been reported that adiponectin also plays a central role in energy homeostasis through its action in the hypothalamus, and a new role for adiponectin as a "starvation gene" has been proposed [29]. Adiponectin stimulates food intake through AdipoR1 in the hypothalamus. The increased serum levels of inflammatory mediators secreted from adipocytes have been shown to be responsible for inhibiting the synthesis and secretion of adiponectin. Adiponectin increases insulin sensitivity through an inhibition of both the production and action of TNF-a. Therefore, an increased serum level of inflammatory mediators might be responsible for the decreased adiponectin production in obesity [15, 30, 31].

Recent studies have indicated that serum levels of progranulin, which is an adipokine expressed from visceral adipose tissue, are elevated in obese patients and that hyperprogranulinemia may be involved in the pathogenesis of obesity-associated IR [32].

Obesity and Insulin Resistance

Insulin is required for the transport of glucose to muscle and adipose tissue, the release of dietary triglycerides from chylomicrons and endogenous triglycerides from very low-density lipoprotein (VLDL), and the proper function of the PPARs that are the receptors of the peroxisomes. Insulin is bound to its receptor. Conformational changes in the receptor lead to tyrosine autophosphorylation of the cytoplasmic domains. Through auto-phosphorylation, the insulin receptor gains tyrosine kinase activity and stimulates tyrosine phosphorylation of the signaling insulin proteins, including insulin receptor substrates (IRS) 1, 2, 3, and 4, and the Src Homology 2 domain, a protein domain. Activation of IRS-1 or IRS-2 starts a kinase signaling cascade that involves metabolic insulin signaling pathways, such as the phosphatidylinositol 3-kinase, molecular target of rapamycin, RAS, and protein kinase B pathways [33, 34]. IR refers to a loss of sensitivity to insulin in the body's tissue cells. The circulating level of insulin increases. IR stimulates the formation of new fatty tissue and accelerates weight gain. It is well known that IR commonly coexists with obesity.

Table 2. Adipocytokines associated with adipose tissue.

Adipocytokine	Characteristics
Leptin	A protein hormone made by adipose cells that helps to regulate energy balance by appetite suppression.
Adiponectin	A protein hormone that modulates a number of metabolic processes, including glucose regulation and fatty acid oxidation.
Resistin	A protein involved in insulin resistance *via* inflammatory responses.
Interleukin-6	A cell signaling protein (cytokine) involved in inflammatory and in auto-immune processes.
Tumor necrosis factor	A cell cytokine involved in systemic inflammation and in acute phase reaction.
Visfatin	A protein secreted by visceral fat that mimics the effects of insulin.
Apelin	A peptide increased during adipocyte differentiation and stimulated by insulin.
Vaspin	An adipocytokine with insulin-sensitizing effects.
Obestatin	A peptide identified as an anorectic.
Ghrelin	A peptide hormone that stimulate growth hormone receptors. It plays a significant role in regulating the distribution and rate of use of energy.
Adipsin	An adipokine as a prime candidate to coordinate adipose tissue inflammation and the ensuing metabolic consequences of obesity and inflammation.
Omentin	A novel adipokine with insulin-sensitizing effects.
Nesfatin	A potent anorexigenic peptide involved in the regulation of homeostatic feeding.

In IR, several mechanisms may be involved in an impaired insulin-signaling pathway. One mechanism is an elevated state of inflammation. Adipose tissue macrophages, including macrophages that have infiltrated the tissue, are a major source of pro-inflammatory cytokines and chemokines in adipose tissue. These proinflammatory molecules (such as TNF-a, IL-6, IL-1) released from adipose tissue are linked to inflammation and insulin resistance. TNF-a was the first pro-inflammatory cytokine related to inflammation-induced IR. TNF-a stimulates IR in adipose tissue *via* disturbance of the IRS-1 protein and activates the nuclear factor-kappa B (NF-Kb) and Jun NH$_2$-terminal kinase (JNK) signaling pathways.

As a result, TNF-a is associated with a defect in insulin receptor phosphorylation and the kinase pathway [35, 36].

Elevated levels of free fatty acids and triglycerides in the blood stream and tissues in obese individuals due to dietary habits contribute to diminished insulin sensitivity and stimulate endoplasmic reticulum stress through sheer intracellular nutrient and energy flux. The JNK pathway is also activated by endoplasmic reticulum stress. IR is closely linked to increased levels of triglycerides in the liver and muscles as a result of mitochondrial dysfunction in obesity due to oxidative stress [37].

Adipose tissue also expresses RAS components, which play an important role in adipogenesis and lipid and glucose metabolism regulation in an auto/paracrine manner. RAS has been found to be over-activated during adipose tissue enlargement; thus, elevated generation of angiotensin II (Ang II) may contribute to the regulation of adipose tissue homeostasis and IR [38].

Obesity, Oxidative Stress, and Inflammation

Reactive oxygen species (ROS) are generated under normal physiological conditions as well as in the presence of diabetes, cancer, atherosclerosis, and obesity. In many diseases, they cause direct or indirect damage to various organs. Oxidative stress indicates an imbalance between ROS production and the antioxidant system. In stress conditions, ROS levels increase and, due to their high reactivity, they participate in a variety of chemical reactions. Oxidative stress is linked to obesity *via* inflammation [39]. It has been shown that adipose tissue cells produce ROS as intensely as adipokines and increase oxidative stress [40, 41]. Increased secretion of Ang II from adipose tissue also increases the activity of nicotinamide adenine dinucleotide phosphate oxidase, which stimulates the production of ROS from adipocytes [38]. Due to excessive ROS production and increased oxidative stress, obesity is also associated with decreased antioxidant capacity. There are also other several factors associated with increased ROS levels in the obese, such as increased mitochondrial and peroxisomal oxidation of fatty acids, excessive oxygen consumption, and a lipid-rich diet [21, 28]. Obese patients usually have high levels of reactive oxygen or nitrogen species, impaired antioxidant defenses, and increased levels of inflammatory adipokines. It has also been suggested that IR elevates oxidative stress in part by increasing the mitochondrial production of ROS and inactivating antioxidant enzymes [42, 43].

Increased adipose tissue mass and adipocyte hypertrophy lead to macrophage infiltration and inflammation. Adipocytes laden with fats can themselves generate oxidants and free radicals, which in turn can initiate cytokine-dependent signals to activate and recruit macrophages and other inflammatory cells. These cells are also deeply involved in the development of various metabolic disorders and more complex vascular diseases. NF-Kb secreted from adipocytes is a molecular receptor for pathogen binding and inflammatory signals. Due to the activation of the receptor, secretion of inflammatory cytokines, including TNF-a and IL-6, is induced from adipocyte tissue (Fig. **2**). Chronic low-grade inflammation is related to the IR involved in the pathogenesis of both obesity and obesity-related disorders (such as cardiovascular diseases). Another pro-inflammatory response is an increased production of unfolded proteins leading to endoplasmic reticulum stress, which further elevates the chemotactic and pro-inflammatory signal [44 - 46].

Behavioral changes in adipocytes are related to endoplasmic reticulum (ER) stress and oxidative stress-induced mitochondrial dysfunction. ER stress in fat tissue, especially due to overfeeding, can be defined as the accumulation of unfolded or misfolded proteins in the ER lumen. This is called the unfolded protein response (UPR). Incorrectly folded proteins, which cannot pass through the Golgi bodies, are released into the cytoplasm. Their degradation takes place in proteasomes. Unfolded proteins and other conditions act on ER homeostasis. Due to UPR activation, ER metabolism changes and ends in apoptosis. A chronic UPR response initiates metabolic inflammation, impaired insulin action, and glucose metabolism. ER suppresses expression at the resistin mRNA-level associated with IR, which is secreted from adipose tissue. ER stress suppresses the signaling of insulin receptors by providing JNK hyper activation and by increasing the phosphorylation of serine residue of IRS-1. Therefore, ER stress results in IR [47, 48]. A high-calorie diet changes the secretion patterns of chemokines from adipocytes, leading to ER stress. This secretion contributes to inflammation by causing phenotypic changes in macrophages. ER stress mediates mitochondrial dysfunction with the production of NO. NO binds to cytochrome C oxidase by competing with oxygen and suppresses its activity. This changes the flow of calcium between the ER and the mitochondria. The NO-mediated calcium flux enhances the activity of the glucose-regulating protein-78 gene, which responds to ER stress. Studies have shown that ER stress and UPR activation inhibit the signals of hypothalamic leptin receptors, resulting in leptin resistance. Hyperhomocysteinemia also causes ER stress by blocking disulfide bond formation and causing protein misfolding. As a result, ER stress is associated with inflammation and apoptosis in adipose tissue [49, 50].

Peroxisomes are subcellular organelles involved in non-ATP producing oxidations. Their functions are glycerolipid synthesis, cholesterol biosynthesis, cholesterol breakdown, and fatty-acid beta-oxidation. PPARs are classified as PPAR-alpha (PPAR-α), PPAR-beta (PPAR-β) and PPAR-gamma (PPAR-γ). PPAR-α is present in tissues with a high capacity for fatty acid oxidation, including the liver, heart, skeletal muscle, brown fat, and the kidneys, and is important for glucose homeostasis. Leptin stimulates fatty acid oxidation and PPAR-α gene expression. PPAR-β is activated by fatty acids, but its functions are not well understood. PPAR-γ is found in white adipose tissue and immune cells, and has been considered the "master regulator" of adipocyte differentiation. It stimulates the storage of fatty acids in adipocytes and enhances insulin sensitivity to channel fatty acids into adipose tissue [51]. PPAR-γ modulates inflammation by inhibiting the expression of proinflammatory genes, such as cytokines and NF Kb. PPAR-γ can enhance insulin resistance by decreasing the production of proinflammatory mediators and NFKB transcriptional activities and up-regulating IRS proteins. In addition, PPAR-γ has inhibitory effects on inflammation *via* the alteration of immune cell phenotypes toward anti-inflammatory M2 macrophage polarization [28, 30, 36, 52].

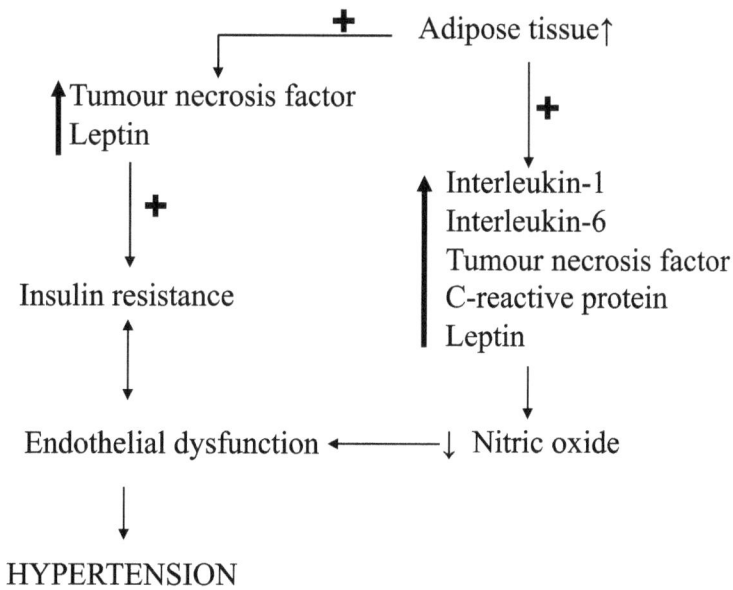

Fig. (2). Molecules involved in the pathogenesis of hypertension by releasing from adipose tissue.

Obesity and Endothelial Dysfunction

The endothelium is endocrine tissue. It has several paracrine functions (vasoactive, inflammatory, vasculoprotective, and angiogenic) and expresses several receptors enrolled in cellular and hormonal events [53]. In healthy endothelial tissues, there is a balance between endothelium-derived relaxing factors and endothelium-derived contracting factors. There are several complex molecular mechanisms in the relationship between obesity and endothelial dysfunction [54, 55]. In endothelial dysfunction, the response of vascular smooth muscle to the vasodilators is impaired, NO bioavailability is decreased, and the elevated sensitivity of endothelial cells to vasoconstrictors is increased. It has been considered that increased oxidative stress may be a major mechanism associated with the pathogenesis of endothelial dysfunction. Disturbance of NO metabolism may be responsible for elevated oxidative stress [42, 56]. Perivascular adipose tissue secretes greater quantities of ROS and adipokines that disrupt NO signaling pathways. Visceral obesity, in particular, induces IR through fat-derived metabolic products, hormones, and adipocytokines. Insulin maintains vascular homeostasis by stimulating production of NO from endothelial cells and limits the growth and migration of vascular smooth muscle cells [57]. When IR appears, the mitogen-activated protein kinase/extracellular signal-regulated kinase pathway is activated, which mediates inflammation, vasoconstriction, and vascular smooth muscle cell proliferation [35, 37]. It has also been indicated that plasma viscosity, an early atherosclerotic risk factor, might be a cardiovascular risk factor in obese patients, along with plasma cholesterol and the atherogenic index [58].

Obesity and Genetics

Monogenic obesity has been associated with a single gene mutation in the leptin gene, the leptin receptor, POMC, and the melanocortin 4 receptor (MC4R). MC4R mutation-linked obesity represents approximately 2% to 3% of obesity cases. In polygenic forms of obesity, gene expression screening can help to identify the key drivers of obesity physiopathology. More than 200 chromosomal regions have been linked to different obesity-related phenotypes, such as fat mass and the distribution of adipose tissue. However, genetic predisposition does not automatically lead to the development of obesity, because eating habits and patterns of physical activity may play a more significant role in weight gain [59, 60]. Even if food intake and exercise are controlled, genetic factors may influence the amount of weight gained through an elevation in energy intake and a reduction in energy consumption. The body of evidence on gene-environment interaction, known as nutrigenomics and nutrigenetics, has grown rapidly [61].

Possible Molecular Link Between Obesity and Hypertension

Obesity and being overweight are conditions that affect body composition and damage and modify aspects of organs. Both are a significant risk factor for hypertension and an indicator of poor response to hypertension treatment [62]. Several molecular mechanisms have been described to explain the association between obesity and hypertension (Figs. **3** and **4**). They include imbalance between pressor/depressor mechanisms (such as RAS) and the sympathetic nervous system (SNS), metabolic dysregulation (such as hyperinsulinemia or adipokine imbalance), and elevated levels of inflammatory cytokines and altered vascular function [63 - 66]. Evidence suggests that abnormal body fat distribution is an important factor in obesity-related morbidity and that visceral adiposity may be related to hypertension, diabetes mellitus, hyperlipidemia, and atherosclerosis. Visceral adipose tissue macrophages produce more proinflammatory cytokines [67, 68]. It has also been indicated that genetic and environmental factors may be important in obesity-related hypertension [69]. However, the exact mechanisms of the relationship between obesity and hypertension are still not fully understood.

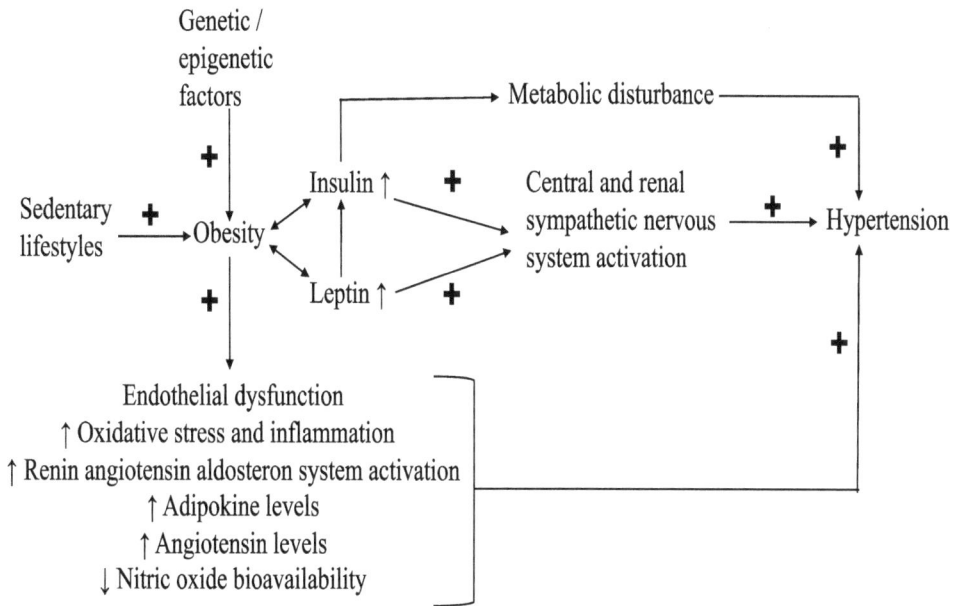

Fig. (3). Causes of obesity and links between obesity and hypertension.

Increased Activity of RAS in Obesity is Related to Hypertension

Obesity increases tissue blood flow and cardiac output and decreases blood flow reserve. Obesity-related increased activity of RAS is an important pathophysiological mechanism for obesity-related hypertension [70]. In the circulation, the majority of the angiotensinogen contents come from the adipose tissue, but Ang I and Ang II are also produced locally and simultaneously taken up from plasma by adipose tissue cells. Ang receptors are overexpressed in the intra-abdominal adipose tissue in obesity [71].

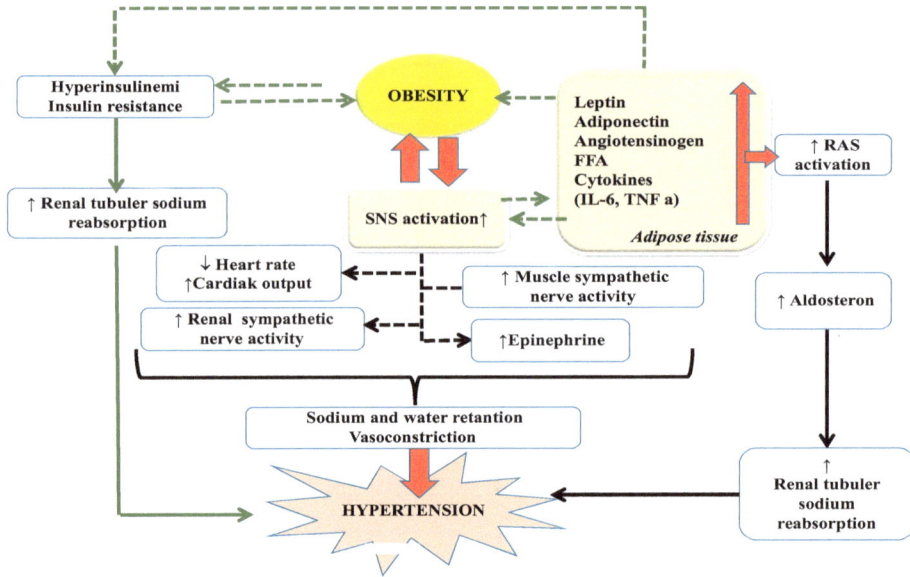

Fig. (4). The relationship between obesity and the pathogenesis of hypertension. SNS, santral nerve system, RAS, renin-angiotensin system, FFA, free fatty acid.

Increased blood pressure, cardiac output, and heart rate due to long-term overactivity of the SNS and RAS and increased renal tubular sodium reabsorption in human obesity are associated with leptin, adiponectin, Ang II, insulin, and cytokines released from adipocytes [72 - 74]. These molecules trigger inflammation, oxidative stress, activation of RAS, and abnormal lipid metabolism. Evidence has suggested that the majority of the alterations of kidney function in obesity are mediated by increased levels of leptin, the stimulation of POMC neurons, and activation of central nervous system MC4Rs [75]. It has been reported that elevated leptin and insulin levels in circulation with decreased ghrelin or adiponectin levels were related to the activation of SNA in obesity [76]. Brain RAS is a necessary prerequisite for leptin-induced sympathetic activation. Due to the overexpression of neuropeptide Y (NPY) in leptin resistance, sympathetic activation occurs and NPY, as a vasoconstrictor, could play a role in obesity-related hypertension [77, 78].

Another mechanism may be an elevated aldosterone level in obesity, but the mechanism by which excess fat may increase aldosterone is as yet unknown [79]. Aldosterone can raise blood pressure in patients who are obese through mineralocorticoid receptors located in different tissues, including the kidneys, the vasculature, and the brain [80, 81]. A recent study suggested that leptin is a direct agonist for aldosterone secretion and that VLDL directly stimulates aldosterone biosynthesis [82].

It has been also reported that the elevated levels and abnormally distributed free-fatty acid levels in obese hypertensives is associated with enhanced vascular alpha-adrenergic sensitivity, and consequently the increase of alpha-adrenergic tone [83]. It has been reported that activity of adipose tissue Na^+-K^+-ATPase in obese patients was decreased and negatively correlated with BMI and blood pressure [84].

In summary, systematic vasoconstriction, direct sodium and water retention, and aldosterone production are greater in obesity-related hypertension and these changes are associated with several fat tissue derived molecules.

Leptin Resistance in Obesity and Effects on Blood Pressure

In obesity, leptin resistance and hyperleptinemia develop. Leptin has sympathetic, vascular, and renal actions that can influence blood pressure, and the SNS-stimulating effects of leptin mainly affect the kidneys, adrenal gland, and brown adipose tissue. Therefore, hyperleptinemia or leptin resistance may be the cause of chronically elevated SNS in obesity. Possible mechanisms of leptin-related hypertension in obesity reported in studies include following [17, 24, 42, 61, 76 - 79, 81 - 90]:

a. Chronic increases in plasma leptin lead to increases in SNS activity.
b. Leptin-induced increases in renal sympathetic activity and blood pressure are mediated by the ventromedial and dorsomedial hypothalamus.
c. In the leptin-resistant state, NPY is overexpressed and it is released from neural sites by sympathetic activation and acts as a vasoconstrictor; thus, it could play a role in obesity-related hypertension.
d. Leptin stimulates the divergent signaling pathways downstream from the leptin receptor. Phosphoinositol-3 kinase is an important intracellular signaling pathway in the control of renal sympathetic outflow because renal sympathoactivation to leptin is prevented by inhibition of this enzyme. The other mechanism is the possible divergent control of cardiovascular function and metabolic functions by the central nervous system (CNS) POMC-MC3/4R pathway.
e. The melanocortin system is an essential downstream mediator of leptin action on renal sympathetic outflow and blood pressure. Chronic activation of the CNS POMC-MC3/4R pathway causes SNS activation and hypertension. Activation of the POMC-MC3/4R pathway mediates the chronic effects of leptin on SNS activation and blood pressure.
f. Elevation in leptin levels triggers oxidative stress in endothelial cells, and

leptin-induced chronic oxidative stress may activate atherogenic processes, contributing to the development of vascular pathology. Additionally, it has been reported that leptin increases the production of endothelial NO in isolated blood vessels, and that leptin has pressor and depressor actions. It has been reported that hypertensive obese women have significantly increased plasma leptin levels when compared with normotensive obese women, and that hyperleptinemia may be responsible for the decreased bioactive mono-nitrogen oxide levels, possibly due to its degradation by ROS in obese hypertensives.

Insulin Resistance-Linked Obesity Triggers Hypertension

It has been suggested that abdominal obesity, in particular, could be an important, complex marker in the IR-hypertension relationship [17, 42, 91 - 97].

a. IR in obesity-related hypertension is associated with both impaired vascular endothelial function and increased SNS activity. Insulin-stimulated renal sodium transport was observed to have a significant role in the pathogenesis of hypertension in IR. Several mechanisms may play a role in this process. In addition, insulin directly increases sympathetic nerve activity.

b. Insulin stimulates all of the transporters involved in sodium absorption, including Na^+-K^+-ATPase, and the sodium bicarbonate cotransporter *via* a signaling cascade involving phosphoinositide 3-kinase, 3-phosphoinosid--dependent protein kinase, and serum/glucocorticoid-kinase 1. Insulin also stimulates sodium chloride reabsorption in Henle's loop.

c. IRS1 signaling defects have been associated with IR in that sodium retention *via* the IRS1-independent pathway is facilitated by hyperinsulinemia.

d. Ang II may increase sodium reabsorption from the proximal tubule in IR. RAS is also related to impaired insulin signaling and systemic IR in various tissues and organs.

e. Vascular effects of insulin include vasoconstriction, vascular smooth muscle cell proliferation and proinflammatory activity by the MAPK pathway.

f. IR is related to an impaired insulin-stimulated NO pathway and an activated MAPK pathway, which may result in vasoconstriction, elevated proinflammation markers, increased sodium and water retention, and elevated blood pressure.

g. Cytokine differences are associated with IR and play an important role in the pathogenesis of endothelial dysfunction.

h. Visceral adipose tissue (VAT) secretes adipokines that act on IR and the vasculature, and the RAS may be more active in VAT than in other adipose tissue.

Obesity Triggers Hypertension *via* Endothelial Dysfunction

Endothelium dysfunction can lead to harmful functional changes in vascular structure. Premature aging and increased turnover of endothelial cells are associated with vasoconstriction. Chronic inflammation can also trigger oxidative stress, which has been associated with hypertension. It has been reported that hypertensives have higher plasma concentrations of pro-inflammatory cytokines. In endothelial dysfunction, NO bioavailability seems to play a central role in the development and progress of hypertension [24, 96 - 99].

It has been well documented that both increased inflammation and oxidative stress induced by fat mass in obesity are involved in the pathogenesis of hypertension. Increased oxidative stress leads to endothelial dysfunction, which, in turn, leads to vascular disruption in obesity [100]. Obesity-induced ROS elevation also promotes vasoconstriction and vascular hypertrophy. Recent evidence suggests that hyperleptinemia may induce systemic oxidative stress and decrease the level of bioactive NO, possibly due to degradation by ROS. This may be one of the most important mechanisms in the generation of hypertension in obesity [101, 102]. Insulin has endothelin-1-dependent vasoconstrictor actions on the vasculature. Endothelin is secreted by endothelial cells and causes vasoconstriction and hypertension. Therefore, IR is related to endothelin-mediated vasoconstriction in the pathogenesis of hypertension [96, 97].

In summary, both hyperleptinemia and hyperinsulinemia in obesity play a role in the pathogenesis of hypertension in relation to endothelial dysfunction.

CONCLUDING REMARKS

Hypertension is one of the major risk factors of cardiovascular disease, but the etiology of this disease is still not fully understood. Obesity and excess weight gain are major causes of human hypertension. Multiple potential mechanisms could play a role in the relationship between obesity and hypertension. These include hyperinsulinemia, activation of the RAS, SNS stimulation, and elevated levels of certain adipokines, such as leptin, or cytokines acting at the vascular endothelial level. Awareness of the link between obesity and hypertension is very important for pharmacological intervention. Early intervention or prevention of obesity can improve the health of the population. In future technological advances in the area of metabolomics have vastly improved the sensitivity and accuracy at which metabolites can be detected and characterized, and metabolomic profiling might help answer these questions.

CONSENT FOR PUBLICATION

Not applicable.

CONFLICT OF INTEREST

The authors declare no conflict of interest, financial or otherwise.

ACKNOWLEDGEMENT

Declared none.

REFERENCES

[1]   World Health Organization. Physical status: The use and interpretation of anthropometry. Report of a WHO Expert Committee. WHO Technical Report Series 854. Geneva: World Health Organization, 1995

[2]   World Health Organization. Obesity: preventing and managing the global epidemic. Report of a WHO Consultation. WHO Technical Report Series 894. Geneva: World Health Organization, 2000.

[3]   James WP. The epidemiology of obesity: the size of the problem. J Intern Med 2008; 263(4): 336-52.
        [http://dx.doi.org/10.1111/j.1365-2796.2008.01922.x] [PMID: 18312311]

[4]   Jung UJ, Choi MS. Obesity and its metabolic complications: the role of adipokines and the relationship between obesity, inflammation, insulin resistance, dyslipidemia and nonalcoholic fatty liver disease. Int J Mol Sci 2014; 15(4): 6184-223.
        [http://dx.doi.org/10.3390/ijms15046184] [PMID: 24733068]

[5]   Tilg H, Moschen AR. Mechanisms behind the link between obesity and gastrointestinal cancers. Best Pract Res Clin Gastroenterol 2014; 28(4): 599-610.
        [http://dx.doi.org/10.1016/j.bpg.2014.07.006] [PMID: 25194178]

[6]   Freedman DS, Kahn HS, Mei Z, *et al.* Relation of body mass index and waist-to-height ratio to cardiovascular disease risk factors in children and adolescents: the Bogalusa Heart Study. Am J Clin Nutr 2007; 86(1): 33-40.
        [http://dx.doi.org/10.1093/ajcn/86.1.33] [PMID: 17616760]

[7]   Seidell JC, Verschuren WM, van Leer EM, Kromhout D. Overweight, underweight, and mortality. A prospective study of 48,287 men and women. Arc Int Med 1996; 156: 958-63.
        [http://dx.doi.org/10.1001/archinte.1996.00440090054006]

[8]   American Diabetes Association. Type 2 diabetes in children and adolescents. Diabetes Care 2000; 23(3): 381-9.
        [http://dx.doi.org/10.2337/diacare.23.3.381] [PMID: 10868870]

[9]   NICE Clinical Guideline. identification assessment and management of overweight and obesity in children young people and adults. 2014.

[10]   Must A, Dallal GE, Dietz WH. Reference data for obesity: 85th and 95th percentiles of body mass index (wt/ht2) and triceps skinfold thickness. Am J Clin Nutr 1991; 53(4): 839-46.
        [http://dx.doi.org/10.1093/ajcn/53.4.839] [PMID: 2008861]

[11]   World Health Organization. Physical status: The use and interpretation of anthropometry. Report of the WHO Expert Committee. WHO Technical Report Series 854. World Health Organization, Geneva, Switzerland, 1995.

[12]   Yumuk V, Tsigos C, Fried M, *et al.* Obesity management task force of the European association for the study of obesity. European guidelines for obesity management in adults. Obes Facts 2015; 8(6):

402-24.
[http://dx.doi.org/10.1159/000442721] [PMID: 26641646]

[13]   Rahmouni K. Cardiovascular regulation by the arcuate nucleus of the hypothalamus: neurocircuitry and signaling systems. Hypertension 2016; 67(6): 1064-71.
[http://dx.doi.org/10.1161/HYPERTENSIONAHA.115.06425] [PMID: 27045026]

[14]   Wynne K, Stanley S, McGowan B, Bloom S. Appetite control. J Endocrinol 2005; 184(2): 291-318.
[http://dx.doi.org/10.1677/joe.1.05866] [PMID: 15684339]

[15]   Maury E, Brichard SM. Adipokine dysregulation, adipose tissue inflammation and metabolic syndrome. Mol Cell Endocrinol 2010; 314(1): 1-16.
[http://dx.doi.org/10.1016/j.mce.2009.07.031] [PMID: 19682539]

[16]   Mishra AK, Dubey V, Ghosh AR. Obesity: An overview of possible role(s) of gut hormones, lipid sensing and gut microbiota. Metabolism 2016; 65(1): 48-65.
[http://dx.doi.org/10.1016/j.metabol.2015.10.008] [PMID: 26683796]

[17]   Ercan M, Konukoglu D. Role of plasma viscosity and plasma homocysteine level on hyperinsulinemic obese female subjects. Clin Hemorheol Microcirc 2008; 38(4): 227-34.
[PMID: 18334777]

[18]   Engin A. The pathogenesis of obesity-associated adipose tissue inflammation. Adv Exp Med Biol 2017; 960: 221-45.
[http://dx.doi.org/10.1007/978-3-319-48382-5_9] [PMID: 28585201]

[19]   Van Zyl M. The effects of drugs on nutrition. South Afr J Clin Nutr 2011; 24(3): S38-4.
[http://dx.doi.org/10.1080/16070658.2011.11734380]

[20]   Timper K, Brüning JC. Hypothalamic circuits regulating appetite and energy homeostasis: Pathways to obesity. Dis Model Mech. 2017,1;10(6):679-89.
[http://dx.doi.org/10.1242/dmm.026609]

[21]   Sominsky L, Spencer SJ. Eating behavior and stress: a pathway to obesity. Front Psychol 2014; 5(5): 434-40.
[http://dx.doi.org/10.3389/fpsyg.2014.00434] [PMID: 24860541]

[22]   Baltatzi M, Hatzitolios A, Tziomalos K, Iliadis F, Zamboulis Ch. Neuropeptide Y and alpha-melanocyte-stimulating hormone: interaction in obesity and possible role in the development of hypertension. Int J Clin Pract 2008; 62(9): 1432-40.
[http://dx.doi.org/10.1111/j.1742-1241.2008.01823.x] [PMID: 18793378]

[23]   Laursen TL, Zak RB, Shute RJ, *et al.* Leptin, adiponectin, and ghrelin responses to endurance exercise in different ambient conditions. Temperature (Austin). 2017;13;4(2):166- 75.
[http://dx.doi.org/10.1080/23328940.2017.1294235] [PMID: 28680932]

[24]   Konukoglu D, Serin O, Turhan MS. Plasma leptin and its relationship with lipid peroxidation and nitric oxide in obese female patients with or without hypertension. Arch Med Res 2006; 37(5): 602-6.
[http://dx.doi.org/10.1016/j.arcmed.2005.12.002] [PMID: 16740429]

[25]   Konukoglu D, Serin O, Ercan M. Plasma leptin levels in obese and non-obese postmenopausal women before and after hormone replacement therapy. Maturitas 2000; 36(3): 203-7.
[http://dx.doi.org/10.1016/S0378-5122(00)00153-5] [PMID: 11063902]

[26]   Ebrahimi-Mamaeghani M, Mohammadi S, Arefhosseini SR, Fallah P, Bazi Z. Adiponectin as a potential biomarker of vascular disease. Vasc Health Risk Manag 2015; 11: 55-70.
[http://dx.doi.org/10.2147/VHRM.S48753] [PMID: 25653535]

[27]   Deepa SS. Role in adiponectin signaling and beyond. Am J Physiol Endocrinol Metab. 2009 ;296 (1):E 22-36.
[http://dx.doi.org/10.1152/ajpendo.90731] [PMID: 18854421]

[28]   Ye JM, Doyle PJ, Iglesias MA, Watson DG, Cooney GJ, Kraegen EW. Peroxisome proliferator-

activated receptor (PPAR)-alpha activation lowers muscle lipids and improves insulin sensitivity in high fat-fed rats: comparison with PPAR-gamma activation. Diabetes 2001; 50(2): 411-7.
[http://dx.doi.org/10.2337/diabetes.50.2.411] [PMID: 11272155]

[29]   Kubota N, Yano W, Kubota T, *et al.* Adiponectin stimulates AMP-activated protein kinase in the hypothalamus and increases food intake. Cell Metab 2007; 6(1): 55-68.
[http://dx.doi.org/10.1016/j.cmet.2007.06.003] [PMID: 17618856]

[30]   Fantuzzi G. Adiponectin in inflammatory and immune-mediated diseases. Cytokine 2013; 64(1): 1-10.
[http://dx.doi.org/10.1016/j.cyto.2013.06.317] [PMID: 23850004]

[31]   Liu C, Feng X, Li Q, Wang Y, Li Q, Hua M. Adiponectin, TNF-α and inflammatory cytokines and risk of type 2 diabetes: A systematic review and meta-analysis. Cytokine 2016; 86: 100-9.
[http://dx.doi.org/10.1016/j.cyto.2016.06.028] [PMID: 27498215]

[32]   Eichelmann F, Rudovich N, Pfeiffer AF, *et al.* Novel adipokines: methodological utility in human obesity research. Int J Obes 2017; 41(6): 976-81.
[http://dx.doi.org/10.1038/ijo.2017.68] [PMID: 28293019]

[33]   Schinner S, Scherbaum WA, Bornstein SR, Barthel A. Molecular mechanisms of insulin resistance. Diabet Med 2005; 22(6): 674-82.
[http://dx.doi.org/10.1111/j.1464-5491.2005.01566.x] [PMID: 15910615]

[34]   Erion KA, Corkey BE. Hyperinsulinemia: a cause of obesity? Curr Obes Rep 2017; 6(2): 178-86.
[http://dx.doi.org/10.1007/s13679-017-0261-z] [PMID: 28466412]

[35]   Belgardt BF, Mauer J, Brüning JC. Novel roles for JNK1 in metabolism. Aging (Albany NY) 2016; 2(9): 621-26.
[http://dx.doi.org/10.18632/aging.100192] [PMID: 20834068]

[36]   Ye J. Mechanisms of insulin resistance in obesity. Front Med 2013; 7(1): 14-24.
[http://dx.doi.org/10.1007/s11684-013-0262-6] [PMID: 23471659]

[37]   Ramalingam L, Menikdiwela K, LeMieux M, *et al.* The renin angiotensin system, oxidative stress and mitochondrial function in obesity and insulin resistance. Biochim Biophys Acta Mol Basis Dis 2017; 1863(5): 1106-14.
[http://dx.doi.org/10.1016/j.bbadis.2016.07.019] [PMID: 27497523]

[38]   Underwood PC, Adler GK. The renin angiotensin aldosterone system and insulin resistance in humans. Curr Hypertens Rep 2013; 15(1): 59-70.
[http://dx.doi.org/10.1007/s11906-012-0323-2] [PMID: 23242734]

[39]   Khan NI, Naz L, Yasmeen G. Obesity: an independent risk factor for systemic oxidative stress. Pak J Pharm Sci 2006; 19(1): 62-5.
[PMID: 16632456]

[40]   Uzun H, Konukoglu D, Gelisgen R, Zengin K, Taskin M. Plasma protein carbonyl and thiol stress before and after laparoscopic gastric banding in morbidly obese patients. Obes Surg 2007; 17(10): 1367-73.
[http://dx.doi.org/10.1007/s11695-007-9242-8] [PMID: 18000722]

[41]   Konukoğlu D, Serin O, Turhan MS. Plasma total homocysteine concentrations in obese and non-obese female patients with type 2 diabetes mellitus; its relations with plasma oxidative stress and nitric oxide levels. Clin Hemorheol Microcirc 2005; 33(1): 41-6.
[PMID: 16037631]

[42]   Konukoglu D, Turhan MS, Ercan M, Serin O. Relationship between plasma leptin and zinc levels and the effect of insulin and oxidative stress on leptin levels in obese diabetic patients. J Nutr Biochem 2004; 15(12): 757-60.
[http://dx.doi.org/10.1016/j.jnutbio.2004.07.007] [PMID: 15607649]

[43]   Konukoglu D, Uzun H, Firtina S, Cigdem Arica P, Kocael A, Taskin M. Plasma adhesion and inflammation markers: asymmetrical dimethyl-L-arginine and secretory phospholipase A2

concentrations before and after laparoscopic gastric banding in morbidly obese patients. Obes Surg 2007; 17(5): 672-8.
[http://dx.doi.org/10.1007/s11695-007-9113-3] [PMID: 17658029]

[44]   Hotamisligil GS, Arner P, Caro JF, Atkinson RL, Spiegelman BM. Increased adipose tissue expression of tumor necrosis factor-alpha in human obesity and insulin resistance. J Clin Invest 1995; 95(5): 2409-15.
[http://dx.doi.org/10.1172/JCI117936] [PMID: 7738205]

[45]   Fantuzzi G. Adipose tissue, adipokines, and inflammation. J Allergy Clin Immunol 2005; 115(5): 911-9.
[http://dx.doi.org/10.1016/j.jaci.2005.02.023] [PMID: 15867843]

[46]   Edsfeldt A, Grufman H, Asciutto G, *et al.* Circulating cytokines reflect the expression of pro-inflammatory cytokines in atherosclerotic plaques. Atherosclerosis 2015; 241(2): 443-9.
[http://dx.doi.org/10.1016/j.atherosclerosis.2015.05.019] [PMID: 26074318]

[47]   Hotamisligil GS. Endoplasmic reticulum stress and the inflammatory basis of metabolic disease. Cell 2010; 140(6): 900-17.
[http://dx.doi.org/10.1016/j.cell.2010.02.034] [PMID: 20303879]

[48]   Ozcan U, Cao Q, Yilmaz E, *et al.* Endoplasmic reticulum stress links obesity, insulin action, and type 2 diabetes. Science 2004; 306(5695): 457-61.
[http://dx.doi.org/10.1126/science.1103160] [PMID: 15486293]

[49]   Ozcan L, Ergin AS, Lu A, *et al.* Endoplasmic reticulum stress plays a central role in development of leptin resistance. Cell Metab 2009; 9(1): 35-51.
[http://dx.doi.org/10.1016/j.cmet.2008.12.004] [PMID: 19117545]

[50]   Zulli A. Endoplasmic stress inhibitors for homocysteine induced cardiovascular disease. Curr Pharm Des 2016; 22(18): 2704-8.
[http://dx.doi.org/10.2174/1381612822666160406121342] [PMID: 27048458]

[51]   Morino K, Petersen K, Shulman GI. "Molecular mechanisms of insulin resistance in humans and their potential links with mitochondrial dysfunction". Diabetes. 2006; 55 Suppl 2 (Suppl 2): S9–15
[http://dx.doi.org/10.2337/db06-S002] [PMID: 17130651]

[52]   Tyagi S, Gupta P, Saini AS, Kaushal C, Sharma S. The peroxisome proliferator-activated receptor: A family of nuclear receptors role in various diseases. J Adv Pharm Technol Res 2011; 2(4): 236-40.
[http://dx.doi.org/10.4103/2231-4040.90879] [PMID: 22247890]

[53]   Cahill PA, Redmond EM. Vascular endothelium - Gatekeeper of vessel health. Atherosclerosis 2016; 248: 97-109.
[http://dx.doi.org/10.1016/j.atherosclerosis.2016.03.007] [PMID: 26994427]

[54]   Meyers MR, Gokce N. Endothelial dysfunction in obesity: etiological role in atherosclerosis. Curr Opin Endocrinol Diabetes Obes. 2007; 14(5):365-9.
[http://dx.doi.org/10.1097/MED.0b013e3282be90a8] [PMID: 17940464]

[55]   Prieto D, Contreras C, Sánchez A. Endothelial dysfunction, obesity and insulin resistance. Curr Vasc Pharmacol 2014; 12(3): 412-26.
[http://dx.doi.org/10.2174/1570161112666140423221008] [PMID: 24846231]

[56]   Papageorgiou N, Androulakis E, Papaioannou S, Antoniades C, Tousoulis D. Homoarginine in the shadow of asymmetric dimethylarginine: from nitric oxide to cardiovascular disease. Amino Acids 2015; 47(9): 1741-50.
[http://dx.doi.org/10.1007/s00726-015-2017-y] [PMID: 26123985]

[57]   Mather K, Anderson TJ, Verma S. Insulin action in the vasculature: physiology and pathophysiology. J Vasc Res 2001; 38(5): 415-22.
[http://dx.doi.org/10.1159/000051074] [PMID: 11561143]

[58]   Ercan M, Konukoglu D, Erdem Yeşim T. Association of plasma viscosity with cardiovascular risk

factors in obesity: an old marker, a new insight. Clin Hemorheol Microcirc 2006; 35(4): 441-6.
[PMID: 17148842]

[59]   Tao YX. Mutations in melanocortin-4 receptor and human obesity. Prog Mol Biol Transl Sci 2009; 88:
173-204.
[http://dx.doi.org/10.1016/S1877-1173(09)88006-X] [PMID: 20374728]

[60]   Kaur Y, de Souza RJ, Gibson WT, Meyre D. A systematic review of genetic syndromes with obesity.
Obes Rev 2017; 18(6): 603-34.
[http://dx.doi.org/10.1111/obr.12531] [PMID: 28346723]

[61]   Huang T, Hu FB. Gene-environment interactions and obesity: recent developments and future
directions. BMC Med Genomics 2015; 8 (Suppl. 1): S2.
[http://dx.doi.org/10.1186/1755-8794-8-S1-S2] [PMID: 25951849]

[62]   Kotchen TA. Obesity-related hypertension: epidemiology, pathophysiology, and clinical management.
Am J Hypertens 2010; 23(11): 1170-8.
[http://dx.doi.org/10.1038/ajh.2010.172] [PMID: 20706196]

[63]   Kang YS. Obesity associated hypertension: new insights into mechanism. Electrolyte Blood Press
2013; 11(2): 46-52.
[http://dx.doi.org/10.5049/EBP.2013.11.2.46] [PMID: 24627704]

[64]   Lambert GW, Straznicky NE, Lambert EA, Dixon JB, Schlaich MP. Sympathetic nervous activation in
obesity and the metabolic syndrome--causes, consequences and therapeutic implications. Pharmacol
Ther 2010; 126(2): 159-72.
[http://dx.doi.org/10.1016/j.pharmthera.2010.02.002] [PMID: 20171982]

[65]   Konukoglu D, Firtina S, Serin O, Cavusoglu C. Relationship among plasma secretory phospholipase
A2, oxidized low density lipoprotein & paraoxonase activities in hypertensive subjects treated with
angiotensin converting enzyme inhibitors. Indian J Med Res 2009; 129(4): 390-4.
[PMID: 19535833]

[66]   Hall JE. The kidney, hypertension, and obesity. Hypertension 2003; 41(3 Pt 2): 625-33.
[http://dx.doi.org/10.1161/01.HYP.0000052314.95497.78] [PMID: 12623970]

[67]   Soto Rodríguez A, García Soidán JL, Arias Gómez MJ, Leirós Rodríguez R, Del Álamo Alonso A,
Pérez Fernández MR. Metabolic syndrome and visceral fat in women with cardiovascular risk factor.
Nutr Hosp 2017; 34(4): 863-8.
[http://dx.doi.org/10.20960/nh.1085] [PMID: 29095010]

[68]   Matsuzawa Y, Funahashi T, Nakamura T. The concept of metabolic syndrome: contribution of visceral
fat accumulation and its molecular mechanism. J Atheroscler Thromb 2011; 18(8): 629-39.
[http://dx.doi.org/10.5551/jat.7922] [PMID: 21737960]

[69]   Skrypnik K, Suliburska J, Skrypnik D, Pilarski Ł, Reguła J, Bogdański P. The genetic basis of obesity
complications. Acta Sci Pol Technol Aliment 2017; 16(1): 83-91.
[http://dx.doi.org/10.17306/J.AFS.2017.0442] [PMID: 28362475]

[70]   Schütten MT, Houben AJ, de Leeuw PW, Stehouwer CD. The link between adipose tissue renin-
angiotensin-aldosterone system signaling and obesity-associated hypertension. Physiology (Bethesda)
2017; 32(3): 197-209.
[http://dx.doi.org/10.1152/physiol.00037.2016] [PMID: 28404736]

[71]   Slamkova M, Zorad S, Krskova K. Alternative renin-angiotensin system pathways in adipose tissue
and their role in the pathogenesis of obesity. Endocr Regul 2016; 50(4): 229-40.
[http://dx.doi.org/10.1515/enr-2016-0025] [PMID: 27941178]

[72]   Rüster C, Wolf G. The role of the renin-angiotensin-aldosterone system in obesity-related renal
diseases. Semin Nephrol 2013; 33(1): 44-53.
[http://dx.doi.org/10.1016/j.semnephrol.2012.12.002] [PMID: 23374893]

[73]   Kovesdy CP, Furth S, Zoccali C. Obesity and kidney disease: Hidden consequences of the epidemic.

Saudi J Kidney Dis Transpl 2017; 28(2): 241-52.
[http://dx.doi.org/10.4103/1319-2442.202776] [PMID: 28352003]

[74]   Sharma K. The link between obesity and albuminuria: adiponectin and podocyte dysfunction. Kidney Int 2009; 76(2): 145-8.
[http://dx.doi.org/10.1038/ki.2009.137] [PMID: 19404275]

[75]   Kotsis V, Nilsson P, Grassi G, *et al.* New developments in the pathogenesis of obesity-induced hypertension. J Hypertens 2015; 33(8): 1499-508.
[http://dx.doi.org/10.1097/HJH.0000000000000645] [PMID: 26103132]

[76]   Hall JE, do Carmo JM, da Silva AA, Wang Z, Hall ME. Obesity-induced hypertension: interaction of neurohumoral and renal mechanisms. Circ Res 2015; 116(6): 991-1006.
[http://dx.doi.org/10.1161/CIRCRESAHA.116.305697] [PMID: 25767285]

[77]   Hilzendeger AM, Morgan DA, Brooks L, *et al.* A brain leptin-renin angiotensin system interaction in the regulation of sympathetic nerve activity. Am J Physiol Heart Circ Physiol 2012; 303(2): H197-206.
[http://dx.doi.org/10.1152/ajpheart.00974.2011] [PMID: 22610169]

[78]   Kotsis V, Stabouli S, Papakatsika S, Rizos Z, Parati G. Mechanisms of obesity-induced hypertension. Hypertens Res 2010; 33(5): 386-93.
[http://dx.doi.org/10.1038/hr.2010.9] [PMID: 20442753]

[79]   Xie D, Bollag WB. Obesity, hypertension and aldosterone: is leptin the link? J Endocrinol 2016; 230(1): F7-F11.
[http://dx.doi.org/10.1530/JOE-16-0160] [PMID: 27252389]

[80]   Dinh Cat AN, Friederich-Persson M, White A, Touyz RM. Adipocytes, aldosterone and obesity-related hypertension. J Mol Endocrinol 2016; 57(1): F7-F21.
[http://dx.doi.org/10.1530/JME-16-0025] [PMID: 27357931]

[81]   Huby AC, Otvos L Jr, Belin de Chantemèle EJ. Leptin induces hypertension and endothelial dysfunction *via* aldosterone-dependent mechanisms in obese female mice. Hypertension 2016; 67(5): 1020-8.
[http://dx.doi.org/10.1161/HYPERTENSIONAHA.115.06642] [PMID: 26953321]

[82]   Tsai YY, Rainey WE, Bollag WB. Very low-density lipoprotein (VLDL)-induced signals mediating aldosterone production. J Endocrinol 2017; 232(2): R115-29.
[http://dx.doi.org/10.1530/JOE-16-0237] [PMID: 27913572]

[82]   Stepniakowski KT, Goodfriend TL, Egan BM. Fatty acids enhance vascular alpha-adrenergic sensitivity. Hypertension 1995; 25(4 Pt 2): 774-8.
[http://dx.doi.org/10.1161/01.HYP.25.4.774] [PMID: 7721431]

[83]   Frayn KN, Karpe F. Regulation of human subcutaneous adipose tissue blood flow. Int J Obes 2014; 38(8): 1019-26.
[http://dx.doi.org/10.1038/ijo.2013.200] [PMID: 24166067]

[84]   Rahmouni K, Haynes WG, Morgan DA, Mark AL. Intracellular mechanisms involved in leptin regulation of sympathetic outflow. Hypertension 2003; 41(3 Pt 2): 763-7.
[http://dx.doi.org/10.1161/01.HYP.0000048342.54392.40] [PMID: 12623993]

[85]   Niswender KD, Schwartz MW. Insulin and leptin revisited: adiposity signals with overlapping physiological and intracellular signaling capabilities. Front Neuroendocrinol 2003; 24(1): 1-10.
[http://dx.doi.org/10.1016/S0091-3022(02)00105-X] [PMID: 12609497]

[86]   Bell BB, Rahmouni K. Leptin as a mediator of obesity-induced hypertension. Curr Obes Rep 2016; 5(4): 397-404.
[http://dx.doi.org/10.1007/s13679-016-0231-x] [PMID: 27665107]

[87]   Hall JE, da Silva AA, do Carmo JM, *et al.* Obesity-induced hypertension: role of sympathetic nervous system, leptin, and melanocortins. J Biol Chem 2010; 285(23): 17271-6.
[http://dx.doi.org/10.1074/jbc.R110.113175] [PMID: 20348094]

[88] Osório J. Obesity: The many faces of leptin-a novel role for leptin signalling in obesity-induced hypertension. Nat Rev Endocrinol 2015; 11(3): 129-40.
[http://dx.doi.org/10.1038/nrendo.2014.231] [PMID: 25534200]

[89] Barzel B, Lim K, Davern PJ, Burke SL, Armitage JA, Head GA. Central proopiomelanocortin but not neuropeptide Y mediates sympathoexcitation and hypertension in fat fed conscious rabbits. J Hypertens 2016; 34(3): 464-73.
[http://dx.doi.org/10.1097/HJH.0000000000000811] [PMID: 26820476]

[90] Redon J, Cifkova R, Laurent S, *et al.* Mechanisms of hypertension in the cardiometabolic syndrome. J Hypertens 2009; 27(3): 441-51.
[http://dx.doi.org/10.1097/HJH.0b013e32831e13e5] [PMID: 19262221]

[91] Rocchini AP, Katch V, Kveselis D, *et al.* Insulin and renal sodium retention in obese adolescents. Hypertension 1989; 14(4): 367-74.
[http://dx.doi.org/10.1161/01.HYP.14.4.367] [PMID: 2676858]

[92] Horita S, Seki G, Yamada H, Suzuki M, Koike K, Fujita T. Insulin resistance, obesity, hypertension, and renal sodium transport. Int J Hypertens 2011; 2011391762
[http://dx.doi.org/10.4061/2011/391762] [PMID: 21629870]

[93] Nizar JM, Dong W, McClellan RB, *et al.* Na$^+$-sensitive elevation in blood pressure is ENaC independent in diet-induced obesity and insulin resistance. Am J Physiol Renal Physiol. 2016 1;310(9):F812-20.
[http://dx.doi.org/10.1152/ajprenal.00265.2015] [PMID: 26841823]

[94] Tasic I, Lovic D. Hypertension and cardiometabolic disease. Front Biosci (Schol Ed) 2018; 10: 166-74.
[http://dx.doi.org/10.2741/s506] [PMID: 28930524]

[95] Zhou MS, Wang A, Yu H. Link between insulin resistance and hypertension: What is the evidence from evolutionary biology? Diabetol Metab Syndr 2014; 6(1): 12.
[http://dx.doi.org/10.1186/1758-5996-6-12] [PMID: 24485020]

[96] Vaněčková I, Maletínská L, Behuliak M, Nagelová V, Zicha J, Kuneš J. Obesity-related hypertension: possible pathophysiological mechanisms. J Endocrinol 2014; 223(3): R63-78.
[http://dx.doi.org/10.1530/JOE-14-0368] [PMID: 25385879]

[97] Crowley SD. The cooperative roles of inflammation and oxidative stress in the pathogenesis of hypertension. Antioxid Redox Signal 2014; 20(1): 102-20.
[http://dx.doi.org/10.1089/ars.2013.5258] [PMID: 23472597]

[98] Yasunari K, Maeda K, Nakamura M, Yoshikawa J. Oxidative stress in leukocytes is a possible link between blood pressure, blood glucose, and C-reacting protein. Hypertension 2002; 39(3): 777-80.
[http://dx.doi.org/10.1161/hy0302.104670] [PMID: 11897762]

[99] Konukoglu D, Uzun H. Endothelial dysfunction and hypertension. Adv Exp Med Biol 2017; 956: 511-40.
[http://dx.doi.org/10.1007/5584_2016_90] [PMID: 28035582]

[100] Konukoğlu D, Serin O, Ercan M, Turhan MS. Plasma homocysteine levels in obese and non-obese subjects with or without hypertension; its relationship with oxidative stress and copper. Clin Biochem 2003; 36(5): 405-8.
[http://dx.doi.org/10.1016/S0009-9120(03)00059-6] [PMID: 12849875]

[101] Leggio M, Lombardi M, Caldarone E, *et al.* The relationship between obesity and hypertension: an updated comprehensive overview on vicious twins. Hypertens Res 2017; 40(12): 947-63.
[http://dx.doi.org/10.1038/hr.2017.75] [PMID: 28978986]

[102] Lin YJ, Juan CC, Kwok CF, *et al.* Endothelin-1 exacerbates development of hypertension and atherosclerosis in modest insulin resistant syndrome. Biochem Biophys Res Commun 2015; 460(3): 497-503.

CHAPTER 12

Significance of Vitamin D Status in Elderly Patients with Systemic Arterial Hypertension

Bahadir Simsek and **Ufuk Çakatay**[*]

Department of Medical Biochemistry, Istanbul University – Cerrahpaşa, Cerrahpaşa Faculty of Medicine, Istanbul, Turkey

Abstract: Hypertension is a significant contributing factor to cardiovascular disease, accounting for a significant mortality and morbidity. The elderly and aging population of our planet, a risk factor for vitamin D deficiency, requires a deeper understanding of the importance of Vitamin D. Musculoskeletal effects of Vitamin D has been well known. Extra-musculoskeletal effects of Vitamin D in cardiovascular health, cancer, diabetes and immunity has been a hot topic for the last decade. Even though Vitamin D deficiency has been shown to play a role in the aggravation of cardiovascular health, understanding of the fundamental mechanisms and the solidity of the data to suggest a causation between Vitamin D deficiency and non-musculoskeletal effects is mostly lacking and these issues have been largely neglected by attending physicians. In this chapter, we explain the proposed mechanisms of the effects of Vitamin D on extra skeletal tissues, summarize complex mechanisms with a special emphasis on hypertension in the elderly and talk about Vitamin D analogues and validity of evidence with regard to non-skeletal effects of Vitamin D in the body.

Keywords: Aging, Apoptosis, Calcitriol, Cardiovascular aging, Cardiovascular disease, Doxercalciferol, Elderly, Hypercalcemia, Hypertension, Klotho, Osteoblast-like cell, Osteoclast-like cell, Paricalcitol, Renin angiotensin aldosterone system, Vascular smooth muscle cell, Vitamin D, Vitamin D analogues, Vitamin D deficiency, Vitamin D receptor, 25-Hydroxyvitamin D.

CARDIOVASCULAR DISEASE AND VITAMIN D

Cardiovascular disease, being one of the leading causes of death, is taking a toll on health care systems and is a major problem worldwide. Cardiovascular diseases represent almost one third of all deaths globally. Systemic arterial hypertension, one of the major culprits in cardiovascular diseases, is closely associated with more than half of the adverse events [1]. Vitamin D, 25(OH)D, insufficiency is highly prevalent among elderly individuals and may contribute to

[*] **Corresponding author Ufuk Çakatay;** Department of Medical Biochemistry, Istanbul University – Cerrahpaşa, Cerrahpaşa Faculty of Medicine, Istanbul, Turkey; Tel: +905307882131; E-mail: ufuk.cakatay@istanbul.edu.tr

Hafize Uzun & Pınar Atukeren (Eds.)

systemic arterial hypertension [2]. A correlation between vitamin D and systemic arterial hypertension is interesting and considering the evidence, causative relationship may exist. It has been noted for decades that Nordic countries with less year-round sunlight, such as those furthest from the equator and at high altitudes, have a higher prevalence of ischemic heart disease and hypertension than those with more sunlight [3]. Interestingly, the incidence of new cardiovascular events is highest during the winter season. Limited sunlight exposure, low dietary intake of vitamin D and cardiovascular disease are all extremely common, implying a possibility of causation between vitamin D status and systemic arterial hypertension and making this issue an interesting topic for investigation and also an important subject for the wellbeing of the elderly. Initially, retrospective studies were performed to test the hypothesis that vitamin D deficiency was responsible for aforementioned disease patterns. A large body of clinical evidence linked vitamin D deficiency with prevalent and incident systemic arterial hypertension. A meta-analysis of cross-sectional studies reported that every 16 ng/mL decrement in blood Vitamin D was associated with a 16% higher risk of hypertension [4]. Similarly, longitudinal studies have shown that low vitamin D status predicts future development of hypertension among individuals with normal blood pressure at baseline [5].

Number of research related to vitamin D and non-skeletal disorders has increased enormously in the last decade. A PubMed search using 'Vitamin D' as a keyword generates around 44.000 papers before 2010. From 2010 to late 2017, the same search generates around 30.000 results. It is clear that vitamin D and its extra-skeletal activity drew significant attention in the last decade. Despite hundreds, if not thousands, of papers on the ideal vitamin D levels and extra-musculoskeletal benefits of vitamin D, this subject has remained largely controversial. Optimum vitamin D levels and alleged extra-musculoskeletal physiological effects of vitamin D evaded us mostly because of study designs being observational rather than causational/randomized controlled cohorts, also the inherent complexity of the topic and multiple comorbidities of the elderly kept aggravating the issue. In this chapter, we will briefly talk about the relevant literature, share some 'controversial' vitamin D reference ranges and studies published by prominent authors and reputable sources such as Institute of Medicine and Endocrine Society, then we will explain and suggest mechanisms by which vitamin D may exert its effect on the system and how it could affect cardiovascular health and shortly mention a few incoming major gold-standard randomized controlled trials, in which the effects of vitamin D on cardiovascular disease/total mortality are investigated.

The Institute of Medicine (The Health and Medicine Division of The National Academy of Sciences, USA) classifies vitamin D levels less than 12 ng/mL as deficient, 12 to 20 ng/mL as inadequate and >20 ng/mL as adequate [6]. The Endocrine Society defines deficiency as vitamin D below 20 ng/mL and insufficiency as 21-29 ng/mL [7]. Although they are mostly overlapping, The Endocrine Society sets the reference limit for higher deficiency (Table 1).

Table 1. Disputed optimum Vitamin D 25(OH)D levels.

Institution	Vitamin D Status		
	Deficient	Insufficient	Adequate
Institute of Medicine (The Health and Medicine Division of the National Academy of Sciences, USA)	<12ng/mL	12-20ng/mL	>20ng/mL
The Endocrine Society	<20ng/mL	21-29ng/mL	>29ng/mL

Although consensus is lacking on the optimum vitamin D levels, the latest expert opinions and major trials use deficiency reference levels as vitamin D less than 20 ng/mL. Various clinical studies and their results indicate that less than 20 ng/mL (50 mmol/L) may be accepted as deficiency and 21-29 ng/mL (52-72 mmol/L) can be considered as insufficiency, parallel with the recommendation of the Endocrine Society. Investigation of the association between systemic arterial hypertension and vitamin D status in elderly hypertensive patients has gained substantial momentum in the last decade, spurred by a large body of experimental and clinical evidence.

Hypertension and Vitamin D

Systemic hypertension is a chronic elevation of blood pressure and it causes debilitating target-organ damage affecting, vascular system, heart, kidney, eye and brain over a long-period of time and causes increased morbidity and mortality. Systemic hypertension is commonly classified as primary and secondary hypertension. Essential/Primary/Idiopathic hypertension, comprising nearly 90-95% of all cases, is when the etiology of hypertension is unknown, but thought to be linked to genetics, lack of exercise, obesity and poor diet [8]. Secondary hypertension, comprising around 5-10% of cases, is when the cause can be determined such as aortic stenosis, coarctation of aorta, renal artery stenosis or by certain endocrine disorders such as Cushing's disease (Table 2).

Although early in childhood, causes of hypertension appear to be secondary, in elderly patients and later in childhood primary hypertension tops the list. While in the youngsters hypertension tends to go with elevated cardiac output due to congenital structural disorders, in the elderly, increased systemic vascular resistance and vascular stiffness may play a dominant role in the etiology of hypertension [8]. A great deal of clinical studies have reported a correlation between vitamin D deficiency and various disorders such as coronary artery disease, heart failure, contrast-induced nephropathy and diabetes mellitus. Vitamin D deficiency is reported to be prevalent in elder population and has been shown to have significant pathophysiological effects on the body, including cardiovascular disorders and overall mortality.

Table 2. Hypertension types, incidences and etiology in elderly.

Type	Incidences	Etiology
Primary/Essential/Idiopathic Hypertension	90-95%	Unknown, attributed to Genetics? Poor diet? Lack of Exercise? Obesity? Stress?
Secondary Hypertension	5-10%	Hyperaldosteronism Coarctation of the aorta Pheochromocytoma Chronic Kidney Diseases Renovascular disease Cushing's Sleep apnea Drugs Endocrine disorders Salt

Vitamin D receptors are extensively expressed by cardiovascular tissues such as endothelial cells, cardiomyocytes and vascular smooth muscle cells (VSMCs). Vitamin D has also been shown to play an important role in renin gene expression. Despite current antihypertensive therapies, in 10-35% of hypertensive patients, blood pressure remains high or is barely controlled with combination therapy [9]. Some of these patients are classified as having resistant hypertension and suffer from a higher risk of complications. Vitamin D and its physiological functions may thus be important to prevent this resistance as there is a strong correlation between vitamin D deficiency, predisposing factors to deficiency and cardiovascular morbidity in elderly.

Vitamin D Metabolism and Signaling Pathways

Vitamin D is widely considered as a prohormone rather than a vitamin, because its synthesis primarily takes place in the epidermis layer of the skin upon exposure of 7-dehydrocholesterol to sunlight. The ability of human skin to synthesize vitamin D declines with age. It may be speculated that the ability of the skin to make vitamin D declines as aging progresses is one reason why cardiovascular health becomes predisposed to age-related degenerative processes [10]. Metabolic activation of vitamin D3 comprises different metabolic stages: Ultraviolet B lights convert 7-dehydrocholesterol to vitamin D3 in epidermis and then, following its 25-hydroxylation, it is finally 1-hydroxylated in the kidneys. Although $1,25(OH)_2D$ is the active metabolite of vitamin D, $25(OH)D$ is the form most commonly used to assess vitamin D status in clinical laboratory. Vitamin D exists in two vitameric forms: D2 (ergocalciferol) and D3 (cholecalciferol). Vitamin D is classically known for its physiological effects in calcium metabolism and bone turnover, but various novel roles have been revealed including its physiological effects in mental health, glucose homeostasis, immune system, and oncogenesis [11].

The antihypertensive effects of vitamin D are mainly attributed to its suppressive effects on renin and parathyroid hormone levels as well as its renoprotective, anti-inflammatory and vasculoprotective properties [12]. Vitamin D poses significant cardiovascular pleiotropic effects by activating its nuclear receptor in both cardiomyocytes and vascular endothelial cells. $1,25(OH)_2D$ is the ligand for vitamin D receptor (VDR), which is expressed in nearly every tissue in the body including cardiomyocytes. $1,25(OH)_2D$-bound VDR translocates to the nucleus, where it interacts with regulatory regions of target genes to regulate their transcription. It functions by regulating the low resting levels of cell signaling components such as Ca^{2+} and the formation of reactive oxygen species (ROS). Optimum regulation of these signaling pathways depends on the ability of vitamin D to control the expression of antiaging protein Klotho and antioxidant sensitive Nfr2 components. Vitamin D binds to the VDR that interacts with the retinoid X receptor (RXR) to form the VDR/RXR heterodimer. Heterodimer binds to the vitamin D response element (VDRE). VDR initiates the expression of a large number of genes located in many different cell types to express various proteins that take role in variety of cellular processes. Many of its actions also depend on its ability to increase the expression of both Klotho and Nrf2 pathways that carry out many of its homeostatic actions [11]. Vitamin D and Klotho deficiency is thought to contribute to the aging process through dysregulation of the Ca^{2+} and redox signaling pathways. The ability of vitamin D to protect the cardiovascular system depends on its ability to maintain the homeostasis of ROS and Ca^{2+} signaling systems, which are known to be dysregulated in hypertension, atrial arrhythmias and cardiac hypertrophy. We have chosen not to deal with the non-cardiovascular roles of vitamin D in this chapter and concentrated on more recently proposed role of vitamin D on systemic arterial hypertension and cardiovascular health in elderly people.

Vitamin D Analogs and Selective Effects

The chemical structure of vitamin D is 25-hydroxycholecalciferol. Even though vitamin D analogs erroneously imply analogs of 25-hydroxycholecalciferol, actually they are meant to refer to calcitriol analogs. Since this common usage is established in the literature, we will refer to them as 'Vitamin D analogs' rather than 'calcitriol analogs'. Calcitriol-1,25(OH)$_2$D, the hormonally active metabolite of vitamin D, is used to treat secondary hyperparathyroidism, hypocalcemia, rickets and osteomalacia. In recent years, vitamin D has shown to be promising in the treatment of extra-musculoskeletal disorders and vitamin D supplementation has been shown to be effective in the treatment of major cardiac disorders such as heart failure as exemplified in the VINDICATE study [13], where patients who received non-calcium based vitamin D tablet had dramatically improved center ventricular ejection fraction, reduced center ventricular end diastolic dimensions after 12 months of supplementation that was not seen in the parallel placebo group. Although conclusive results will require replication of these results and large scale clinical trials that are yet to published, this study opens new horizons to the possibly therapeutic vitamin D supplements. Although vitamin D analogs seem to have various significant therapeutic effects ranging from cancer to cardiovascular disease, in some cases they also cause undesirable effects such as hypercalcemia, hyperphosphatemia and vitamin D toxicity, and although rare, are associated with increased cardiovascular mortality. Due to these problems, many vitamin D analogues, without these unsought effects are developed. To explain the differing effects of calcitriol analogs and to develop even more precise potentially therapeutic agents, we need to understand molecular mechanisms better.

25(OH)D uptake in renal proximal tubular cells, occurs *via* receptor mediated endocytosis of 25(OH)D bound to vitamin D binding protein of plasma (DBP). After 1α-hydroxylation in the kidney, calcitriol is formed and it is released back into the blood. Calcitriol binds to VDR, a nuclear receptor, and activates it. Activated VDR translocates to the nucleus where it heterodimerizes with RXR. VDR-RXR heterodimer then binds specific promotor sequences of vitamin D responsive genes, called VDRE. Recent findings show that vitamin D receptor is found nearly in every tissue and probably it has binding sites widely distributed throughout the genome. This finding spawned a huge effort to develop calcitriol analogs that could, possibly, exert different effects -preferably single/distinct- rather than already utilized effects of calcitriol on calcium and phosphate homeostasis. It has been shown that differing effects of these analogs may partly be explained by differences in their pharmacokinetics: their affinity for DBP, their affinity for VDR, clearance rates, their bioavailability-catabolism, and also the conformational alterations they trigger. Evidence suggests that vitamin D analogs exert their effects through the same VDR, but their downstream effects differ [14]. This difference was attributed to the transcriptional factors / coactivators they recruit after the formation of VDR-RXR heterodimer in the nucleus. Different coactivators / corepressors / transcriptional factors are recruited to the heterodimer-VDRE and this complex, by inducing allosteric effects exerts its genomic activity, explaining cell and tissue specific actions of calcitriol and its analogs [15]. In their 2010 review [16], Pike and Meyer names six main principles with which the differences in actions of thousands of synthesized analogs on different tissues could be explained. Some are edited for brevity and clarity.

I-The number of VDR binding sites on the genome is cell type-specific.
II-The active transcription unit is not exclusively the VDR/RXR heterodimer.
III-VDR binding sites are not always the same.
IV-Enhancers are located at varying distances from the transcriptional start sites. Enhancers are located promoter-proximal (near), promoter distal (far) or a combination thereof, relative to transcriptional start sites: many enhancers are located in clusters hundreds of kilobases from their target genes.
V-Enhancers are modular in nature, containing binding sites for a number of different transcription factors
VI-Enhancers that populate a genome are cell type-unique and highly dynamic.

From the cardiac point of view, throughout the cardiovascular system, vitamin D receptors are known to exist. It is known that cardiomyocytes and fibroblasts in the heart, both, express VDR and subsequent to hypertrophic stimuli, these receptors are shown to increase both *in vitro* and *in vivo*. Cardiac ventricular tissue is also known to express 1α-hydroxylase, which means those cardiomyocytes could convert circulating 25(OH)D to 1,25(OH)$_2$D, the same ligand that binds to VDR [17]. Ligand bound VDR has been shown to have anti-hypertrophic effects, a probable evidence for the negative feedback process [18]. It is known that calcitriol and some of its analogs have appreciably different therapeutic uses. We will exemplify this with a few analogs and explain what different downstream effects they exert than the effects of calcitriol (Table **3**).

Falecalcitriol is an analog of calcitriol, from Japan. It has been shown to be effective in a double-blind study which enrolled 121 patients for the treatment of secondary hyperparathyroidism due to chronic kidney disease. Despite the absence of concrete human clinical studies on the effects of analogs, the study of Morii *et al.* is one of few showing its clinical effects with a gold-standard method. This analog is important and is clinically used in Japan. It decreased i-PTH levels around 33% and similar effects were observed with m-PTH and c-PTH without a concurrent surge in calcium levels [19]. 22-Oxacalcitriol, (OCT, maxacalcitol) was shown to have significantly less calcemic side effects compared to calcitriol and this difference was attributed to differences in their pharmacokinetics [20]. To give a few examples, OCT is found to be rapidly cleared from the circulation, limiting its effects on the intestines. Another one is calcipotriol and it has shown some promise in the treatment of psoriasis because it can be applied topically and metabolized locally, limiting its systemic activity [21]. In end stage renal disease, calcitriol synthesis is known to be diminished. A study comparing the effects of calcitriol and its analog, paricalcitol, supplementation found that calcitriol, but not paricalcitol, increased VSMC calcification *in vivo*, independent of calcium and phosphate levels [22]. Even though analogs have some adverse effects too, they exemplify that tissue specific, personalized therapeutic agents could revolutionize pharmacotherapy.

Table 3. Clinically utilized calcitriol analogs.

Calcitriol Analogs	Indications	Calcitriol Analogs	Indications
Calcifediol	Secondary Hyperparathyroidism associated with vitamin D insufficiency CKD 3,4	Calcipotriol	Psoriasis
Maxacalcitol	Psoriasis, Secondary hyperparathyroidism and psoriasis (Japan)	Tacalcitol	Psoriasis
Falecalcitriol	Secondary hyperparathyroidism(Japan)	22-Oxacalcitriol	Secondary hyperparathyroidism (Japan)
Doxercalciferol	Dialysis, Secondary hyperparathyroidism	Eldecalcitol	Osteoporosis (Japan)
Paricalcitol	Secondary hyperparathyroidism CKD stage 3,4,5	Alfacalcidol	Osteoporosis, Hyperparathyroidism, Renal osteodystophy

In some cases there are animal studies showing benefits of some analogs over others, but most are limited and we would caution extrapolating direct results from animal studies.

Vitamin D Deficiency and Cardiovascular Morbidities

Vitamin D deficiency has been shown to be a culprit for age-related cardiovascular disease which is still a huge cause of mortality and morbidity in the elderly [23]. Low 25-hydroxyvitamin D levels are an independent risk factor for the pathogenesis of systemic arterial hypertension. Meta-analyses of randomized controlled trials showed that vitamin D supplementation reduces systolic blood pressure [12]. The Centers for Disease Control and Prevention (CDC) attributes the growing size of elderly population primarily to the developments in the treatment of age-related cardiovascular disease and stroke, emphasizing that early diagnosis and prevention may decrease mortality and morbidity rates in addition to reducing health care costs.

The prevalence of vitamin D insufficiency in elderly individuals varies widely based on the highly disputed cut-off values. Serum 25-hydroxyvitamin D levels less than 20 ng/mL are generally considered to be vitamin D deficiency (Table **1**). Despite lacking consensus on what the optimum systemic vitamin D levels should be, significant relationship has been found between below-average levels of vitamin D and cardiovascular morbidities such as high blood pressure, vascular dysfunction, arterial stiffening, deranged renin-angiotensin-aldosterone system, left ventricular hypertrophy, heart failure, hyperlipidemia, myocardial infarction, stroke [23 - 26]. Its cardiac effect is closely related to the regulation of renin-angiotensin-aldosterone system (Fig. **1**).

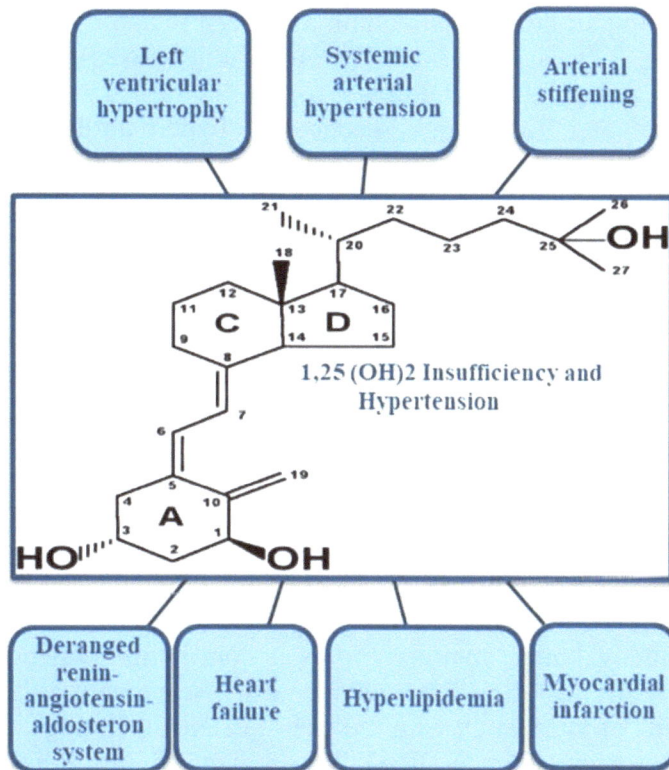

Fig. (1). Relationship vitamin D deficiency, hypertension and age-related cardiovascular morbidities.

In the elderly, cardiovascular disease is rarely non-concomitant to the involvement of other systems. Renal diseases and musculoskeletal disorders are major comorbidities, effecting cardiovascular health and precluding effective treatments in most cases. Studies on the sustainability of health systems and improvements in personalized medicine have decisively showed that exercise and prevention are the key factors [27]. In recent years, it has been shown that even in patients with New York Heart Association (NYHA) heart failure class II-III, exercise could improve hemodynamics. Also, 2016 European Society of Cardiology (ESC) guidelines for the diagnosis and treatment of acute and chronic heart failure recommends regular aerobic exercise and endurance training in patients with heart failure to improve functional capacity, symptoms and to reduce the risk of hospitalization (Class I recommendation) [28]. What this means is musculoskeletal system should always be kept in mind when cardiovascular health and treatment options are considered. Renal involvement affects pharmacotherapy options and the kidneys too, has the autonomy to disturb hemodynamics mainly through renin angiotensin aldosteron system (RAAS) on which the effects of vitamin D are outlined in this chapter earlier. Renal system could therefore impair heart failure commonly seen in elderly. The vicious cycle, as shown in Fig. (**2**), is as follows: Chronic kidney disease commonly causes reduced levels of $1,25(OH)_2D$ (active metabolite of vitamin D) and causes hyperphosphatemia, triggering secondary hyperparathyroidism, causing debilitating musculoskeletal disorders, which in turn increases polypharmacy, musculoskeletal weakness, limited mobility and bedridden-indoor lifestyle and significantly limited quality of life. Limiting mobility, musculoskeletal and hemodynamic impairment further effect cardiovascular system and patients become unable and unwilling to exercise. Impaired hemodynamics trigger even larger renal involvement starting the cycle again (Fig. **2**). Polypharmacy is recently proposed in a Dutch cross-sectional study as a significant risk factor predisposing to vitamin D deficiency where sulfonamides and urea derivatives, metformin, vitamin K antagonists, loop diuretics in >80 age group were found to be associated with vitamin D deficiency [29]. In the same study, number of drugs used was also associated with the severity of vitamin D deficiency. However, a potential undesirable outcome with vitamin D supplements, hypercalcemia and high phosphate levels cautions its use in chronic kidney disease. It is known that hypercalcemia is a risk factor for coronary atherosclerosis, calcification of the aortic valve and valvular annulus and is a contributing factor to dystrophic calcification. While avoiding these adverse effects, it might still be possible to reap the benefits of vitamin D, with the use of calcitriol analogs, in other words, vitamin D receptor activators (VDRA) [30]. In many studies, it has been observed that patients with chronic kidney disorders undergoing dialysis therapy with vitamin D analogs are less likely to die [31]. It is shown that being elderly, female, non-white ethnicity are all independently associated with vitamin D deficiency. On the other hand, physical activity and vitamin D supplementation were inversely associated with vitamin D deficiency [32]. In the same study, multivariate models adjusted for demographics, season, and cardiovascular disease risk factors showed 26% increased rate of all-cause mortality, vitamin D levels of less than 17.8 ng/mL were independently associated with all-cause mortality in the general population with an attributable risk of 3.1% [32].

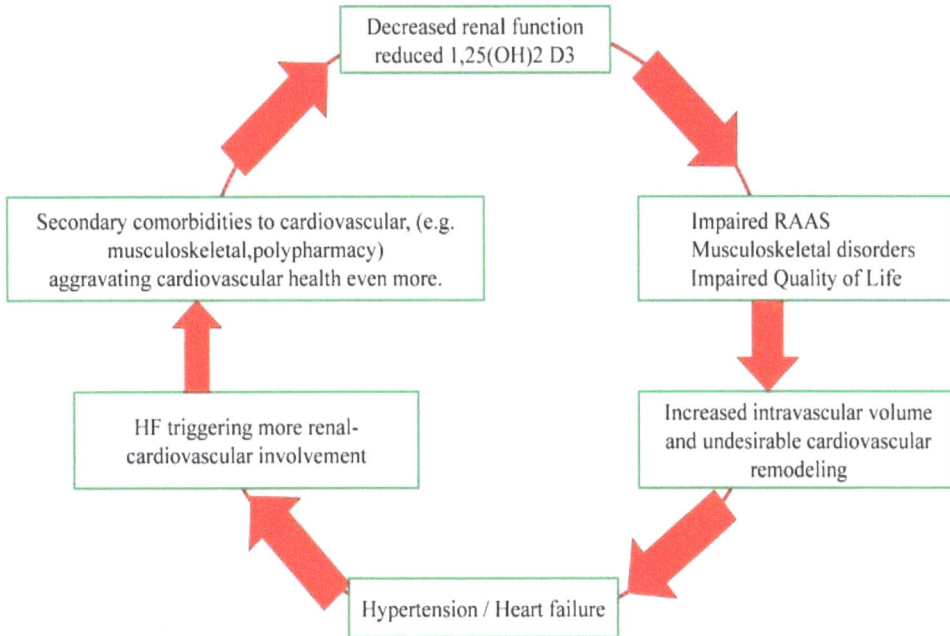

Fig. (2). The vicious cycle involving renal dysfunction, vitamin D deficiency and musculoskeletal system, HF; Heart Failure, RAAS; Renin Angiotensin Aldosteron System, 1,25(OH)$_2$D3; Active Vitamin D.

Vitamin D and Renin-Angiotensin-Aldosterone System

The RAAS maintains vascular resistance through angiotensin II synthesis and the subsequent release of aldosterone to regulate extracellular fluid volume homeostasis. Angiotensinogen – a serpin family protein mainly produced by the hepatocytes is systematically processed by proteases of the RAAS, generating peptide hormones. Specific cell surface receptors for at least three different form of angiotensin peptides produce distinct cellular signals that regulate system-wide physiological response to RAAS. Two well characterized membrane receptors are angiotensin type 1 receptor (AT1 receptor) and type 2 receptor (AT2 receptor). Both type of receptors respond to the octapeptide hormone angiotensin II. The MAS oncogene is shown to encode receptors for Ang (1–7). While these are G-protein coupled receptors, the *in vivo* angiotensin IV binding sites may be type

2 transmembrane proteins. All these receptors together regulate cardiovascular, hemodynamic, neurological, renal, and endothelial functions; as well as cell proliferation, survival, matrix-cell interactions and inflammation. Angiotensin receptors are important pharmacological targets for several different types of disorders. Thus, researchers and pharmaceutical companies are focusing on drugs targeting AT1 receptor rather than AT2 receptor, MAS and Ang IV binding sites. AT1 receptor blockers are currently the cornerstone of treatment for hypertension, heart failure, renal failure and many types of vascular diseases including atherosclerosis. AT1 receptor signaling pathway is mediated through G-proteins, G-protein independent β-arrestin, ROS, non-receptor type tyrosine kinases, small G-proteins, transactivation of receptor tyrosine kinases. Abnormal activation of AT1 receptor causes a number of pathophysiologies including cardiovascular remodeling and hypertrophy, vascular inflammation and atherosclerosis, endothelial dysfunction, oxidative damage, extracellular matrix deposition. The AT2 receptor shares amino acid sequence homology with AT1 receptor. Physiological functions of AT2 receptor are not yet exactly defined, but 15 years of research devoted to this protein have further detailed physiological modulations by AT2 receptor, including those promoted by discovery of small molecule agonists and antagonists. Beneficial effects of AT2 receptor have long been unclear due to its low expression levels in adults. The intracellular signal transduction process of AT2 receptor is unique among the G-protein coupled receptors and is different from the AT1 receptor mediated signaling. AT2 receptor signaling involves G-protein, protein phosphatases. Beneficial AT2 receptor functions from the knock out mouse study could be protective, counteracting blood pressure regulation by the AT1 receptor [33]. $1,25(OH)_2D$ regulates the genes involved in renin production, through a cis-DNA element in the renin gene promoter, downregulating the renin-angiotensin-aldosterone system [34]. It has been demonstrated in both animals and humans that vitamin D decreases renin-angiotensin-aldosterone system activity by suppressing the gene expression of renin (Fig. **3**).

Vitamin D Analogs and Renin-Angiotensin-Aldosterone System

The finding that 1,25-dihydroxyvitamin D is a negative regulator of renin expression also provides a molecular basis to explore the use of vitamin D analogs as novel therapeutic renin inhibitors. Recent data have demonstrated that vitamin D analogs used in combination with the classic RAAS inhibitors can block the undesired compensatory renin activity and thus markedly increase the therapeutic efficacy. This combination strategy has been applied to a number of renal and cardiovascular diseases [36]. Left ventricular hypertrophy is a maladaptive response to chronic pressure overload and an important risk factor for atrial fibrillation, systolic heart failure, diastolic heart failure, and may cause sudden

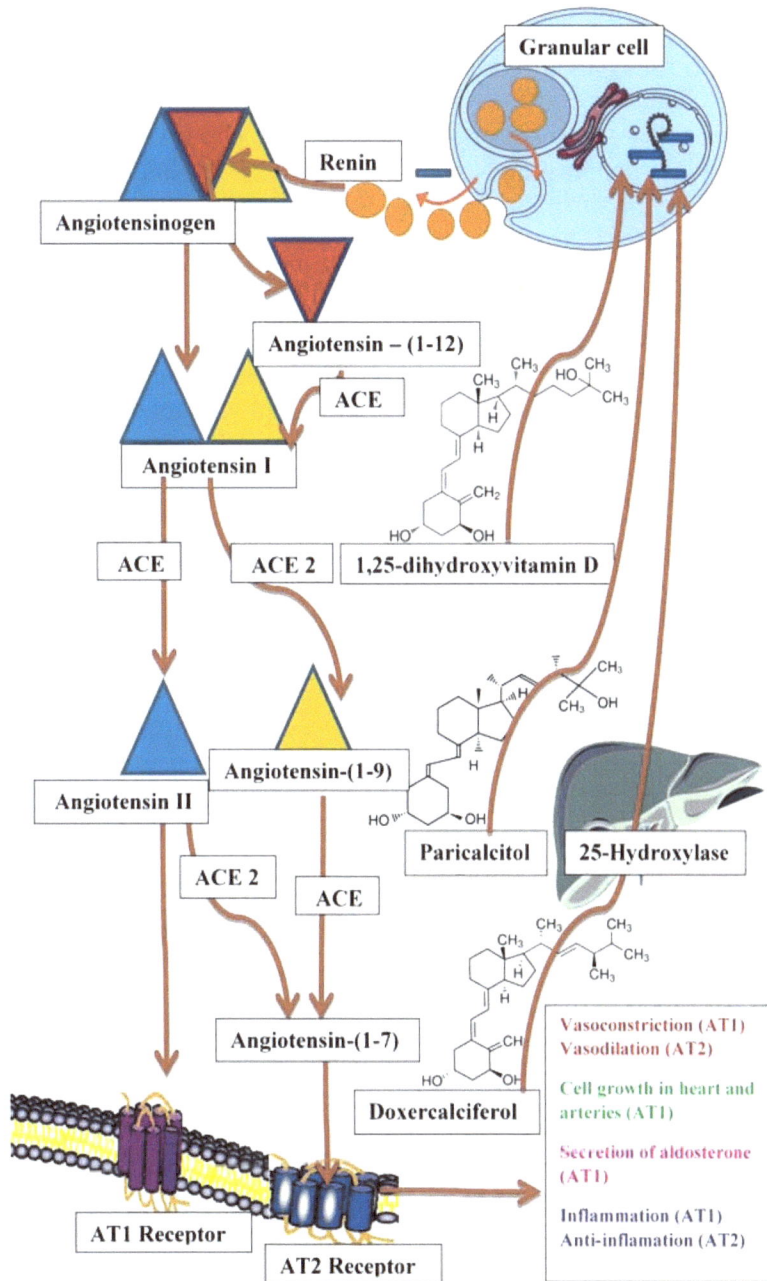

Fig. (3). The antihypertensive therapeutic efficacy of vitamin D analogs on renin-angiotensin-aldosterone system in hypertensive elderly individuals.
ACE; Angiotensin Converting Enzyme, AT1; Angiotensin 1, AT2; Angiotensin 2.

death in patients with hypertension [37]. Vitamin D analogs commonly used in the United States, paricalcitol (19-nor-1α, 25-dihydroxyvitamin D2) and doxercalciferol (1α-hyroxyvitamin D2) have strong anti-hypertrophic activity when given either as mono-therapy or in combination with the angiotensin 1 receptor blocker losartan. Paricalcitol is an activated vitamin D analog and doxercalciferol is a prodrug and is activated *in vivo* by hepatic 25-hydroxylase. Paricalcitol, like calcitriol, activates vitamin D receptor directly, while doxercalciferol is inactive until it is metabolized in the liver to form 1,25-dihydroxyvitamin D2 and 1,24-dihydroxyvitamin D2 (Fig. **3**).

Combination treatment with angiotensin 1 receptor blockade and vitamin D analogs represents remarkable therapeutic improvement against the development of left ventricular hypertrophy, as a result of blockage of the compensatory induction of renin expression leading to improved renin-angiotensin-aldosterone system inhibition [38]. Preclinical studies also support a role for vitamin D deficiency in the development of left ventricular hypertrophy. Vitamin D receptor knockout rodents develop cardiomyocyte hypertrophy with increases in activation of the renin-angiotensin system as well as elevated expression of matrix proteins involved in cardiac remodeling process. Induction of cardiomyocyte hypertrophy leads to an increase in vitamin D receptor levels implying that vitamin D may be a part of a regulatory mechanism to limit cardiac hypertrophy in the setting of hypertrophic stimuli. Treatment with a vitamin D analog reduced cardiac hypertrophy in a rodent model, supporting an important role for vitamin D in the regulation of left ventricular hypertrophy. In particular, elderly patients have an increased prevalence of left ventricular hypertrophy and chronic kidney disease, both of which predict increased cardiovascular morbidity and mortality [39].

Vitamin D and Osteoblast-like Transformation of Vascular Smooth Muscle Cells

The coexistence of aforementioned pathophysiological factors, acting mainly on cardiomyocytes and arterial media-intima layer, leads to high levels of ventricular and vascular stiffness, phenomena closely related to the cardiovascular aging process. The relationships of vitamin D with atherosclerotic calcification and with aortic medial calcification are strong and most likely involve multiple mechanisms within the complex, bone-vascular-renal endocrine axis. Vitamin D is also involved in the regulation of growth and proliferation of VSMCs and cardiomyocytes. Low and high serum vitamin D are both associated with vascular calcification, implying an U shaped risk graph. In the arterial bed, the major structural and functional changes originated from calcification can be summarized as follows: wall diameter increase and elasticity loss, increased collagen deposition and elastin degradation in the media layer [1]. Matrix metalloproteinase-2 (MMP-2) activity induces elastin degradation and vascular calcification. In cultured VSMCs, vitamin D and its analogues inhibits expression of MMP-2 [40]. Pathogenesis of vascular calcification is complex but it seems to be similar to normal bone osteogenesis that involves the transformation of VSMCs into osteoblast-like VSMCs (o-VSMCs) [41]. The initiation of vascular calcification is an active process involving o-VSMC apoptosis, trans-differentiation into calcifying cells and deposition of an osteogenic extracellular matrix [42]. o-VSMC produces matrix vesicles that contain calcium and phosphorus. Matrix vesicles also contain various proteins such as alkaline phosphatase, annexins, osteoprotegerin and fetuin-A (Fig. **4**). A ubiquitous serum glycoprotein fetuin-A is also produced by liver and adipose tissue and is considered to be a systemic inhibitor of vascular calcification. Osteoprotegerin is a soluble glycoprotein which was initially found in bone tissue cells, but is also produced by cardiovascular system cells such as VSMCs. In animal studies, osteoprotegerin plays a protective role for vascular system and variation in its systemic levels is associated with cardiovascular disease. On the other hand, human clinical studies suggest a positive correlation between disease and serum osteoprotegerin levels [43, 44]. Several overlapping mechanisms involving VSMCs have been implicated in the pathogenesis of vascular intimal and medial calcification, including reprogramming and differentiation of VSMC to an osteoblast-like phenotype and deposition of smooth muscle cell-generated calcifying matrix vesicles in the arterial wall. These processes are facilitated by loss of calcification inhibitors such as osteoprotogerin, osteopontin, pyrophosphate, matrix GLA protein and fetuin-A, (Fig. **4**). Increased VSMC oxidant and/or endoplasmic reticulum stress, DNA damage response signaling, apoptosis, and disorders of calcium-phosphate homeostasis may also occur as a result of perturbed hormonal regulation of the cellular system [45]. Inflammatory cytokines such as, tumor necrosis factor-α (TNF-α) accelerates osteogenic process in VSMCs (Fig. **4**). TNF-α also activates Cbfa1 /Runx2 transcription factors for osteoblastic transformation. VSMCs express (25-hydroxyvitamin) 1α-hydroxylase and VDR [40]. Vitamin D also inhibits proliferation of VSMCs by modulating influx of calcium into the intracellular environment. The Notch signaling pathway is a highly conserved cell-cell signaling mechanism that plays a central role in the development and maturation of most vertebrate organs. Notch signaling in the cardiovascular system is important during embryonic development, vascular repair of injury, and vascular pathology in humans. VSMC expresses multiple membrane-bound Notch receptors throughout its life cycle, and responds to vascular endothelial Notch ligands as a regulatory mechanism of differentiation, recruitment to growing vessels, and maturation [46]. Vitamin D inhibits myoblast proliferation and differentiation by altering expression of cell cycle regulators and myogenic regulatory factors with associated changes in Notch signaling pathways. Differentiation of human osteoblasts with vitamin D and dexamethasone distinctly affects the expression of Notch receptor family members.

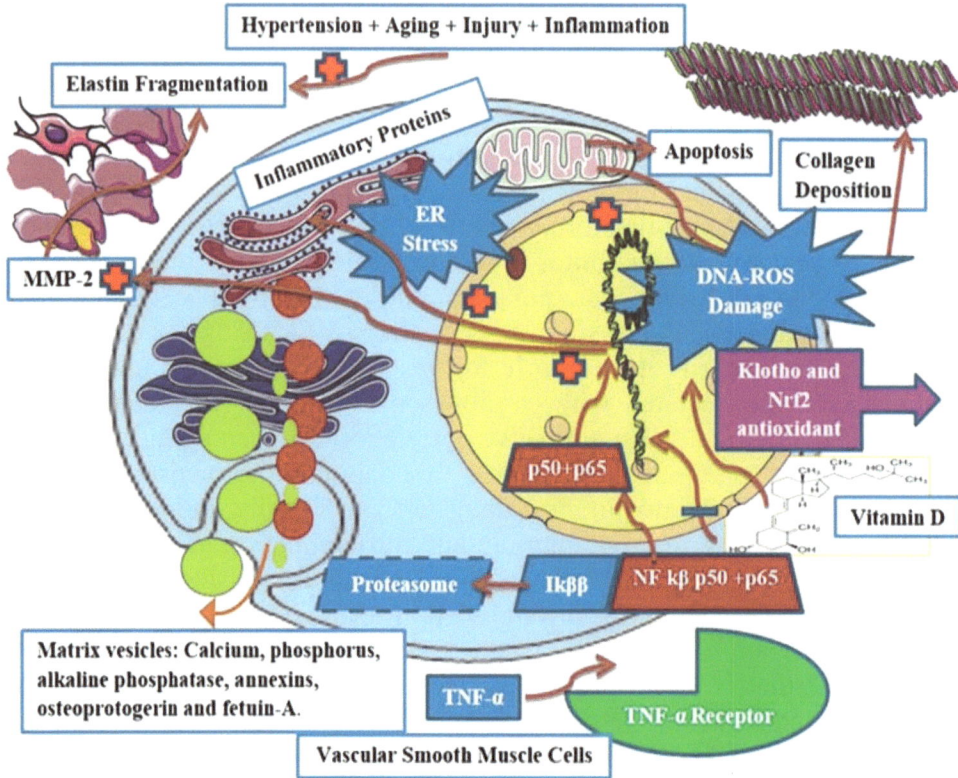

Fig. (4). The effects of Vitamin D on differentiation of vascular smooth muscle cell to an osteoblast-like phenotype and deposition of smooth muscle cell-generated calcifying matrix vesicles. MMP-2; Matrix metalloproteinase-2, TNF-α; tumor necrosis factor-α, NFκβ; Nuclear factor κβ.

Vitamin D and Differentiation of Monocytes to Osteoclast-like Cells

Vitamin D affects atherosclerotic calcification *via* effects on osteoprotegerin or its target, the ligand for receptor activator of NF-κB, a critical osteoclast differentiation factor [47]. It has been suggested that dietary calciol and vitamin D may be carried by low density lipoprotein particles into cells of the artery wall and atherosclerotic plaque where it may be transformed to its active form by monocyte-macrophages (Fig. **5**). Calcitriol; $1,25(OH)_2D$, is also carried by LDL particles and internalized by vascular cells *via* the LDL receptor. VSMCs, monocytes and endothelial cells express receptors for vitamin D, enabling conversion of calcidiol to calcitriol. Osteoclast differentiation is tightly coupled with the presence of intercellular contacts between the osteoclast precursors and osteoblasts in the bone tissue (the receptor activator of NF-κB, (RANK) / RANK ligand (RANKL) / osteoprotegerin system). VSMCs that have osteoblast-like phenotype and secrete factors such as RANKL and macrophage colony stimulating factor (M-CSF) are involved in osteoclast differentiation (Fig. **5**). In the calcified vascular wall the presence of monocyte / macrophage cell types are able to differentiate directly into osteoclasts. Vitamin D is also known to promote cell differentiation.

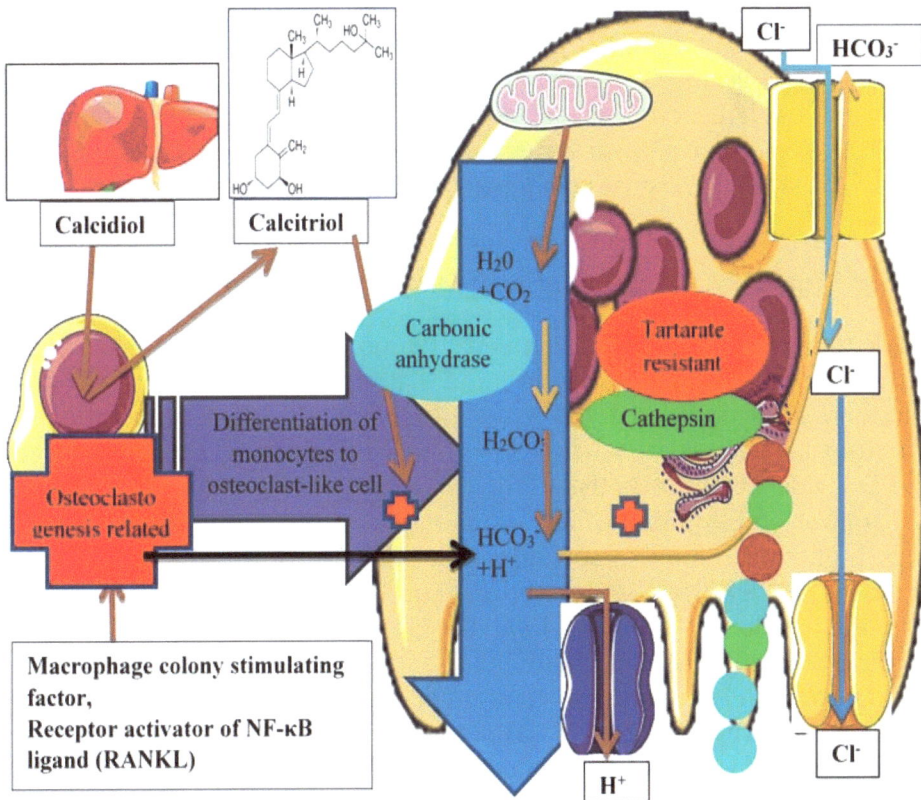

Fig. (5). The effects of Vitamin D on differentiation of monocytes to osteoclast-like cell and degradation of extracellular matrix.

A treatment with 1,25-hydroxyvitamin D can induce the differentiation of monocytes to osteoclast-like cells. Carbonic anhydrases play a crucial role in osteoclast function and bone remodeling by catalyzing the formation of bicarbonate and proton from carbon dioxide. According to previous histochemical studies, advanced atherosclerotic plaques share significant similarities with bone. An imbalance between osteoblast-like and osteoclast-like cell activities would therefore favor the occurrence of a pathological calcification process in vessel walls [42]. Osteoclast-like cells have been found in the artery wall, and their resorptive activity is driven by carbonic anhydrase, which has VDRE in its gene promoter. It is plausible that osteoclast-like cells in calcified arteries originate from circulating or locally present macrophages, particularly in inflammation-driven vascular calcification, as both cell types are derived from mononuclear precursors. As in normal bone turnover, where RANKL secreted by osteoblasts induces osteoclast differentiation and activation by binding on its RANK receptor to stimulate bone resorption, high RANKL expression by vascular cells in calcified vessels might stimulate transdifferentiation of monocytes/macrophages into bone-resorbing cells. Receptor activator of NF-κB (RANK) signaling triggered by RANKL activates the downstream signaling pathways, including NF-κB, Erk, JNK, and p38, to induce expression of osteoclastogenesis-related genes, such as tartrate-resistant acid phosphatase, cathepsin K, carbonic anhydrase (Fig. **5**).

Validity of Evidence for Extra-Skeletal Effects of Vitamin D

Although it is still early to recommend vitamin D supplementation for extra-skeletal disorders, we should keep in mind that vitamin D status that is barely at the currently recommended level may not necessarily mean that patients will benefit from the alleged extra-skeletal effects of vitamin D. Given suggested vitamin D levels, at least 40-50% of the US population, around 50-60% of South Korean population [48], 30% of the UK [49], is vitamin D deficient and numbers are even higher according to several studies. The VINDICATE study enrolled patients with cholecalciferol levels of less than 20 ng/mL and supplemented daily oral vitamin D3 for 12 months, 4000 IU/day. After 12 months, patients with chronic heart failure due to left ventricular systolic dysfunction showed improved ejection fraction and reduced left ventricular end systolic diameters. Vitamin D has also been shown to inhibit NF-κB signaling and linked to anti-inflammation [50]. VDR (-/-) knockout animals have been shown to have significant cardiac hypertrophy and moderately elevated blood pressure [35]. This has been attributed to both the systemic and cardiac increased expression of renin angiotensin aldosterone system (RAAS) we explained earlier in this chapter. Cardiomyocyte-specific deletion of the vitamin D receptor study, published in Circulation 2011, hypothesized that VDR, independent of RAAS, has a direct antihypertrophic effects on cardiomyocytes. The authors attributed this to the suppression of the prohypertrophic calcineurin/NFAT/MCIP1 pathway [51]. A meta-analysis involving 10170 Danish, published in Atherosclerosis, Thrombosis and Vascular Biology in 2012, an American Heart Association (AHA) journal, observed an association between lower 25(OH)D levels and increased risk of ischemic heart disease, myocardial infarction, and early death [23]. The 2013 JAMA study where prospective cohort of 6436 patients from Multi-Ethnic Study of Atherosclerosis (MESA) were evaluated for vitamin D deficiency and cardiovascular events showed increased risk for white race and Chinese participants, but results were unable to be generalized to black and Hispanic patients, leaving the door open for racial differences in the metabolism [52]. A 2014 BMJ study where meta-analysis of 26018 patients from eight prospective cohort studies from the US and Europe with follow up between 4.2 and 15.9 years consistently showed that lower 25(OH)D levels were associated with increased all cause and cause specific cardiovascular mortality [53]. 2017 EVITA study, where 400 patients were randomized to placebo or 4000 IU daily vitamin D to observe the effects of oral vitamin D supplementation to patients with vitamin D levels less than <16 ng/mL on advanced heart failure was sought did not show any improvements in mortality and was associated with higher mechanical support device implantation [54]. A randomized, double-blind, placebo controlled clinical trial including 5110 patients, investigating monthly high dose vitamin D supplementation published in JAMA in 2017 did not observe the claimed inverse relationship between 25(OH)D levels and cardiovascular events [55]. In this study, vitamin D supplementation was monthly and median follow up time (3.3 years) was relatively too short observe, if any, difference in cardiovascular events considering the relatively good health of enrolled patients [56, 57]. Another confounding factor was only around 30% of the enrolled patients had vitamin D deficiency, further lowering the power of the study to show any difference. Ludwigshafen Risk and Cardiovascular Health study showed increased mortality for patients in the 7.6 ng/mL – 13.3 ng/mL compared with 28.4 ng/mL of 25(OH)D. These results imply that the effects of vitamin D deficiency on non-musculoskeletal system may be detectible only when vitamin D is dramatically deficient in patients -considering patient age group and confounding factors-detecting relatively small differences probably would require large samples and long term follow ups. Recent evidence supports the existence of a biphasic relationship of serum vitamin D with cardiovascular disease, deficiency effects are observed in below-around 15 ng/mL, no clear benefit observed over 20 ng/mL and possibly increased risk over 40 ng/mL. In the Framingham Offspring Study, involving more than 1700 individuals without symptoms and previous cardiovascular disease and a mean follow-up of 5.4 year, the relationship between serum vitamin D and cardiovascular disease was found to increase at levels below 15 ng/mL and no clear benefit observed at levels higher than guideline 25(OH)D levels. Though accumulating evidence supports the biphasic hypothesis with risk increasing at levels <15 ng/mL and >40 ng/mL, considering the evidence for extra-skeletal benefits of Vitamin D, we think 40 ng/mL could be low for effects of toxicity to be observed. In the ViDA study, a large randomized placebo controlled trial, results of which published in JAMA in June 2017, monthly vitamin D supplementation did not result in decreased cardiovascular disease (Table **4**) and [55, 58 - 61].

Table 4. Major studies investigating vitamin D and its claimed extra musculoskeletal effects on a large scale, randomized, placebo controlled way.

Study Name	Relevant Outcome Measures	Enrollment(n)	Age	Link
VITAL[58]	MI, Stroke, CVD Mortality	25.871	>50	https://clinicaltrials.gov/ct2/ show/NCT01169259
D-Health [59]	All cause mortality, including total cardiovascular events	21315	60-79	https://www.anzctr.org.au/Trial/Registration/ TrialReview.aspx?id=364534
VIDAL[60]	Overall mortality reduction	1615*	60-84	http://www.isrctn.com/ ISRCTN46328341
FIND[61]	Cardiovascular Risk	2500	>60	https://clinicaltrials.gov/ct2/show/ NCT01463813
ViDA[55]	Resulted, 2017, "Monthly high-dose vitamin D supplementation does not prevent CVD."	5108	50-84	https://www.anzctr.org.au/Trial/Registration/ TrialReview.aspx?id=336777

[58]*VIT*amin D and Omeg*A*-3 Tria*L* (VITAL), [59] The D-Health Trial: A trial of vitamin D for prevention of mortality and cancer in older Australian adults. [60]Vitamin D and Longevity (VIDAL) Trial, [61]Finnish Vitamin D Trial (FIND), [55]The Vitamin D Assessment (ViDA) Study, [60]VIDAL is a feasibility study for a larger 20.000 enrollment study.

This non-significance of vitamin D supplementation in the ViDA study could be, as the authors pointed out, due to supplementations being monthly rather than daily/weekly. Still, considering the data and the complexity of health status of the elderly, it can be suggested that only patients whose 25(OH)D levels less than <20 ng/mL are expected to receive clear benefits from vitamin D supplementation. Thus, both vitamin D deficiency and vitamin D excess could increase the risk for cardiovascular disease. These biphasic findings and conflicting studies raise interesting questions regarding the effects of vitamin D intake, daily-weekl--monthly supplementation and their effects on atherosclerotic calcification and cardiovascular risk. It has been proposed that with optimum systemic vitamin D levels, reversing or slowing the progression of most of the aforementioned age-related cardiovascular disorders is possible *via* decreasing blood pressure. Meta-analyses also show that low levels of systemic vitamin D are associated with peripheral artery disease and myocardial infarction [62, 63].

CONCLUDING REMARKS

The relationship of vitamin D with atherosclerotic calcification and with systemic hypertension seems strong and most likely involve multiple mechanisms within the complex, vascular-renal endocrine axis. Overall, clear evidence is still lacking to say that vitamin D supplementation would reduce cardiovascular events and mortality. Hopefully the D-Health, VIDAL studies which are all randomized, double blinded and placebo controlled and the Vitamin D and Omega-3 Trial (VITAL) study from Harvard, which is also a randomized double blinded, placebo controlled trial involving more than 25.000 people to investigate the effects of vitamin D and fish oil in the prevention of cardiovascular disease and cancer will hopefully shed light on these issues soon.

CONSENT FOR PUBLICATION

Not applicable.

CONFLICT OF INTEREST

The authors declare no conflict of interest, financial or otherwise.

ACKNOWLEDGEMENTS

Declare none.

REFERENCES

[1]   Mikael LR, Paiva AMG, Gomes MM, *et al.* Vascular aging and arterial stiffness. Arq Bras Cardiol 2017; 109(3): 253-8.
[PMID: 28678931]

[2]   Hassan-Smith ZK, Hewison M, Gittoes NJ. Effect of vitamin D deficiency in developed countries. Br Med Bull 2017; 122(1): 79-89.
[http://dx.doi.org/10.1093/bmb/ldx005] [PMID: 28334220]

[3]   Grimes DS, Hindle E, Dyer T. Sunlight, cholesterol and coronary heart disease. QJM 1996; 89(8): 579-89.
[http://dx.doi.org/10.1093/qjmed/89.8.579] [PMID: 8935479]

[4]   Burgaz A, Orsini N, Larsson SC, Wolk A. Blood 25-hydroxyvitamin D concentration and hypertension: a meta-analysis. J Hypertens 2011; 29(4): 636-45.
[http://dx.doi.org/10.1097/HJH.0b013e32834320f9] [PMID: 21191311]

[5]   Wang TJ. Vitamin D and cardiovascular disease. Annu Rev Med 2016; 67: 261-72.
[http://dx.doi.org/10.1146/annurev-med-051214-025146] [PMID: 26768241]

[6]   ods.od.nih.gov. [homepage on the Internet]. National Institutes of Health, Office of Dietary Supplements. [updated February 11th 2016; cited: 19th November 2017]. Available from: https://ods.od.nih.gov/factsheets/VitaminD-HealthProfessional/

[7]   Holick MF, Binkley NC, Bischoff-Ferrari HA, *et al.* Evaluation, treatment, and prevention of vitamin D deficiency: an Endocrine Society clinical practice guideline. J Clin Endocrinol Metab 2011; 96(7): 1911-30.

[http://dx.doi.org/10.1210/jc.2011-0385] [PMID: 21646368]

[8]   Viera AJ, Neutze DM. Diagnosis of secondary hypertension: an age-based approach. Am Fam
        Physician 2010; 82(12): 1471-8.
        [PMID: 21166367]

[9]   Calhoun DA, Jones D, Textor S, *et al.* Resistant hypertension: diagnosis, evaluation, and treatment: a
        scientific statement from the American Heart Association Professional Education Committee of the
        Council for High Blood Pressure Research. Circulation 2008; 117(25): e510-26.
        [http://dx.doi.org/10.1161/CIRCULATIONAHA.108.189141] [PMID: 18574054]

[10]   Berridge MJ. Vitamin D deficiency accelerates ageing and age-related diseases: a novel hypothesis. J
        Physiol 2017; 595(22): 6825-36.
        [http://dx.doi.org/10.1113/JP274887] [PMID: 28949008]

[11]   Berridge MJ. Vitamin D, reactive oxygen species and calcium signalling in ageing and disease. Philos
        Trans R Soc Lond B Biol Sci. 2016; Aug 5; 371(1700).

[12]   Pilz S, Tomaschitz A. Role of vitamin D in arterial hypertension. Expert Rev Cardiovasc Ther 2010;
        8(11): 1599-608.
        [http://dx.doi.org/10.1586/erc.10.142] [PMID: 21090935]

[13]   Witte KK, Byrom R, Gierula J, *et al.* Effects of vitamin D on cardiac function in patients with chronic
        HF: The VINDICATE study. J Am Coll Cardiol 2016; 67(22): 2593-603.
        [http://dx.doi.org/10.1016/j.jacc.2016.03.508] [PMID: 27058906]

[14]   Issa LL, Leong GM, Eisman JA. Molecular mechanism of vitamin D receptor action. Inflamm Res
        1998; 47(12): 451-75.
        [http://dx.doi.org/10.1007/s000110050360] [PMID: 9892040]

[15]   Haussler MR, Jurutka PW, Mizwicki M, Norman AW. Vitamin D receptor (VDR)-mediated actions of
        1α,25(OH)$_2$vitamin D$_3$: genomic and non-genomic mechanisms. Best Pract Res Clin Endocrinol Metab
        2011; 25(4): 543-59.
        [http://dx.doi.org/10.1016/j.beem.2011.05.010] [PMID: 21872797]

[16]   Pike JW, Meyer MB. The vitamin D receptor: new paradigms for the regulation of gene expression by
        1,25-dihydroxyvitamin D(3). Endocrinol Metab Clin North Am 2010; 39(2): 255-69.
        [http://dx.doi.org/10.1016/j.ecl.2010.02.007] [PMID: 20511050]

[17]   Chen S, Glenn DJ, Ni W, *et al.* Expression of the vitamin d receptor is increased in the hypertrophic
        heart. Hypertension 2008; 52(6): 1106-12.
        [http://dx.doi.org/10.1161/HYPERTENSIONAHA.108.119602] [PMID: 18936343]

[18]   Gardner DG, Chen S, Glenn DJ. Vitamin D and the heart. Am J Physiol Regul Integr Comp Physiol
        2013; 305(9): R969-77.
        [http://dx.doi.org/10.1152/ajpregu.00322.2013] [PMID: 24026071]

[19]   Morii H, Ogura Y, Koshikawa S, *et al.* Efficacy and safety of oral falecalcitriol in reducing
        parathyroid hormone in hemodialysis patients with secondary hyperparathyroidism. Bone Miner
        Metab 1998; 16: 34.
        [http://dx.doi.org/10.1007/s007740050026]

[20]   Brown AJ, Finch J, Grieff M, *et al.* The mechanism for the disparate actions of calcitriol and 22-
        oxacalcitriol in the intestine. Endocrinology 1993; 133(3): 1158-64.
        [http://dx.doi.org/10.1210/endo.133.3.8396012] [PMID: 8396012]

[21]   Bikle DD. Vitamin D metabolism, mechanism of action, and clinical applications. Chem Biol 2014;
        21(3): 319-29.
        [http://dx.doi.org/10.1016/j.chembiol.2013.12.016] [PMID: 24529992]

[22]   Zheng Z, Shi H, Jia J, Li D, Lin S. Vitamin D supplementation and mortality risk in chronic kidney
        disease: a meta-analysis of 20 observational studies. BMC Nephrol 2013; 14: 199.
        [http://dx.doi.org/10.1186/1471-2369-14-199] [PMID: 24066946]

[23]   Brøndum-Jacobsen P, Benn M, Jensen GB, Nordestgaard BG. 25-hydroxyvitamin d levels and risk of ischemic heart disease, myocardial infarction, and early death: population-based study and meta-analyses of 18 and 17 studies. Arterioscler Thromb Vasc Biol 2012; 32(11): 2794-802.
[http://dx.doi.org/10.1161/ATVBAHA.112.248039] [PMID: 22936341]

[24]   Al Mheid I, Quyyumi AA. Vitamin D and cardiovascular disease: controversy unresolved. J Am Coll Cardiol 2017; 70(1): 89-100.
[http://dx.doi.org/10.1016/j.jacc.2017.05.031] [PMID: 28662812]

[25]   Li YC. Vitamin D regulation of the renin-angiotensin system. J Cell Biochem 2003; 88(2): 327-31.
[http://dx.doi.org/10.1002/jcb.10343] [PMID: 12520534]

[26]   Yuan W, Pan W, Kong J, *et al.* 1,25-dihydroxyvitamin D3 suppresses renin gene transcription by blocking the activity of the cyclic AMP response element in the renin gene promoter. J Biol Chem 2007; 282(41): 29821-30.
[http://dx.doi.org/10.1074/jbc.M705495200] [PMID: 17690094]

[27]   Gilford DM. Health Promotion and Disease Prevention. In: Gilford DM, Ed. The Aging Population in the Twenty-First Century: Statistics for Health Policy National Research Council (US) Panel on Statistics for an Aging Population Washington (DC): National Academies Press (US). 1988; pp. 108-25.

[28]   Escardio.org. Health Promotion and Disease Prevention. In: Gilford DM, Ed. The Aging Population in the Twenty-First Century: Statistics for Health Policy https://www.escardio.org/Journals/E-Journal--f-Cardiology-Practice/Volume-14/Exercise-training-as-therapy-for-chronic-heart-failure

[29]   van Orten-Luiten ACB, Janse A, Dhonukshe-Rutten RAM, Witkamp RF. Vitamin D deficiency as adverse drug reaction? A cross-sectional study in Dutch geriatric outpatients. Eur J Clin Pharmacol 2016; 72(5): 605-14.
[http://dx.doi.org/10.1007/s00228-016-2016-2] [PMID: 26873590]

[30]   Şimşek B, Çakatay U. Vitamin D supplementation, polypharmacy and cardiovascular health in elderly. Edorium J Aging Res 2017; 2: 1-3.

[31]   Jean G, Souberbielle JC, Chazot C. Vitamin D in chronic kidney disease and dialysis patients. Nutrients 2017; 9(4)E328
[http://dx.doi.org/10.3390/nu9040328] [PMID: 28346348]

[32]   Lutsey PL, Michos ED. Vitamin D, calcium, and atherosclerotic risk: evidence from serum levels and supplementation studies. Curr Atheroscler Rep 2013; 15(1): 293.
[http://dx.doi.org/10.1007/s11883-012-0293-5] [PMID: 23232985]

[33]   Singh KD, Karnik SS. Angiotensin receptors: structure, function, signaling and clinical applications. J Cell Signal 2016; 1(2): 111.
[PMID: 27512731]

[34]   Mozos I, Marginean O. Links between vitamin D deficiency and cardiovascular diseases. Biomed Res Intern 2015; vol. 2015; Article ID 109275; 12 pages
[http://dx.doi.org/10.1155/2015/109275]

[35]   Xiang W, Kong J, Chen S, *et al.* Cardiac hypertrophy in vitamin D receptor knockout mice: role of the systemic and cardiac renin-angiotensin systems. Am J Physiol Endocrinol Metab 2005; 288(1): E125-32.
[http://dx.doi.org/10.1152/ajpendo.00224.2004] [PMID: 15367398]

[36]   Li YC. Vitamin D, renin, and blood pressure.Vitamin D Nutrition and Health. Humana Press 2010; pp. 937-53.

[37]   Katholi RE, Couri DM. . Left ventricular hypertrophy: Major risk factor in patients with hypertension: Update and Practical Clinical Applications. Int J Hypertens vol. 2011; Article ID 495349, 10 pages.

[38]   Kong J, Kim GH, Wei M, *et al.* Therapeutic effects of vitamin D analogs on cardiac hypertrophy in

spontaneously hypertensive rats. Am J Pathol 2010; 177(2): 622-31.
[http://dx.doi.org/10.2353/ajpath.2010.091292] [PMID: 20616348]

[39]   Leibowitz D. Left ventricular hypertrophy and chronic renal insufficiency in the elderly. Cardiorenal Med 2014; 4(3-4): 168-75.
[http://dx.doi.org/10.1159/000366455] [PMID: 25737681]

[40]   Aoshima Y, Mizobuchi M, Ogata H, *et al.* Vitamin D receptor activators inhibit vascular smooth muscle cell mineralization induced by phosphate and TNF-α. Nephrol Dial Transplant 2012; 27(5): 1800-6.
[http://dx.doi.org/10.1093/ndt/gfr758] [PMID: 22287655]

[41]   Schmidt N, Brandsch C, Kühne H, Thiele A, Hirche F, Stangl GI. Vitamin D receptor deficiency and low vitamin D diet stimulate aortic calcification and osteogenic key factor expression in mice. PLoS One 2012; 7(4)e35316
[http://dx.doi.org/10.1371/journal.pone.0035316] [PMID: 22536373]

[42]   Massy ZA, Mentaverri R, Mozar A, Brazier M, Kamel S. The pathophysiology of vascular calcification: are osteoclast-like cells the missing link? Diabetes Metab 2008; 34(1) (Suppl. 1): S16-20.
[http://dx.doi.org/10.1016/S1262-3636(08)70098-3] [PMID: 18358422]

[43]   Kiechl S, Schett G, Wenning G, *et al.* Osteoprotegerin is a risk factor for progressive atherosclerosis and cardiovascular disease. Circulation 2004; 109(18): 2175-80.
[http://dx.doi.org/10.1161/01.CIR.0000127957.43874.BB] [PMID: 15117849]

[44]   Van Campenhout A, Golledge J. Osteoprotegerin, vascular calcification and atherosclerosis. Atherosclerosis 2009; 204(2): 321-9.
[http://dx.doi.org/10.1016/j.atherosclerosis.2008.09.033] [PMID: 19007931]

[45]   Leopold JA. Vascular calcification: Mechanisms of vascular smooth muscle cell calcification. Trends Cardiovasc Med 2015; 25(4): 267-74.
[http://dx.doi.org/10.1016/j.tcm.2014.10.021] [PMID: 25435520]

[46]   Boucher J, Gridley T, Liaw L. Molecular pathways of notch signaling in vascular smooth muscle cells. Front Physiol 2012; 3: 81.
[http://dx.doi.org/10.3389/fphys.2012.00081] [PMID: 22509166]

[47]   Zhou S, Fang X, Xin H, Li W, Qiu H, Guan S. Osteoprotegerin inhibits calcification of vascular smooth muscle cell *via* down regulation of the Notch1-RBP-Jκ/Msx2 signaling pathway. PLoS One 2013; 8(7)e68987
[http://dx.doi.org/10.1371/journal.pone.0068987] [PMID: 23874840]

[48]   Choi HS, Oh HJ, Choi H, *et al.* Vitamin D insufficiency in Korea-a greater threat to younger generation: the Korea National Health and Nutrition Examination Survey (KNHANES) 2008. J Clin Endocrinol Metab 2011; 96(3): 643-51.
[http://dx.doi.org/10.1210/jc.2010-2133] [PMID: 21190984]

[49]   Hassan-Smith ZK, Hewison M, Gittoes NJ. Effect of vitamin D deficiency in developed countries. Br Med Bull 2017; 122(1): 79-89.
[http://dx.doi.org/10.1093/bmb/ldx005] [PMID: 28334220]

[50]   Vanoirbeek E, Krishnan A, Eelen G, *et al.* The anti-cancer and anti-inflammatory actions of 1,25(OH)$_2$D$_3$. Best Pract Res Clin Endocrinol Metab 2011; 25(4): 593-604.
[http://dx.doi.org/10.1016/j.beem.2011.05.001] [PMID: 21872801]

[51]   Chen S, Law CS, Grigsby CL, *et al.* Cardiomyocyte-specific deletion of the vitamin D receptor gene results in cardiac hypertrophy. Circulation 2011; 124(17): 1838-47.
[http://dx.doi.org/10.1161/CIRCULATIONAHA.111.032680] [PMID: 21947295]

[52]   Robinson-Cohen C, Hoofnagle AN, Ix JH, *et al.* Racial differences in the association of serum 25-hydroxyvitamin D concentration with coronary heart disease events. JAMA 2013; 310(2): 179-88.

[http://dx.doi.org/10.1001/jama.2013.7228] [PMID: 23839752]

[53] Schöttker B, Jorde R, Peasey A, *et al.* Vitamin D and mortality: meta-analysis of individual participant data from a large consortium of cohort studies from Europe and the United States. BMJ 2014; 348: g3656.
[http://dx.doi.org/10.1136/bmj.g3656] [PMID: 24938302]

[54] Zittermann A, Ernst JB, Prokop S, *et al.* Effect of vitamin D on all-cause mortality in heart failure (EVITA): a 3-year randomized clinical trial with 4000 IU vitamin D daily. Eur Heart J 2017; 38(29): 2279-86.
[http://dx.doi.org/10.1093/eurheartj/ehx235] [PMID: 28498942]

[55] Scragg R, Stewart AW, Waayer D, *et al.* Effect of monthly high-dose vitamin D supplementation on cardiovascular disease in the vitamin D assessment study : A randomized clinical trial. JAMA Cardiol 2017; 2(6): 608-16.
[http://dx.doi.org/10.1001/jamacardio.2017.0175] [PMID: 28384800]

[56] Anagnostis P, Paschou SA, Goulis DG, Vitamin D. Vitamin D supplementation and cardiovascular disease risk. JAMA Cardiol 2017; 2(11): 1281-2.
[http://dx.doi.org/10.1001/jamacardio.2017.2938] [PMID: 28854312]

[57] Scragg R, Camargo CA Jr, Vitamin D. Vitamin D supplementation and cardiovascular disease risk-reply. JAMA Cardiol 2017; 2(11): 1282.
[http://dx.doi.org/10.1001/jamacardio.2017.2941] [PMID: 28854307]

[58] Pradhan AD, Manson JE. Update on the vitamin D and OmegA-3 trial (VITAL). J Steroid Biochem Mol Biol 2016; Jan; 155(Pt B); 252-6

[59] Neale RE, Armstrong BK, Baxter C, *et al.* The D-Health Trial: A randomized trial of vitamin D for prevention of mortality and cancer. Contemp Clin Trials 2016; 48: 83-90.
[http://dx.doi.org/10.1016/j.cct.2016.04.005] [PMID: 27086041]

[60] http://vidal.lshtm.ac.uk [homepage on the Internet].

[61] clinicaltrials.gov. [homepage on the Internet]. [updated: 8th November 2017; cited: 19th November 2017]. Available from: https://clinicaltrials.gov/ct2/show/NCT01463813

[62] Nsengiyumva V, Fernando ME, Moxon JV, *et al.* The association of circulating 25-hydroxyvitamin D concentration with peripheral arterial disease: A meta-analysis of observational studies. Atherosclerosis 2015; 243(2): 645-51.
[http://dx.doi.org/10.1016/j.atherosclerosis.2015.10.011] [PMID: 26554715]

[63] Huang J, Wang Z, Hu Z, Jiang W, Li B. Association between blood vitamin D and myocardial infarction: A meta-analysis including observational studies. Clin Chim Acta 2017; 471: 270-5.
[http://dx.doi.org/10.1016/j.cca.2017.06.018] [PMID: 28645551]

CHAPTER 13

Emerging and Routine Biomarkers in Hypertension, Current Aspects and Future Directions

Mustafa Erinç Sitar[1] and **Pınar Atukeren[2,*]**

[1] *Department of Medical Biochemistry, Faculty of Medicine, Maltepe University, Istanbul, Turkey*

[2] *Department of Medical Biochemistry, Faculty of Medicine, Istanbul Cerrahpasa University, Istanbul, Turkey*

Abstract: Hypertension is an insidious and silent disease that is diagnosed relatively late due to its asymptomatic course. It is considered one of the most substantial major risk factor for fatal cardiovascular diseases in entire world especially people who live in developed communities. Epidemiological statistics and public health concerns are resulting in a need for an objective biomarker for this remedy. This necessity is quite crucial for hypertension due to available treatment options, silent clinical outcome progressing and discrepancy between blood pressure measurement methods. The use of biomarkers can contribute not only to pre-diagnosis but also to disease follow-up, treatment success, and prognosis estimation and complication analysis as a whole. As a general concept, biological markers can be located at various sites like systemic circulation, urine, pleural fluid, pericardial fluid, peritoneal cavity, synovial fluid, aqueous humor and even cerebrospinal fluid. Researchers are steadily trying to develop new markers to medical usage or pre-existing ones are being modified for new or enlarged purposes. Analysis methods are also becoming more accessible with less intense labor and less expensive thanks to high technology. Regardless of the tissue from which the biomarker is taken and difficulty in measurement procedures, it will always be a serious target to contribute new, more sensitive and more specific biomarkers on hypertension in clinical biochemistry.

Keywords: Aldosterone, Analysis, Biomarker, Cardiovascular, Decision threshold, Differential diagnosis, Essential hypertension, Fibrinogen, Laboratory, Metanephrine, Microalbumin, Normetanephrine, Oxidized LDL, Pre-hypertension, Prognosis, Prostocycline, Renin, Screening, Silent clinic, Sphygmomanometer.

---

* **Corresponding author Pinar Atukeren:** Department of Medical Biochemistry, Cerrahpaşa Faculty of Medicine, Istanbul University-Cerrahpasa, Istanbul, Turkey; Tel: +902124143056; Fax: +902126332987; E-mail: p_atukeren@yahoo.com

Hafize Uzun & Pınar Atukeren (Eds.)

INTRODUCTION

For today's medical era, measuring different aspects of the human organism is becoming more crucial every day. Measurement of different biological aspects is needed at different levels of physiologic incidences, pathologic states, during assessment of potential risks, analyzing responses to therapies, estimation of prognosis, population screening programs and/or finally as an outcome for clinical decision making. Researchers and clinicians need objective tools as decision thresholds.

These measurable tools can be as simple as a medical history question, measurement of blood temperature, calculation of body mass index, pulse rate or as complicated as a state of art, sophisticated, expensive and time consuming laboratory result.

Any type of biologically defining measurement that is accurate, objective, reproducible and informative can be called as "marker" or more precisely "biomarker". Key word search for publications as "biomarker" in Pubmed, performed on March 2018, yielded over 750.000 results, which enlights the significance more. The argument of our chapter will be conventional and specific biochemical tests to appoint diagnose and make assumptions about hypertension in different populations. Cardiovascular diseases (CVD) are one of the most common reasons that cause death worldwide in 21st century especially in high income countries. Actually they can be considered as the most common non communicable killer of all time as a whole. There are lots of modifiable and non-modifiable risk factors for CVD tendency. Even the etiology is not clear totally, essential hypertension is considered to be one of the most significant modifiable risk factors for stroke, myocardial infarction, heart failure, chronic kidney failure and retinopathy. It is reported that %30 of grown-ups have definitive hypertension diagnosis and an extra %8 of the whole population is unaware of their self-hypertensive states in USA [1]. For this reason, one of the first definitions that come to mind for high blood pressure is to call it a deep and silent killer. Lewington *et al.* performed a meta-analysis and revealed that every 20 mmHg increase in systolic blood pressure (SBP) and 10 mmHg increase in diastolic blood pressure (DBP) are doubling overall cardiovascular risk for patients at the ages between 40-69 [2]. The biggest portion of hypertensive population remains unaware of their clinical risks. In a multinational, systematic and population based analysis including almost 1 million people, researchers estimated hypertension prevalence 31% for men and 30% for women. Very interestingly, the same study showed that hypertension frequency was declining in high-income countries, but rising in low and middle-income countries [3]. Clinicians in the field of cardiovascular diseases were hesitant during laboratory analysis due to properties of surrogate hypertension markers. Due to its silent clinic before any major complication, remaining untreated for a long time and high frequency in the society, screening, detection, diagnosis, prevention, treatment and follow-up of hypertension is quite significant. Even timing, frequency and location of measurements are becoming controversial topics among clinicians; screening programs for hypertension can reduce cardiovascular mortalities. Health care workers desire to decrease hypertension related morbidities and mortalities to improve public health. Several markers instead of one biomarker would certainly increase the accuracy of clinical outcome. It is obvious that several indirectly related biological pathways take important roles in hypertension development.

DIAGNOSIS OF HYPERTENSION

In medical history, Stephan Hales was the first scientist who mentioned about blood pressure measurement in 18th century [4]. A battle surgeon, Nikolai Sergeevich Korotkoff, proposed a different and new blood pressure measurement method unexpectedly and it made a huge effect on blood pressure monitoring [5]. Blood pressure assessment requires delicate measurements on different time intervals using correct positioning of appropriate sized cuffs according to individual's arm perimeter. Readings can be applied by different methods or at different places like hospitals, clinical offices, homes and/or using ambulatory tools. An accurately calibrated sphygmomanometer or an automated tool can be used to make two consecutive readings with minimum 5 minutes' interval. Mean of two systolic and diastolic blood pressures are used in terms to define high blood pressure. More than 90% of arterial hypertension cases are arranged as essential hypertension which occurs without any known pathology. There are multiple classification patterns for hypertension in different medical communities [6]. In 2017, American College of Cardiology categorized blood pressure in adults;

I- elevated (120-129 mmHg systolic and <80 mmHg diastolic blood pressure),

II- stage 1 (130-139 mmHg systolic or 80-89 mmHg diastolic blood pressure) and

III- stage 2 ($\geq$140 mmHg systolic or $\geq$ 90 mmHg diastolic blood pressure) [7].

Once diagnosed, detailed examination together with follow-up and treatment are essential. Although similar treatment and follow-up guidelines may be used in different countries, recommended markers to be used can be separated into three categories: general screening phase, definitive diagnosis phase, follow-up phase biomarkers (Fig. **1**) . For any kind of research or clinical institute, it is impossible to examine all suspected hypertension biomarkers in all these three phases due to cost effective, labor intense and time based issues. Instead of this approach, choosing selective parameters in different states should be considered more wisely. Three different scales of panels should be set up: (i) early prediction of hypertension in normotensive individuals, (ii) diagnosis of new onset hypertension and (iii) follow up of hypertensive patients. Those all can be re-considered according to accessibility, coverage of insurance companies, policy of the institution and patient compliance. Clinicians must be aware that they are not absolute categories but a cost-effective and frequency dependent evaluation of the disease is logical.

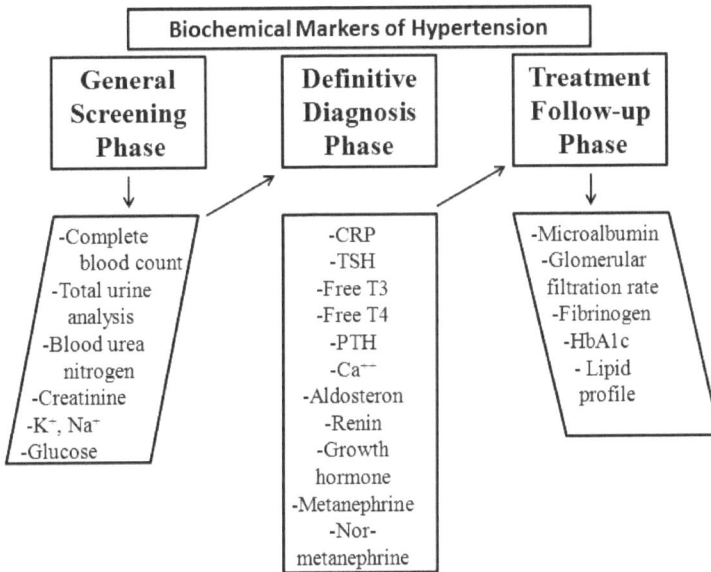

Fig. (1). Detailed laboratory analysis for hypertension screening, diagnosis and follow-up.

General Screening Tests

One of the most significant contributions to clinicians would be solving this question: "who should we examine more closely for hypertension development among pre-hypertensive population?" In addition to aforementioned query "Who are carrying the biggest risk and what can we do to prevent it?" questions come to mind. The answer can be simple: by using biomarkers. Even the answer seems easy and plain; it is actually very complicated to find less expensive, less laborious and less time-consuming tests than pre-existing ones. It should be always kept in mind that following confirmation of correct measurement, drug and diet related causes should all be excluded for hypertension diagnosis [8]. After a detailed medical history, physical examination and initial diagnosis of hypertension, other diagnostic procedures can be performed to analyze primary hypertension. Investigation of common co-morbidities should begin with simple & fast routine tests and then relatively rare disease search can be continued. Those primary tests, which can be chosen by primary care physicians, are listed (Table 1).

Table 1. Basic routine biomarkers analyzed systematically for hypertensive individuals.

Biomarker	Suspicion or Aim for the Physician	Acquired Clinical Information about Hypertension	References
High sensitive C reactive protein (hs- CRP)	Vascular inflammation	Predictor of hypertension	[9]
Fibrinogen	Predictor for cardiovascular outcome	Presence of strong association between high plasma levels and prevalent hypertension in males	[10]
Urine protein (micro-albumin)	Renal impairment in 1/5 of hypertensive patients	Progression risk to end stage renal impairment requiring dialysis	[11]
Serum albumin	General screening test	Decreased levels are associated with high risk	[12]
BUN (Blood urea nitrogen)	Renal function analysis	Acute and chronic kidney failure progression and hypertension	[13]
Creatinine	Renal function analysis	Acute and chronic kidney failure progression	[13]
GFR (Glomerular filtration rate)	Renal function analysis - gold standard	Reduction in GFR is a risk factor for incident hypertension	[14]
Ca^{+2}	General screening	Hyperparathyroidism, nephrolithiasis, paraneoplastic syndrome detection	[15]
TSH, free T3, free T4,	Dry or warm skin, cold or heat intolerance, GIS disturbances	Hypothyroidism or hyperthyroidisms detection	[7]
Growth hormone	Characteristic facial appearance	Acromegaly investigation	[7]
Plasma aldosterone/renin levels	Hypertension together with unexplained hypopotassemia	To detect primary hyperaldosteronism	[16]
Metanephrine and normetanephrine	Episodic catecholamine excess, palpitations, headaches,	To detect primary phaeochromocytoma or paraganglioma	[17, 18]

Even screening is a matter of debate for many clinicians; we can start with C reactive protein (CRP) which shows the presence of systemic inflammation in human organism. Comprehensive studies has established the information that atherosclerosis is a primordial inflammatory process [19]. Large scale cohort studies showed a very significant interaction between high CRP levels and future cardiovascular risk [20]. Woman's Health Study, which contained more than twenty thousand health care provider volunteer women with no history of hypertension, showed that CRP levels were modestly associated with hypertension or hypertension related maladies [21]. It was the first cohort prospective study which resulted a very noteworthy report regarding prediction of future CVD events. Actually, high-sensitive CRP (hs-CRP) is a more delicate test than traditional and ordinary CRP test. Even it is accepted as an inexpensive and highly available test, it must be always kept in mind that hs-CRP has to be united with other traditional risk factors and routine laboratory tests to asses CVD risk [22]. For example, complete blood count (CBC) can be joined with hs-CRP to detect inflammation. CBC is a very basic tool to overview general health status of the individuals. High WBC (white blood cells) and erythrocyte sedimentation rate (ESR) levels can show the presence of inflammation very closely [23, 24]. WBC and hs-CRP are nonspecific markers of vascular inflammation, so it is controversial to use them as screening tools for CVD on different populations and time intervals [24].

Definitive Diagnosis and Secondary Hypertension

Ruling out secondary causes of hypertension, detection of end organ damage due to hypertension and presence of other cardiovascular risk factors together with hypertension need enlightment for the benefit of the patient. Secondary hypertension is not a primary disease but a result of another disease which is usually treatable generally by surgery. Possible reversible causes of secondary hypertension vary with age and gender. It may cause high blood pressure in unexpected early ages and initial treatment is often difficult in spite of polypharmacotherapy. Renal artery occlusion, coarctation of aorta, side effect of nonsteroidal anti-inflammatory agents, renal parenchymal diseases, exogenous or endogenous glucocorticoid excess, Cushing Syndrome, Cushing Disease, thyroid pathologies, hyperparathyroidism, pregnancy, obesity, pheochromacytoma, hypokalemia due to aldosteronism, and other medications can lead to high blood pressure formation [8]. For relatively young patients, cases which do not respond to multidrug treatment and also for rapidly progressing clinical states, secondary hypertension should always be suspected.

Treatment and Follow-up Phase

High blood pressure damages waste and water excretion or disposal function of the kidneys and also most chronic renal failure patients have hypertension outcome [25]. Hypertension often can be seen at the same time with CKD (chronic kidney disease), and the opposite is true as well just like a vicious circle. It is like a chicken and egg issue. In other words kidneys are not only the target of hypertension but they can be the cause of hypertension [26]. Due to these reasons, renal functions are having pivotal roles for follow-up phase. Microalbuminuria is accepted as a very important early diagnostic and predictor criterion for CKD development for diabetic patients [27]. Prevalence of hypertension correlates very well with high degree of albuminuria and low glomerular filtration rates (GFR) [28]. For this reason, regular follow-up of renal function tests plays a very important role. Controlling and lowering microalbuminuria could reduce the effect of hypertension and renavascular related morbidities [27]. Other CVD risk factors such as hypercholesterolemia and hypertriglyceridemia should be reviewed in treatment and follow up phase as well. Lipid profile and HbA1c should be investigated routinely for this purpose.

EMERGING BIOMARKERS

Thanks to high technology and scientific researches, the test panels are expanding and the precision of existing tests are increasing. There may be different instances where different clinical conditions can be exemplified (Table **2**).

Table 2. Emerging biomarkers and their role for hypertension management.

Emerging Biomarker	Physiological or Pathological Importance/Definition	Clinical Information for Hypertension	References
Asymmetric dimethylarginine	Inhibitor of nitric oxide synthase	High concentration in non-complicated essential hypertensive cases	[29, 30]
Galectin-3	Cardiac remodeling	Aldosterone mediated fibrosis	[31]
Prostocycline	Antagonizes endothelial dysfunction	Regulation of vascular homeostasis by vasorelaxation and inhibition of platelet aggregation	[32]
Oxidized LDL	Oxidative stress related origin	Progression for atherosclerosis	[32]
IL-6	Vascular stress	Nitric oxide pathway blockade	[33]
8-iso-PGF2α	Stable end product of first line reactive oxidative stress damage	Highly reliable and self-sufficient risk factor for atherosclerotic diseases	[34]

Hypertensive cardiac remodeling is attended on molecular inflammation and fibrosis, and one of the main intermediary agents of cardiac remodeling is aldosterone. Galectin-3 could be one of the new emerging marker for hypertension linking cardiac inflammation and fibrosis in situations with high-aldosterone levels. Galectin-3 inhibition could block aldosterone-induced cardiac inflammation and fibrosis [31]. It is a process of "inhibition of inhibition". Calvier *et al.* also found that Galectin-3 is requested for inflammatory and fibrotic responses to aldosterone in vascular smooth muscle cells *in vitro* and *in vivo*. They proposed that Galectin-3 has a key role in vascular fibrosis in rats [35]. Monocytes may have a substantial lead role in hypertension by involving differentiation into macrophages and monocyte-derived dendritic cells. Monocyte transformation can be effected by endothelium, that can be activated in hypertension by mechanical stretch [33]. De Ciuceis *et al.* found that macrophage colony-stimulating factor is necessary for the stimulation of macrophage differentiation from monocytes and mice lacking macrophage colony-stimulating factor are preserved against blood pressure rise [36]. Loperena *et al.* investigated the role of increased endothelial stretch and hypertension on monocyte function. They found that monocytes are activated by vascular endothelium due to hypertension. This is probably because of a loss of NO (nitric oxide) signaling and raised release of IL-6. IL-6 could be considered as another potential emerging biomarker in hypertension as a result of these studies. F2-isoprostane 8-is--prostaglandin (8-iso-PGF2α), asymmetric dimethyl arginine (ADMA) and oxidized LDL can be included into this list due to their deleterious end effects on cardiovascular system. These effects are limitedly based on free radical formation [29]. ADMA can function as a bridge between dysfunctional endothelial layer and inflammation together with oxidized LDL helping us understand the process of atherosclerosis [37]. This enlightened important link may cause new strategies to use this route for therapeutic applications [38]. But the main issue is difficult and expansive measurement tools. For example stable and more certain determination of F2-isoprostane 8-iso-prostaglandin (8-iso-PGF2α) require analytical tools like tandem mass spectrometry [39]. ADMA measurement require derivatization process and mass spectrometry, as well [40].

CONCLUDING REMARKS

In conclusion, alternative panel testing can be chosen instead of one single test for approaching to hypertension. Thanks to state of art technology, personalized medicine and molecular diagnostic tools are the new lights seen from horizon of hypertension diagnosis. There is always great hope for new and better test parameters in clinical chemistry.

CONSENT FOR PUBLICATION

Not applicable.

CONFLICT OF INTEREST

The authors declare no conflict of interest, financial or otherwise.

ACKNOWLEDGEMENTS

Declare none.

REFERENCES

[1] Olives C, Myerson R, Mokdad AH, Murray CJ, Lim SS. Prevalence, awareness, treatment, and control of hypertension in United States counties, 2001-2009. PLoS One 2013; 8(4)e60308
[http://dx.doi.org/10.1371/journal.pone.0060308] [PMID: 23577099]

[2] Lewington S, Clarke R, Qizilbash N, Peto R, Collins R. Age-specific relevance of usual blood pressure to vascular mortality: a meta-analysis of individual data for one million adults in 61 prospective studies. Lancet 2002; 360(9349): 1903-13.
[http://dx.doi.org/10.1016/S0140-6736(02)11911-8] [PMID: 12493255]

[3] Mills KT, Bundy JD, Kelly TN, *et al.* Global disparities of hypertension prevalence and control: a systematic analysis of population-based studies from 90 countries. Circulation 2016; 134(6): 441-50.
[http://dx.doi.org/10.1161/CIRCULATIONAHA.115.018912] [PMID: 27502908]

[4] Parker KH. A brief history of arterial wave mechanics. Med Biol Eng Comput 2009; 47(2): 111-8.
[http://dx.doi.org/10.1007/s11517-009-0440-5] [PMID: 19198914]

[5] Estañol B, Delgado G, Borgstein J. Korotkoff sounds - the improbable also occurs. Arq Bras Cardiol 2013; 101(5): e99-e105.
[PMID: 24343557]

[6] Abel N, Contino K, Jain N, *et al.* Eighth joint national committee (JNC-8) guidelines and the outpatient management of hypertension in the African-American population. N Am J Med Sci 2015; 7(10): 438-45.
[http://dx.doi.org/10.4103/1947-2714.168669] [PMID: 26713289]

[7] Whelton PK, Carey RM, Aronow WS, Casey DE, Collins KJ, Dennison Himmelfarb C, *et al.* ACC/AHA/AAPA/ABC/ACPM/AGS/APhA/ASH/ASPC/NMA/PCNA Guideline for the Prevention, Detection, Evaluation, and Management of High Blood Pressure in Adults A Report of the American College of Cardiology/American Heart Association Task Force on Clinical Practice Guidelines 2017.

[8] Viera AJ, Neutze DM. Diagnosis of secondary hypertension: an age-based approach. Am Fam Physician 2010; 82(12): 1471-8.
[PMID: 21166367]

[9] Wang TJ, Gona P, Larson MG, *et al.* Multiple biomarkers and the risk of incident hypertension. Hypertension 2007; 49(3): 432-8.
[http://dx.doi.org/10.1161/01.HYP.0000256956.61872.aa] [PMID: 17242302]

[10] Shankar A, Wang JJ, Rochtchina E, Mitchell P. Positive association between plasma fibrinogen level and incident hypertension among men: population-based cohort study. Hypertension 2006; 48(6): 1043-9.
[http://dx.doi.org/10.1161/01.HYP.0000245700.13817.3c] [PMID: 17000922]

[11] Sharma R, Kamalakar S, McCarthy E, Fields TA, Gupta K, Barua R, *et al.* Proteinuria in hypertensive nephropathy: a review. Open J Nephrol 2014; 4(02): 92.
[http://dx.doi.org/10.4236/ojneph.2014.42013]

[12] Oda E. Decreased serum albumin predicts hypertension in a Japanese health screening population. Intern Med 2014; 53(7): 655-60.
[http://dx.doi.org/10.2169/internalmedicine.53.1894] [PMID: 24694472]

[13] Pandya D, Nagrajappa AK, Ravi KS. Assessment and correlation of urea and creatinine levels in saliva and serum of patients with chronic kidney disease, diabetes and hypertension - a research study. J Clin Diagn Res 2016; 10(10): ZC58-62.
[http://dx.doi.org/10.7860/JCDR/2016/20294.8651] [PMID: 27891460]

[14]   Brands MW, Labazi H. Role of glomerular filtration rate in controlling blood pressure early in diabetes. Hypertension 2008; 52(2): 188-94.
       [http://dx.doi.org/10.1161/HYPERTENSIONAHA.107.090647] [PMID: 18606911]

[15]   Cupisti A, D'Alessandro C, Samoni S, Meola M, Egidi MF. Nephrolithiasis and hypertension: possible links and clinical implications. J Nephrol 2014; 27(5): 477-82.
       [http://dx.doi.org/10.1007/s40620-014-0068-x] [PMID: 24577680]

[16]   Australia NHFo. Guideline for the diagnosis and management of hypertension in adults Melbourne, Australia: National Heart Foundation of Australia National Heart Foundation of Australia; 2016.

[17]   Gabb GM, Mangoni A, Anderson CS, Cowley D, Dowden JS, Golledge J, *et al.* Guideline for the diagnosis and management of hypertension in adults—2016 mortality 2016; 3: 4.

[18]   Leung AA, Daskalopoulou SS, Dasgupta K, *et al.* Hypertension Canada's 2017 guidelines for diagnosis, risk assessment, prevention, and treatment of hypertension in adults. Can J Cardiol 2017; 33(5): 557-76.
       [http://dx.doi.org/10.1016/j.cjca.2017.03.005] [PMID: 28449828]

[19]   Libby P. Inflammation in atherosclerosis. Arterioscler Thromb Vasc Biol 2012; 32(9): 2045-51.
       [http://dx.doi.org/10.1161/ATVBAHA.108.179705] [PMID: 22895665]

[20]   Legarth C, Grimm D, Wehland M, Bauer J, Krüger M. The impact of vitamin D in the treatment of essential hypertension. Int J Mol Sci 2018; 19(2)E455
       [http://dx.doi.org/10.3390/ijms19020455] [PMID: 29401665]

[21]   Sesso HD, Buring JE, Rifai N, Blake GJ, Gaziano JM, Ridker PM. C-reactive protein and the risk of developing hypertension. JAMA 2003; 290(22): 2945-51.
       [http://dx.doi.org/10.1001/jama.290.22.2945] [PMID: 14665655]

[22]   Diederichsen MZ, Diederichsen SZ, Mickley H, *et al.* Prognostic value of suPAR and hs-CRP on cardiovascular disease. Atherosclerosis 2018; 271: 245-51.
       [http://dx.doi.org/10.1016/j.atherosclerosis.2018.01.029] [PMID: 29402404]

[23]   Madjid M, Awan I, Willerson JT, Casscells SW. Leukocyte count and coronary heart disease: implications for risk assessment. J Am Coll Cardiol 2004; 44(10): 1945-56.
       [http://dx.doi.org/10.1016/j.jacc.2004.07.056] [PMID: 15542275]

[24]   Madjid M, Fatemi O. Components of the complete blood count as risk predictors for coronary heart disease: in-depth review and update. Tex Heart Inst J 2013; 40(1): 17-29.
       [PMID: 23467296]

[25]   Bromfield S, Muntner P. High blood pressure: the leading global burden of disease risk factor and the need for worldwide prevention programs. Curr Hypertens Rep 2013; 15(3): 134-6.
       [http://dx.doi.org/10.1007/s11906-013-0340-9] [PMID: 23536128]

[26]   Abe K, Ito S. The kidney and hypertension. Hypertens Res 1997; 20(2): 75-84.
       [http://dx.doi.org/10.1291/hypres.20.75] [PMID: 9220270]

[27]   Yadav D, Kang DR, Koh SB, Kim JY, Ahn SV. Association between urine albumin-to-creatinine ratio within the normal range and incident hypertension in men and women. Yonsei Med J 2016; 57(6): 1454-60.
       [http://dx.doi.org/10.3349/ymj.2016.57.6.1454] [PMID: 27593874]

[28]   Mahmoodi BK, Matsushita K, Woodward M, *et al.* Associations of kidney disease measures with mortality and end-stage renal disease in individuals with and without hypertension: a meta-analysis. Lancet 2012; 380(9854): 1649-61.
       [http://dx.doi.org/10.1016/S0140-6736(12)61272-0] [PMID: 23013600]

[29]   Sitar ME. Asymmetric dimethylarginine and its relation as a biomarker in nephrologic diseases. Biomark Insights 2016; 11: 131-7.
       [http://dx.doi.org/10.4137/BMI.S38434] [PMID: 27980388]

[30]   Surdacki A, Nowicki M, Sandmann J, *et al.* Reduced urinary excretion of nitric oxide metabolites and increased plasma levels of asymmetric dimethylarginine in men with essential hypertension. J Cardiovasc Pharmacol 1999; 33(4): 652-8.
[http://dx.doi.org/10.1097/00005344-199904000-00020] [PMID: 10218738]

[31]   Martínez-Martínez E, Calvier L, Fernández-Celis A, *et al.* Galectin-3 blockade inhibits cardiac inflammation and fibrosis in experimental hyperaldosteronism and hypertension. Hypertension 2015; 66(4): 767-75.
[http://dx.doi.org/10.1161/HYPERTENSIONAHA.115.05876] [PMID: 26238446]

[32]   Kuklinska AM, Mroczko B, Musial WJ, *et al.* Diagnostic biomarkers of essential arterial hypertension: the value of prostacyclin, nitric oxide, oxidized-LDL, and peroxide measurements. Int Heart J 2009; 50(3): 341-51.
[http://dx.doi.org/10.1536/ihj.50.341] [PMID: 19506338]

[33]   Loperena R, Van Beusecum JP, Itani HA, *et al.* Hypertension and increased endothelial mechanical stretch promote monocyte differentiation and activation: roles of STAT3, interleukin 6 and hydrogen peroxide. Cardiovasc Res 2018; 114(11): 1547-63.
[http://dx.doi.org/10.1093/cvr/cvy112] [PMID: 29800237]

[34]   Schwedhelm E, Bartling A, Lenzen H, *et al.* Urinary 8-iso-prostaglandin F2alpha as a risk marker in patients with coronary heart disease: a matched case-control study. Circulation 2004; 109(7): 843-8.
[http://dx.doi.org/10.1161/01.CIR.0000116761.93647.30] [PMID: 14757688]

[35]   Calvier L, Miana M, Reboul P, *et al.* Galectin-3 mediates aldosterone-induced vascular fibrosis. Arterioscler Thromb Vasc Biol 2013; 33(1): 67-75.
[http://dx.doi.org/10.1161/ATVBAHA.112.300569] [PMID: 23117656]

[36]   De Ciuceis C, Amiri F, Brassard P, Endemann DH, Touyz RM, Schiffrin EL. Reduced vascular remodeling, endothelial dysfunction, and oxidative stress in resistance arteries of angiotensin II-infused macrophage colony-stimulating factor-deficient mice: evidence for a role in inflammation in angiotensin-induced vascular injury. Arterioscler Thromb Vasc Biol 2005; 25(10): 2106-13.
[http://dx.doi.org/10.1161/01.ATV.0000181743.28028.57] [PMID: 16100037]

[37]   Sitar ME, Kayacelebi AA, Beckmann B, Kielstein JT, Tsikas D. Asymmetric dimethylarginine (ADMA) in human blood: effects of extended haemodialysis in the critically ill patient with acute kidney injury, protein binding to human serum albumin and proteolysis by thermolysin. Amino Acids 2015; 47(9): 1983-93.
[http://dx.doi.org/10.1007/s00726-015-1991-4] [PMID: 25921952]

[38]   Chobanyan-Jürgens K, Pham VV, Stichtenoth DO, Tsikas D. Asymmetrical dimethylarginine, oxidative stress, and atherosclerosis. Hypertension 2011; 58(5): e184-5.
[http://dx.doi.org/10.1161/HYPERTENSIONAHA.111.180984] [PMID: 21968759]

[39]   Tsikas D, Schwedhelm E, Suchy MT, *et al.* Divergence in urinary 8-iso-PGF(2alpha) (iPF(2alpha)-III, 15-F(2t)-IsoP) levels from gas chromatography-tandem mass spectrometry quantification after thin-layer chromatography and immunoaffinity column chromatography reveals heterogeneity of 8-is--PGF(2alpha). Possible methodological, mechanistic and clinical implications. J Chromatogr B Analyt Technol Biomed Life Sci 2003; 794(2): 237-55.
[http://dx.doi.org/10.1016/S1570-0232(03)00457-4] [PMID: 12954376]

[40]   Tsikas D, Schubert B, Gutzki F-M, Sandmann J, Frölich JC. Quantitative determination of circulating and urinary asymmetric dimethylarginine (ADMA) in humans by gas chromatography-tandem mass spectrometry as methyl ester tri(N-pentafluoropropionyl) derivative. J Chromatogr B Analyt Technol Biomed Life Sci 2003; 798(1): 87-99.
[http://dx.doi.org/10.1016/j.jchromb.2003.09.001] [PMID: 14630363]

CHAPTER 14

Medical Nutrition in Hypertension

M. Emel Alphan[1] and **Pınar Atukeren**[2,*]

[1] *Department of Nutrition and Dietetics, Institute of Health Sciences, Okan University, Istanbul, Turkey*

[2] *Department of Medical Biochemistry, Cerrahpasa Medical Faculty, Istanbul University-Cerrahpasa, Istanbul, Turkey*

Abstract: High blood pressure is the most common cause of death worldwide. The goal of treatment should be lowering blood pressure to reduce the risk of heart disease and to reduce the risk of heart attack and stroke. Hypertension is treated with drugs and in addition the person's lifestyle and nutrition should be paid attention. Lifestyle changes are needed to control LDL-cholesterol, lipids and BP which are the cardiovascular risk factors. Lifestyle changes; nutrition recommendations involving the control of salt intake and weight loss, regular physical activity, avoiding alcohol/cigarette consumption, *etc.* are summarized in this chapter. It was shown that with DASH diet, which recommends reducing saturated fat, total fat and cholesterol, and increasing consumption of low-fat dairy products with vegetables and fruits, BP is reduced. Sodium, sugar, sugary drinks, fats and ready to eat meat are less involved in the DASH diet.

Keywords: Alcohol consumption, Blood pressure, Cardiovascular diseases, Calcium, Cholesterol, Diet, Exercise, Fruits, Hypertension, Lifestyle management, Nutrition, Sodium intake, Salt-sensitive hypertensive, Salt-resistant hypertension, Sodium, Potassium, Magnesium, Weight loss, DASH diet, Vegetables.

INTRODUCTION

Raised blood pressure (BP); hypertension, is the leading global risk factor for cardiovascular diseases such as heart failure and renal diseases such as chronic kidney disease [1]. In 2000, the prevalence of raised BP was 26.4% of the population (26.6% in men and 26.1% in women) and predicted to be 29.2% of the population (29.0% in men and 29.5% in women) in 2015 [2]. During the last 40 years, it was reported that the number of hypertensive patients has been raised

* **Corresponding author Pinar Atukeren:** Department of Medical Biochemistry, Cerrahpaşa Faculty of Medicine, Istanbul University-Cerrahpasa, Istanbul, Turkey; Tel: +902124143056; Fax: +902126332987; E-mail: p_atukeren@yahoo.com

upto two times and men have higher BP when compared with women. In 2015, there were 1.13 billion people with high BP worldwide mostly seen in countries with low-income and middle-income [1]. People with prehypertension are more prone to hypertension development and have higher risk of having cardiovascular diseases compared to normal healthy persons (systolic BP;<120 mmHg, diastolic BP; <80 mmHg). The risk of hypertension progress is known to be around 90% in Americans who are over 50 years old [3]. Due to the WHO assembly in 2013, the most important target should be reducing the increasing prevalence of hypertension worldwide. Every year, deaths due to the complications of hypertension account for 9.4 million people worldwide [4]. Studies on the prevalence of hypertension in Turkey have been performed since 1960, both regional and in a large scale. In 2003, the Turkish Society of Hypertension and Renal Diseases carried out a population based cross-sectional epidemiological survey, determining the distribution of blood pressure, namely PatenT-1 study (Prevalence, awareness and treatment of hypertension in Turkey), and due to this study, the prevalence of hypertension in our country is 31.8% and higher in women (36.1%) than in men (27.5%) [5] In 2012, due to PatenT-2 study, although the prevalence of hypertension was lower as 30.3%, still it was seen higher in women (32.3%) than in men (28.4%) [6]. Hypertension is the most common risk factor for stroke, congestive heart failure, myocardial infarction, periferal vascular disease and last stage renal failure [1, 4].

Elevations in BP is due to genetic factors, environmental factor or both of them. "Environmental factors (nutrition, physical activity and psychosocial factors) play an important role in blood pressure homeostasis [1, 2, 4]. Nutritional modifications potentially prevent hypertension and reduce BP, thus diminishing the risk of clinical complications related to BP in prehypertensive people and in people who do not have hypertension. In INTERSALT study, it was implied that a 3mmHg reduction in systolic BP reduces the mortality due to stroke by 8% and coronary heart disease by 5% [7]. When hypertensive patients having drug therapy change their diet, especially reduce salt intake, their BP is reduced and they lower their drug doses too. Generally, the nutrition therapy performed by hypertensive patients is more effective in reducing BP when compared to people without hypertension [1]. The only therapy of mild hypertension in the elderly is lifestyle changes. Quiting smoking, weight loss, reducing mental stress, reducing excess intake of sodium and alcohol, and enhancing physical activity reduces the doses of antihypertensive drugs. In 2013, AHA/ACC Lifestyle Management Guideline, it was shown that, in people who are mildly overweight, the reduced sodium intake combined with weight loss is very effective in hypertension and preventing and controlling cardiovascular diseases. The lifestyle changes needed to control LDL-cholesterol, lipids and BP which are the cardiovascular risk factors, which are shown in (Table **1**). in "2013 AHA/ACC Lifestyle Management Guideline" (Nutrition/Activity recommendations) [8].

Table 1. 2013 AHA/ACC Lifestyle Management Guideline (Nutrition/Activity recommendations) [8].

Nutrition	
LDL-Cholesterol	Advises to adults who would benefit lowering LDL cholesterol

	1. Consume a dietary pattern that emphasizes intake of vegetables, fruits, and whole grains; includes low-fat dairy products, poultry, fish, legumes, nontropical vegetable oils, and nuts; and limits intake of sweets, sugar-sweetened beverages, and red meats.
	    a. Adapt this dietary pattern to appropriate calorie requirements, personal and cultural food preferences, and nutrition therapy for other medical conditions (including diabetes).
	    b. Achieve this pattern by following plans such as the DASH dietary pattern, the USDA Food Pattern, or the AHA.

	2. Aim for a dietary pattern that achieves 5% to 6% of calories from saturated fat.
	3. Reduce percentage of calories from saturated fat.
	4. Reduce percentage of calories from trans fat.
Blood Pressure	Advises to lower BP in adults
Sodium Intake	1. Reducing sodium intake

	2. Advise adults who would benefit from BP lowering to:
	    a. Consume no more than 2400 mg of sodium/d
	    b. Further reduction of sodium intake to 1500 mg/d can result in even greater reduction in BP
	    c. Even without achieving these goals, reducing
	    sodium intake by at least 1000 mg/d lowers BP.

	3. Combine the DASH dietary pattern with lower sodium intake.
Physical Activity	
Lipids	1. Advise adults to engage in aerobic physical activity to reduce LDL-C and non–HDL-C: 3 to 4 sessions per week, lasting on average 40 minutes per session, and involving moderate- to vigorous-intensity physical activity.
Blood Pressure	1. 1. Advise adults to engage in aerobic physical activity to lower BP: 3 to 4 sessions per week, lasting on average 40 minutes per session, and involving moderate- to vigorous-intensity physical activity.

Restricting sodium intake in elder hypertension patients is more effective when compared with younger patients. Increasing potassium intake with vegetables and fruits, lowers BP especially in people who have high sodium intake. If 1 and/or 2 units/day alcohol limit is exceeded, it is inevitable for BP rise and reducing alcohol intake lowers BP especially in the elderly. Moderate exercise also lowers BP similar to strict diets [9].

The Effects of Lifestyle Modification on Reducing BP

Lifestyle modification, complementary to drug treatment, is generally recommended to all patients who have high BP. It is especially important to apply lifestyle modifications to whom the drug treatment is not recommended with mild and/or normal BP. Lifestyle changes not only reduce BP, but also delay starting pharmacological therapy, and also prevent complications and cardiovascular risk factors via lowering the doses and amount of antihypertensive drugs [8, 10]. The lifestyle modification strategies which are effective on systolic BP levels are shown in (Table **2**).

Table 2. The BP lowering effects on improvement in life style behaviour [8, 9].

Changes in Life Style	Recommendations	Lowering in Systolic BP ($\approx$) (mmHg)
Weight loss	Achieving the normal Body Mass Index (BMI) and maintaining this	5–20 mm Hg/ (Weight loss as 10 kgs)
DASH Diet	Increasing vegetable and fruits consumption and having low fat milk products and reducing the consumption of saturated fats.	8-14 mmHg
Lowering salt intake	Reducing salt consumption (1.5 gram/d sodium = 3.8 gram/d salt)	2-8 mmHg
Physical activity	Regular aerobic physical activity (3-4 days/week 40 min/day)	4-9 mmHg
Moderate alcohol consumption	Limiting alcohol consumption as $\leq$1 unit for women, $\leq$2 unit for men	2-4 mmHg
	Decrease in BP in Total	**21-55 mmHg**

The Diet Factors Lowering Blood Pressure

Lifestyle changes are the nutritional recommendations involving the control of salt intake and weight loss, regular physical activity, avoiding alcohol/cigarette consumption, *etc.* [8, 9, 11, 12]. The summary of lifestyle changes related to BP reducing diet is shown in (Table **3**).

Weight Loss

Observational and clinical study results implied that body weight is directly proportional with BP. This relationship is supported by the increase in the prevalence of mild overweight and obesity both in United States of America and in the entire world. The BMI of 65% of American people is 25kg/m² because of them being mildly overweight or obese.

Table 3. The changes in lifestyle related to the BP lowering diet.

Lifestyle Changes	Recommendations
Weight loss	Reducing the BMI to lower <25kg/m2 and ensuring the mild overweight and overweight people lose weight >%3
Lowering salt intake	Reducing the salt intake as lower as possible (1.5 g/d sodium = 3.8 g/d salt), can be reduced to 1 g/d sodium incase needed
DASH diet	Increasing vegetable and fruits consumption (8-10 portion/d) and having low fat milk products (2-3 portion/d) and reducing the consumption of lipids, saturated fats and cholesterol.
Increasing potassium, calcium and magnesium intake	Increasing potassium intake (4.7 g/d), calcium intake (1250 g/d) and magnesium intake (500 mg/d) (These amounts of potassium, calcium and magnesium are supplied via DASH diet)
Moderate alcohol consumption	Limiting alcohol consumption as ≤ 1 unit for women, ≤ 2 unit for men (1 unit=12-15 g alcohol containing beverage)
Lowering the levels of saturated and trans lipids in diet	Reducing the percentage of the calories taken from saturated fat to %5-6, and trans fat lower than %1

Due to OECD, obesity levels are expected to be particularly high in the United States, Mexico and England, where 47%, 39% and 35% of the population, respectively, are projected to be obese (≥ 30 kg/m^2) in 2030 [11, 13]. According to the World Health Organization data, over 400 million are obese and over 1.6 billion are overweight (BMI=25-29.9 kg/m^2) and it is estimated this will reach 700 million and 2.3 billion, respectively, in 2015 [14]. In the studies implying the relationship between obesity and hypertension, it was found that the risk of hypertension was three times higher in overweight individuals with BMI >27 kg/m^2 than in individuals with normal weight. In the last 10 years, the prevalence of overweight in children and adolescents in the USA has increased, and accordingly, increases in the BP levels have been recorded [14 - 16]. The prevalence of obesity in Turkey is not different than the developed Western countries, and reaches to high levels as 30% especially in women. According to the results of the TURDEP-II study where 24,788 people were screened, obesity prevalence was detected to be 30% in women, 13% in men, and 23,3% in general [17]. Epidemiological studies have shown that there is a relationship between body weight and arterial hypertension. In the Framingham Study, a 10% increase in body weight was found to increase systolic BP by 7 mmHg and a 1 kg decrease in weight was found to decrease BP by 0.3-0.4 mmHg. 78% of hypertensive men and 65% of women are obese. In 70% of hypertensive men and in 60% of hypertensive women, hypertension was found to be related with excess adiposity and this relation is more effective in abdominal obesity [18, 19].

Individuals with high BP should lose weight in such a way that their BMI will be in the normal range (18.5-24.9 kg/m2) and they should maintain their body weight at this level [2, 8, 9].

Weight loss is the first option in people with hypertension and abdominal obesity. Weight loss and weight protection can be achieved by restricting energy intake, increasing physical activity, and implementing behavioural changes. Weight loss should not exceed 7-10% of the person's initial weight within a period of 6-12 months. The recommended amount of weight loss is reduced by all or most of the metabolic risk factors. The most important point in maintaining weight loss is long-term follow-up and monitoring. According to current information, the effect of weight-loss drugs on the treatment of obesity is very low. However, medications can help some individuals lose weight [11, 19, 20].

The Effect of Salt (Sodium) on Blood Pressure

The role of kidneys and sodium metabolism is very important for the occurrence of hypertension although there are also other factors. There is strong and consistent clinical trial evidence that daily sodium intake is related with the frequency of hypertension [21 - 24]. The prevalence of hypertension is elevated in high sodium consuming populations whereas it declines in low sodium consuming populations [4, 9]. Due to DASH (Dietary Approaches to Stop Hypertension) research published in 1998 and updated in April 2006, it was implied that reducing sodium intake is parallel with decline in BP. Interestingly, this situation is also valid for normotansives [25]. Reducing salt intake in controlling hypertension is very important [4, 9]. Because salt sensitive blood pressure is more common especially in people with abdominal obesity, salt restriction has great importance in the treatment. In SALTURK study, performed by Turkish Society of Hypertension and Renal Diseases, it was detected that salt intake is very high in Turkey as 18 g/day [26].

This subject should be given importance in the populations having high salt intake similar to Turkey. According to the Turkish Hypertension prevalence study, the mean hypertension prevalence in the country is 31.8% and considering about one in every three adults has hypertension; the importance of salt restriction arises.

In the dash study, the effect of three different amounts of sodium intake (1500 mg, 2300 mg and 3300 mg) was tested in combination with a typical American diet or Step 1 diet [1, 20, 25]. In both DASH and typical American diet, with the diet containing 1,500 mg of sodium which is the lowest level, the lowest BP level is achieved. These findings prove that sodium should be reduced to 1500 mg in order to achieve optimal BP. In order to achieve a normal BP value, it is stated in the American guidelines that sodium should be taken less than 2300 mg (equivalent to 6 grams of salt) [27]. This salt goal determined in DASH study was included in the American Dietetic Association's practical guide (2009) [28] and Turkey Nutrition Guide 2015 [30], and it was also supported by the Australian National Heart Association [29], American Heart Association [8] and other by organizations around the world.

The main factor which raises BP was asserted to be sodium chloride other than sodium itself [30]. The individual responses which people give to sodium intake are very heterogeneous. The BPs of some hypertensives may respond more to the reduction of sodium than others. For these people, the definition **"salt-sensitive hypertensive"** is used. On the other hand, patients with **"salt-resistant hypertension"** do not respond to reduced sodium intake. Because of the sensitivity to salt, the degree of decrease in BP will be more or less. People who are more sensitive to salt and sodium often are negro or older adults with obesity, diabetes, metabolic syndrome, chronic kidney failure or hypertension. It may be necessary for people to follow the other advices of a DASH diet except salt to control their hypertension [31, 32]. It is important to note that there is no practical way to differentiate between **"salt-sensitive hypertension"** and **"salt-resistant hypertension"** [20]. If bread is consumed too much, the amount of salt and sodium intake will increase. The most sodium-containing foods are; baking powder, olive, cheese, salted butter, ready-to-eat food, ready-to-eat soup, bouillon, dill, biscuits and similar foods, eggs, liver, kidney, heart, brain, lamb meat, beef, chicken meat, *etc.* [20, 30].

What Should Be Done to Reduce Sodium Intake [8, 15, 20, 25, 30]?

In order to raise awareness about the sodium content of food, a source showing the sodium content of food should be kept under hand, the nutrients eaten, their quantities and sodium content should be recorded.

- Sodium consumption should be limited to 2300 mg per day (2300 mg Na=1 teaspoon salt). If you need to consume 1500 mg/day, you need to specify the amount (1500 mg Na=3/4 teaspoon salt). When the desired BP targets are not achieved, the amount of sodium can be reduced to 1000 mg per day to reduce the BP.
- All food labels should be read and this behavior should become a habit.
- Food containing 5% or less of the daily sodium requirement should be preferred (this ratio is usually available from labels).
- 20% of the daily sodium requirement and more sodium-containing food should be avoided.
- Canned food, ready to eat meat and fast-food food should be avoided.
- Care should be taken to use unsalted sauces in the preparation of meals.

- When food is eaten in restaurants outside the home, the food to be eaten should be made less salty by avoiding condiments, *etc.*

The Effect of Calcium on Blood Pressure

In the Framingham Study, which examined 10,000 people, there was a negative correlation between calcium intake and hypertension incidence. The risk of developing hypertension increases with age [11]. In a study conducted by Wang and colleagues, taking calcium as dairy products reduced the risk of hypertension compared to taking it as a supplement [33]. In the studies implying the effects of calcium treatment on blood pressure, systolic and diastolic blood pressure were decreased by 1 and 2 mmHg, respectively [34 - 46]. In a recent study, it was found that high levels of calcium intake as a component of a healthy diet in the general population resulted in significantly lower systolic BP [37]. 13 studies, consisting of randomized controlled studies on calcium, meta-analysis and systemic review articles, were reviewed in Cochrane Library, where 485 participants were monitored for eight to fifteen weeks [38]. According to this article, the volunteers were given a calcium supplement of 0.4 to 2 g/day and compared with the control group, as a result a significant decrease of 2.5 mmHg in systolic BP was seen statistically, but it was also noted that there were heterogeneity that could not be explained due to the dose of calcium or the initial values of the BP. The mechanism of calcium in reducing blood pressure; high calcium intake increases intracellular calcium concentration and this causes increase in 1.25 vitamin D_3 and parathyroid hormone levels, calcium to pass into vascular smooth muscle cells, and vascular resistance develops more. Alternatively, milk proteins, especially peptides obtained from some fermented products such as milk, can function like ACE and therefore lower blood pressure [19]. A diet that does not contain low-fat dairy products, but contains vegetables and fruits, has also been found to reduce blood pressure by about half [38]. Calcium taken with diet should be at a level for adults to meet the DRI values [20].

The best sources of calcium are milk, yogurt, cheese, coriander, white cheese, molasses, sesame, hazelnut, peanuts, lettuce, greens, green vegetables, dried fruits, eggs, orange, lemon, strawberries, *etc.* [30].

The Effects of Magnesium on Blood Pressure

Magnesium is a potential inhibitor of vascular smooth muscle contractions and may play a role in blood pressure regulation as vasodilator. High blood pressure is the most common cause of death in the United States [20, 29, 39]. A contraindication was found between serum magnesium levels and BP [8, 29]. However, the findings of the studies with magnesium supplementation are contradictory with each other. Inconsistent evidence has prevented magnesium from being a major component that is effective on the BP and has prevented making recommendations for lower magnesium supplementation for BP. In some studies, magnesium was shown to have no effect on the BP [40, 41]. A systemic study of randomized controlled trials suggested that magnesium was not effective in preventing hypertension or lowering BP [42]. In a review involving observational studies, it was suggested that there was a significant inverse relationship between dietary magnesium and BP, and in the recent Cochrane article, magnesium supplementation decreased diastolic BP significantly [43]. The DASH diet consists of magnesium-rich food such as green leafy vegetables, hard shell food, whole grain bread and cereals. It has been suggested that the consumption of magnesium-rich food should be recommended to control hypertension or to prevent hypertension. Food rich in magnesium include whole wheat bread, raisins, green leafy vegetables, almonds, peanuts, milk, yogurt, potatoes, oranges, *etc.* [20, 30, 43].

The Effects of Potassium on Blood Pressure

In epidemiological studies, blood pressure was found to be associated with potassium intake oppositely [44, 45]. The findings such as high levels of potassium in the diet decreased BP are contradictory. Randomised studies on potassium supplementation were evaluated being collected in a pool of four meta-analyses [29, 44 - 49]. Three of these studies suggested that increasing potassium intake with diet lowered BP. Especially, in a meta-analysis of 33 studies, performed by Whelton and his colleagues, it was found that potassium excretion increased (50 mmol/day), an average decrease of 4.4 mmHg in BP of hypertensives and an average decrease of 1.8 mm Hg in normotensives [29, 47]. In a meta-analysis,which is a 4 randomized controlled study, the potassium supplementation in the diets of participants who were followed for 8 weeks did not significantly lower BP, but it was also reported that there was heterogeneity among the findings of different studies [29]. In a study, it was reported that potassium intake between 1900 and 4700 mg/day reduced the BP by 2 to 6 mmHg [48]. In this study, the effect of potassium is largely due to the initial BP and the excessive intake of sodium. High potassium intake also reduces the risk of stroke. It has also been found that the regulation of nutrition, the regular aerobic exercise, alcohol and sodium restriction and the use of fish oil supplements are much more effective than the usage of potassium supplementation [29, 49]. Higher blood potassium levels and lower sodium-potassium ratio have greater effects rather than the effects of sodium and potassium levels each alone [50, 51]. High-potassium diet protects endothelial cells due to high BP and thus its preventing brain hemorrhage and failure has been suggested [50, 52]. 4700 mg/day potassium is not difficult to be provided via the DASH diet which recommends increased amounts of vegetables and fruits [28]. It should also be noted that if people with chronic kidney failure, diabetes and congestive heart failure, *etc.* need to take less potassium, it should be taken care of [20]. Food rich in potassium are: dried egg, lettuce, nuts, spinach, bananas, potatoes, parsley, dill, artichokes, carrots, fresh beans, cabbage, tomato, eggplant, liver, beef, lamb, brain, heart, kidney, eggs, milk, yogurt, *etc.* [20, 30].

The Effects of Physical Activity on Blood Pressure

The risk of developing hypertension is 30% to 50% higher for inactive persons than those who are active. Although it is known that being physically active and exercising reduce the the risk of disease, yet many people still remain inactive. According to the American Heart Association (AHA), the sedentary lifestyle in general has been determined (inactivity; 20-40%) [53]. Exercise is useful for blood pressure. In most days of the week, 30-45 minutes/day low-to-moderate intensity exercise is known to be beneficial for health and is an important strategy for lifestyle change [8, 20, 54].

The Effects of Alcohol Consumption on Blood Pressure

Excessive alcohol consumption is a 5-7% of hypertension cause in the population [8, 20]. The hypertensive effect of alcohol consumption is seen higher in men. Drinking 30 grams of alcohol three times a day causes a 3 mmHg increase in systolic BP [54]. There is information that it is not harmful to drink alcohol once a day for women and twice a day for men containing 15 grams of alcohol. It is also suggested that alcohol taken in these amounts reduces the risk of cardiovascular disease [8, 20]. People with normal BMI should drink alcohol in the specified amounts to prevent hypertension [20]. It should be noted that excessive amounts and regular alcoholic beverages can raise blood pressure and also cause serious diseases such as cirrhosis, stroke, and pancreatitis [8, 28, 53, 54].

The Effects of Lipids on Blood Pressure

The recommendations for the lipid composition of the diet are the recommendations that help to control weight and reduce the risk of cardiovascular disease (CVH) [20]. Scientists at the National Heart, Lung, and Blood Institute (NHLBI) have adopted and supported two key studies. As a result, it was shown that reducing total fat and saturated fat and cholesterol and raising the consumption of vegetables and fruit and low fat milk lower BP [55]. However, the American Dietetic Association 2009 guidelines suggest that the knowledge of the effect of omega-3 fatty acids' in the dietary fat on reducing blood pressure, is not adequate [28]. The incidence of hypertension in vegetarians is lower than that of meat consuming people. This may be because saturated fatty acids in the vegetarian diet are lower than unsaturated fatty acids, and potassium and magnesium levels are higher [27, 28]. In a study conducted by Li and colleagues in 2015, it was found that the type of carbohydrate plays a critical role in reducing the risk of coronary heart disease (CHD). It was found that consuming polyunsaturated fats instead of saturated fats lowered the risk of CHD diseases and replacing saturated fats with refined carbohydrates increased the risk of CHD diseases. In the study, 5% of energy from saturated fats were replaced by polyunsaturated fatty acids, monounsaturated fatty acids, or whole grain carbohydrates, respectively, and 25%, 15% and 9% were associated with lower CHD risk [56]. According to the American Heart Association (AHA), saturated fats should not exceed 5-6% of total energy [8]. In this case, the decrease in LDL will be 11-30 mg/dL. However, in American diet, saturated fat is recommended to be less than 10% of the energy [27]. The DASH diet plan, accepted for use in hypertension treatment, consists of vegetables, fruits, whole grains, fish and chicken, nuts and raisins, and low-fat dairy products. These food are rich in nutrients such as potassium, magnesium, calcium, pulp and protein [20, 55, 57]. It is a known fact that trans fats have negative effects on human health. Trans fatty acids also increase LDL cholesterol, such as saturated fatty acids, while lowering HDL cholesterol and raising the risk of heart disease. Trans fatty acids are high in margarines. There is no trans fat in our country since the hydrogenation system which causes the formation of trans fat in margarine production has been used instead of the interpolation method, especially in soft margarines. Trans fatty acids are found in small amounts in the composition of the butter obtained from goat, sheep and cow's milk, but when exposed to high heat, the amount of trans fatty acids may rise. Partially hydrogenated oils used to prepare cakes, biscuits, crackers cookies, popcorn, mayonnaise, chips, mildew dough, pizza, waffles, *etc.* and in the preparation of high-fat fried fast-food food that have high trans-fatty content [15, 30, 58].

DASH NUTRITION PLAN

The original DASH (Dietary Approaches to Stop Hypertension) study which is sponsored by NHLBI is a multi-center study to test the effect of different diets on blood pressure. The study was performed on 459 adults with systolic BP 160 mmHg and diastolic BP 80-95 mmHg. 27% of the participants had high BPs and 50% were female and 60% were African American. Participants were included in one of the following three diets for eight weeks after the control period [20, 57, 59].

1. **Control diet:** The American diet with average macronutrient and pulp content; 4 servings of vegetables and fruits/day, 0.5 servings of dairy products/day;

potassium, magnesium and calcium levels which are in 25. percentile of American' consumption.

2. **Vegetable and fruit diet:** 8.5 servings of vegetables and fruits/day; potassium, magnesium and calcium levels in the 75. percentile of American consumption. The other nutrition items were similar to the control diet.

3. **Combined (DASH) diet:** 10 servings of and fruits and vegetables/day, 2.7 servings of low-fat milk and milk products/day, fat, saturated fat and cholesterol less than in the control diet, potassium, magnesium and calcium consumption levels in the 75. percentile of American consumption.

The sodium content of all diets were 3000 mg/day. Patients who received antihypertensive drugs were excluded from the study until the physician informed consent [60]. According to the results of this study, in all of the participants and in subgroups separated by gender, ethnicity, being hypertensive /normotensives; in participants who applied the vegetable and fruit diet and the combination diet (DASH), their BP were found to be lower [59, 60]. The BPs of the dash-combination diet applied patients were as low as those who were using antihypertensive drugs. Adaptation to the DASH diet plan has been quite high throughout the world and it has been thought that the diet can be useful in reducing the incidence of serious diseases. To reduce mortality due to stroke, kidney disease, and heart failure and heart disease, NHLBI recommended that not only for those with hypertension but also all Americans should use the DASH diet [59].

In the dash-sodium study, which was done by reducing sodium intake with DASH diet, different amounts of sodium restriction were made. According to this, the DASH diet and vegetable and fruit diet plans were applied to 412 participants, including 3300 mg, 2400 mg and 1500 mg of sodium for a period of 1 month. 41% of the participants had hypertension. Those who applied both nutrition plans have reduced their BPs, yet the most decrease in BP was seen with the DASH diet containing 1500 mg of sodium, however it was noted that this decrease was seen more in prehypertensives than hypertensives [57, 61].

The DASH diet plan should have high potassium levels in order to maintain healthy levels of calcium. A diet rich in potassium reduces high blood pressure, but in the DASH diet, potassium must be obtained from food rather than from supplements. Fruits and vegetables, some dairy products and fish are rich sources of potassium. The DASH diet plan is rich in antioxidants (phytochemicals) and pulp because of its vegetable and fruit content. The DASH diet plan may also be considered a healthy heart guide because it reduces the amount of saturated fat and total fat. The DASH diet plan aims to increase the essential minerals (potassium, calcium and magnesium), protein and nutrient rich elements needed to lower blood pressure [20, 57, 62]. These nutrients will compensate the daily recommended amounts according to the Institute of Medicine. The DASH diet plan has also been shown to reduce the incidence of Type 2 diabetes and the rate of heart failure [57, 63, 64]. The DASH diet plan has been suggested to reduce the risk of cancer and osteoporosis [57, 65].

(Table **4**) lists the daily food items and quantities that should be taken in the dash nutrition plan.

Table 4. Daily nutrients in DASH diet [62] (Calculated for a 2100 calorie eating plan).

Total Fat	% 27 (of Total Calories)	Sodium	2300 mg
Saturated Fat	% 6 (of total calories)	Potassium	4700 mg
Protein	% 18 (of total calories)	Calcium	1250 mg
Carbohydrate	% 55 (of total calories)	Magnesium	500 mg
Cholesterol	150 mg/d	Fiber	30 mgr

The initial DASH trial was a 4-site, randomized controlled feeding study. Compared with a control diet typical of US consumption, the DASH diet produced reductions in systolic blood pressure (SBP) and diastolic blood pressure (DBP) of 5.5 and 3.0 mm Hg, respectively—with results evident as early as 2 weeks after baseline [66]. The DASH diet represents a potentially affordable and scalable intervention that could almost immediately produce considerable improvements in population health, however, adherence to DASH on a national level is poor [67].

As a result, it was shown that with DASH diet which recommends reducing saturated fat, total fat and cholesterol, and increasing consumption of low-fat dairy products with vegetables and fruits, BP is reduced. The DASH diet plan consists of vegetables, fruits, whole grains, fish and chicken, hard-shell nuts and raisins and low-fat dairy products. These food are rich in nutrients such as potassium, magnesium, calcium, pulp and protein. Sodium, sugar, sugary drinks, fats and ready to eat meat are less involved in the DASH diet. The nutrition groups and quantities that need to be eaten in DASH diet are given in (Table **5**).

CONCLUDING REMARKS

The DASH diet encourages to reduce the sodium intake and eat a variety of food rich in nutrients that help treat or prevent high BP. Those with high blood pressure and prehypertension may benefit especially from following the DASH eating plan and reducing their sodium intake. The lower the salt intake is, the lower BP will be. The DASH eating plan also has other benefits, such as lowering LDL

Table 5. Nutrient groups and their daily amounts in DASH diet.

Nutrient Groups	Daily Portions	Portion Sizes
Grains	7-8 portion	1 slice cereal bread
		120 g cooked rice/pasta
		30 g cereal (for breakfast)
Vegetables	4-5 portion	240 g raw leafy vegetable
		120 g cooked vegetable
		120 g vegetable juice
Fruits	4-5 portion	1 apple
		120 g fresh fruit
		120 g frozen fruit
		60 g dried fruit
		180 g fruit juice
Low fat or fat free milk products	2-3 portion	240 g milk or yoghurt
		45-50 g cheese
Lean meat, fish, chicken	2 portion	90 g cooked red meat, fish, chicken
		1 egg
Nuts, seed and legumes	4-5 portion/week	45 g nuts
		2 Tbs fatty seeds
		120 g cooked legumes
		120 g pea
Fats	2-3 portion	1Tbs liquid oil
		1Teasp margarine
		1 Tbs low fat mayonnaise
		2 Tbs light salad sauce
Sweets	5 portion/in less then 5 weeks	1 Tbs sugar
		1 Tbs jam/gelatine
		120 g sorbet or gelatine
		240 g lemonade
Consume no more than 2300 mg of sodium/d (Approx. 1 tsp.). In low sodium diets, limiting sodium intake to 1500 mg/d (2/3 tsp.) would be appropriate. Sodium intake can be lowered even to 1000 mg daily when BP is not reduced as itwas wished.		
Abbreviations: g;gram, Tbs;table spoon, Teasp;teaspoon		

cholesterol, which, along with lowering blood pressure, can reduce the risk for getting heart disease. DASH is a balanced dietary strategy that could be adopted to achieve a healthier diet and lifestyle.

CONSENT FOR PUBLICATION

Not applicable.

CONFLICT OF INTEREST

The authors declare no conflict of interest, financial or otherwise.

ACKNOWLEDGEMENTS

Declare none.

REFERENCES

[1]   NCD Risk Factor Collaboration (NCD-RisC). Worldwide trends in blood pressure from 1975 to 2015: a pooled analysis of 1479 population-based measurement studies with 19·1 million participants. Lancet 2017; 389(10064): 37-55.
[http://dx.doi.org/10.1016/S0140-6736(16)31919-5] [PMID: 27863813]

[2]   Çakmak HA, Arslan E, Erdine S. Hipertansiyonda karşılanmamış gereksinimler Türk kardiyol dern arş - arch turk soc cardiol 2009; 37 (Suppl 7): 1-4.

[3]   Wang Y, Wang QJ. The prevalence of prehypertension and hypertension among US adults according to the new joint national committee guidelines: new challenges of the old problem. Arch Intern Med 2004; 164(19): 2126-34.
[http://dx.doi.org/10.1001/archinte.164.19.2126] [PMID: 15505126]

[4]   A Global Brief on Hypertension World Health Day 2013 Publications of the World Health Organization are available on the WHO web site (wwwwhoint) or can be purchased from WHO Press, World Health Organization 2013.A Global Brief on Hypertension www.who.int.

[5]   Altun B, Arici M, Nergizoğlu G, *et al.* Prevalence, awareness, treatment and control of hypertension in Turkey (the PatenT study) in 2003. J Hypertens 2005; 23(10): 1817-23.
[http://dx.doi.org/10.1097/01.hjh.0000176789.89505.59] [PMID: 16148604]

[6]   2012.Türk Hipertansiyon Prevalans Çalışması PatenT2 http:// www.turkhipertansiyon.org / prevelans_calismasi_2.php.

[7]   Stamler R. Implications of the INTERSALT study. Hypertension 1991; 17(1) (Suppl.): I16-20.
[http://dx.doi.org/10.1161/01.HYP.17.1_Suppl.I16] [PMID: 1986996]

[8]   Eckel RH, Jakicic JM, Ard JD, *et al.* 2013 AHA/ACC guideline on lifestyle management to reduce cardiovascular risk: a report of the American College of Cardiology/American Heart Association Task Force on Practice Guidelines. Circulation 2014; 129(25) (Suppl. 2): S76-99.
[http://dx.doi.org/10.1161/01.cir.0000437740.48606.d1] [PMID: 24222015]

[9]   Aronow WS, Fleg JL, Pepine CJ, *et al.* ACCF/AHA 2011 expert consensus document on hypertension in the elderly: a report of the American College of Cardiology Foundation Task Force on Clinical Expert Consensus Documents. Circulation 2011; 123(21): 2434-506.
[http://dx.doi.org/10.1161/CIR.0b013e31821daaf6] [PMID: 21518977]

[10]   Sağlam M, Boşnak-Güçlü M, İnal İnce D, Savcı S, Arıkan H. Hipertansiyon ve EgzersizAnkara: TC Sağlık Bakanlığı Yayın No: 730. 2008.

[11]   Moore LL, Visioni AJ, Qureshi MM, Bradlee ML, Ellison RC, D'Agostino R. Weight loss in overweight adults and the long-term risk of hypertension: the Framingham study. Arch Intern Med

2005; 165(11): 1298-303.
[http://dx.doi.org/10.1001/archinte.165.11.1298] [PMID: 15956011]

[12]   Hedayati SS, Elsayed EF, Reilly RF. Non-pharmacological aspects of blood pressure management: what are the data? Kidney Int 2011; 79(10): 1061-70.
[http://dx.doi.org/10.1038/ki.2011.46] [PMID: 21389976]

[13]   Obesity Update. 2017. www.oecd.org/health/obesity-update.htm

[14]   Obesity Statistics Update. Canada and the World. USA 2015.

[15]   Samur G, Yıldız E. Obezite Kardiyovasküler Hastalıklar ve Hipertansiyon TC Sağlık Bakanlığı Temel Sağlık Hizmetleri Genel Müdürlüğü Beslenme ve Fiziksel Aktiviteler Daire Başkanlığı Sağlık Bakanlığı Yayın No: 729, 2008-Ankara 2008.

[16]   Muntner P, He J, Cutler JA, Wildman RP, Whelton PK. Trends in blood pressure among children and adolescents. JAMA 2004; 291(17): 2107-13.
[http://dx.doi.org/10.1001/jama.291.17.2107] [PMID: 15126439]

[17]   Türkiye Diyabet Prevalansı Çalışmaları: TURDEP-I ve TURDEP-II 47 Ulusal Diyabet Kongresi, 11-15 Mayıs. Antalya: Rixos Sungate Hotel 2011.

[18]   Xavier Pi-Sunyer F. Obesity and Hypertension. Obes Manag 2009; 5(2): 57-61.
[http://dx.doi.org/10.1089/obe.2009.0204]

[19]   Elias MF, Elias PK, Sullivan LM, Wolf PA, D'Agostino RB. Lower cognitive function in the presence of obesity and hypertension: the Framingham heart study. Int J Obes Relat Metab Disord 2003; 27(2): 260-8.
[http://dx.doi.org/10.1038/sj.ijo.802225] [PMID: 12587008]

[20]   Raymond JL, Couch SC. Medical Nutrition Therapy for Cardiovascular Diseases (Chap 31)Krause's Food and the Nutrition Care Process. 13th edition. Philadelphia, London, Toronto, Mexico City, Rio de Janeiro, Sydney, Tokyo: Elsevier WB Saunders Company 2012; pp. 743-81.

[21]   Erdem Y. Hipertansiyon Patofizyolojisi. 2002.

[22]   Intersalt: an international study of electrolyte excretion and blood pressure. Results for 24 hour urinary sodium and potassium excretion. BMJ 1988; 297(6644): 319-28.
[http://dx.doi.org/10.1136/bmj.297.6644.319] [PMID: 3416162]

[23]   Takase H, Sugiura T, Kimura G, Ohte N, Dohi Y. Dietary sodium consumption predicts future blood pressure and incident hypertension in the Japanese normotensive general population. J Am Heart Assoc 2015; 4(8)e001959.
[http://dx.doi.org/10.1161/JAHA.115.001959] [PMID: 26224048]

[24]   Strazzullo P, D'Elia L, Kandala NB, Cappuccio FP. Salt intake, stroke, and cardiovascular disease: meta-analysis of prospective studies. BMJ 2009; 339: b4567.
[http://dx.doi.org/10.1136/bmj.b4567] [PMID: 19934192]

[25]   Vollmer WM, Sacks FM, Ard J, *et al.* Effects of diet and sodium intake on blood pressure: subgroup analysis of the DASH-sodium trial. Ann Intern Med 2001; 135(12): 1019-28.
[http://dx.doi.org/10.7326/0003-4819-135-12-200112180-00005] [PMID: 11747380]

[26]   Erdem Y, Arici M, Altun B, *et al.* The relationship between hypertension and salt intake in Turkish population: SALTURK study. Blood Press 2010; 19(5): 313-8.
[http://dx.doi.org/10.3109/08037051003802541] [PMID: 20698734]

[27]   U.S. Department of Agriculture, U.S. Department of Health and Human Services. Dietary Guidelines for Americans 2010.www.dietaryguidelines.gov

[28]   American Dietetic Association. Hypertension. Chicago, IL: ADA Evidence Analysis Library 2009.

[29]   Summary of Evidence Statement on The Relationships Between Dietary Electrolytes and Cardiovascular Disease 2006. .www.heartfoundation.com.au.

[30]   Türkiye beslenme rehberi "TÜBER 2015", TC Sağlık Bakanlığı Yayın No: 1031, Ankara 2016.

[31]   Sanada H, Jones JE, Jose PA. Genetics of salt-sensitive hypertension. Curr Hypertens Rep 2011; 13(1): 55-66.
[http://dx.doi.org/10.1007/s11906-010-0167-6] [PMID: 21058046]

[32]   Elijovich F, Weinberger MH, Anderson CAM, *et al.* American heart association professional and public education committee of the council on hypertension; council on functional genomics and translational biology; and stroke council. Salt sensitivity of blood pressure: A scientific statement from the American heart association. Hypertension 2016; 68(3): e7-e46.
[http://dx.doi.org/10.1161/HYP.0000000000000047] [PMID: 27443572]

[33]   Wang L. >Blood Pressure Response to Calcium Supplementation: A Meta-Analysis of Randomized Controlled Trials. J Hum Hypertens 2008; 20: 571.

[34]   Griffith LE, Guyatt GH, Cook RJ, Bucher HC, Cook DJ. The influence of dietary and nondietary calcium supplementation on blood pressure: an updated metaanalysis of randomized controlled trials. Am J Hypertens 1999; 12(1 Pt 1): 84-92.
[http://dx.doi.org/10.1016/S0895-7061(98)00224-6] [PMID: 10075392]

[35]   Reid IR, Horne A, Mason B, Ames R, Bava U, Gamble GD. Effects of calcium supplementation on body weight and blood pressure in normal older women: a randomized controlled trial. J Clin Endocrinol Metab 2005; 90(7): 3824-9.
[http://dx.doi.org/10.1210/jc.2004-2205] [PMID: 15827103]

[36]   van Mierlo LA, Arends LR, Streppel MT, *et al.* Blood pressure response to calcium supplementation: a meta-analysis of randomized controlled trials. J Hum Hypertens 2006; 20(8): 571-80.
[http://dx.doi.org/10.1038/sj.jhh.1002038] [PMID: 16673011]

[37]   Ruidavets JB, Bongard V, Simon C, *et al.* Independent contribution of dairy products and calcium intake to blood pressure variations at a population level. J Hypertens 2006; 24(4): 671-81.
[http://dx.doi.org/10.1097/01.hjh.0000217849.10831.16] [PMID: 16531795]

[38]   Dickinson HO, Nicolson DJ, Cook JV, *et al.* Calcium supplementation for the management of primary hypertension in adults. Cochrane Database Syst Rev 2006; 19(2)CD004639
[http://dx.doi.org/10.1002/14651858.CD004639.pub2] [PMID: 16625609]

[39]   Sontia B, Touyz RM. Role of magnesium in hypertension. Arch Biochem Biophys 2007; 458(1): 33-9.
[http://dx.doi.org/10.1016/j.abb.2006.05.005] [PMID: 16762312]

[40]   Hajjar IM, Grim CE, George V, Kotchen TA. Impact of diet on blood pressure and age-related changes in blood pressure in the US population: analysis of NHANES III. Arch Intern Med 2001; 161(4): 589-93.
[http://dx.doi.org/10.1001/archinte.161.4.589] [PMID: 11252120]

[41]   Jee SH, Miller ER III, Guallar E, Singh VK, Appel LJ, Klag MJ. The effect of magnesium supplementation on blood pressure: a meta-analysis of randomized clinical trials. Am J Hypertens 2002; 15(8): 691-6.
[http://dx.doi.org/10.1016/S0895-7061(02)02964-3] [PMID: 12160191]

[42]   Mizushima S, Cappuccio FP, Nichols R, Elliott P. Dietary magnesium intake and blood pressure: a qualitative overview of the observational studies. J Hum Hypertens 1998; 12(7): 447-53.
[http://dx.doi.org/10.1038/sj.jhh.1000641] [PMID: 9702930]

[43]   Dickinson HO, Nicolson DJ, Campbell F, *et al.* Magnesium supplementation for the management of essential hypertension in adults. Cochrane Database Syst Rev 2006; 19(3)CD004640
[PMID: 16856052]

[44]   Dickinson HO, Nicolson DJ, Campbell F, Beyer FR, Mason J. Potassium supplementation for the management of primary hypertension in adults. Cochrane Database Syst Rev 2006; 19(3)CD004641
[http://dx.doi.org/10.1002/14651858.CD004641.pub2] [PMID: 16856053]

[45]   Kieneker LM, Gansevoort RT, Mukamal KJ, *et al.* Urinary potassium excretion and risk of developing hypertension: the prevention of renal and vascular end-stage disease study. Hypertension 2014; 64(4): 769-76.
[http://dx.doi.org/10.1161/HYPERTENSIONAHA.114.03750] [PMID: 25047575]

[46]   Cappuccio FP, MacGregor GA. Does potassium supplementation lower blood pressure? A meta-analysis of published trials. J Hypertens 1991; 9(5): 465-73.
[http://dx.doi.org/10.1097/00004872-199105000-00011] [PMID: 1649867]

[47]   Whelton PK, He J, Cutler JA, *et al.* Effects of oral potassium on blood pressure. Meta-analysis of randomized controlled clinical trials. JAMA 1997; 277(20): 1624-32.
[http://dx.doi.org/10.1001/jama.1997.03540440058033] [PMID: 9168293]

[48]   Geleijnse JM, Kok FJ, Grobbee DE. Blood pressure response to changes in sodium and potassium intake: a metaregression analysis of randomised trials. J Hum Hypertens 2003; 17(7): 471-80.
[http://dx.doi.org/10.1038/sj.jhh.1001575] [PMID: 12821954]

[49]   Dickinson HO, Mason JM, Nicolson DJ, *et al.* Lifestyle interventions to reduce raised blood pressure: a systematic review of randomized controlled trials. J Hypertens 2006; 24(2): 215-33.
[http://dx.doi.org/10.1097/01.hjh.0000199800.72563.26] [PMID: 16508562]

[50]   Vinceti M, Filippini T, Crippa A, de Sesmaisons A, Wise LA, Orsini N. Meta-analysis of potassium intake and the risk of stroke. J Am Heart Assoc 2016; 5(10)e004210
[http://dx.doi.org/10.1161/JAHA.116.004210] [PMID: 27792643]

[51]   Rodrigues SL, Baldo MP, Machado RC, Forechi L, Molina MdelC, Mill JG. High potassium intake blunts the effect of elevated sodium intake on blood pressure levels. J Am Soc Hypertens 2014; 8(4): 232-8.
[http://dx.doi.org/10.1016/j.jash.2014.01.001] [PMID: 24524886]

[52]   Cook NR, Obarzanek E, Cutler JA, *et al.* Joint effects of sodium and potassium intake on subsequent cardiovascular disease: the Trials of Hypertension Prevention follow-up study. Arch Intern Med 2009; 169(1): 32-40.
[http://dx.doi.org/10.1001/archinternmed.2008.523] [PMID: 19139321]

[53]   Lloyd-Jones D, Adams RJ, Brown TM, *et al.* Heart disease and stroke statistics-2010 update: a report from the American Heart Association. Circulation 2010; 121(7): e46-e215.
[PMID: 20019324]

[54]   Artinian NT, Fletcher GF, Mozaffarian D, *et al.* American Heart Association Prevention Committee of the Council on Cardiovascular Nursing. Interventions to promote physical activity and dietary lifestyle changes for cardiovascular risk factor reduction in adults: a scientific statement from the American Heart Association. Circulation 2010; 122(4): 406-41.
[http://dx.doi.org/10.1161/CIR.0b013e3181e8edf1] [PMID: 20625115]

[55]   Your guide to lowering your blood pressure with DASH 2006. .http:// nhlbi.nih.gov/health / public/ hearth/ hbp/ dash/new_dash.pdf.

[56]   Li Y, Hruby A, Bernstein AM, *et al.* Saturated fats compared With unsaturated fats and sources of carbohydrates in relation to risk of coronary heart disease: A prospective cohort study. J Am Coll Cardiol 2015; 66(14): 1538-48.
[http://dx.doi.org/10.1016/j.jacc.2015.07.055] [PMID: 26429077]

[57]   Chapter 15, Hypertension. In: Insel P, Ross D, McMahon K, Bernstein M, Eds. Nutrition Fourth edition. Canada, London: Jones and Bartlett Publishers 2011; pp. 636-42.

[58]   Taşan Ö, Dağlıoğlu O. Trans Yağ Asitlerinin Yapısı Oluşumu ve Gıdalarla Alınması. Tekirdag Ziraat Fak Derg 2005; 2(1): 79-88.

[59]   Harsha DW, Lin PW, Obarzanek E, *et al.* Dietary approaches to stop hypertension: A summary of study results. J Am Diet Assoc 1999; 99(8) (Suppl.): S5-S39.
[http://dx.doi.org/10.1016/S0002-8223(99)00414-9]

[60] Vog TM, Appel LJ, Obarzenek E. *et al.* Dietary approaches to stop hypertension: Rationale, design, and methods. J Am Diet Assoc 1999; 99 (8suppl): S2-S18.

[61] Sacks FM, Svetkey LP, Vollmer WM, *et al.* Effects on blood pressure of reduced dietary sodium and the Dietary Approaches to Stop Hypertension (DASH) diet. N Engl J Med 2001; 344(1): 3-10.
[http://dx.doi.org/10.1056/NEJM200101043440101] [PMID: 11136953]

[62] US Department of Health abd Human Services National Institutes of Health National Heart, Lung, and Blood Institute Your Guide to Lowering Your Blood Pressure With DASH NIH Publication No 06-4082 Originally Printed 1998 2006.

[63] Liese AD, Nichols M, Sun X, D'Agostino RB Jr, Haffner SM. Adherence to the DASH Diet is inversely associated with incidence of type 2 diabetes: the insulin resistance atherosclerosis study. Diabetes Care 2009; 32(8): 1434-6.
[http://dx.doi.org/10.2337/dc09-0228] [PMID: 19487638]

[64] Levitan EB, Wolk A, Mittleman MA. Consistency with the DASH diet and incidence of heart failure. Arch Intern Med 2009; 169(9): 851-7.
[http://dx.doi.org/10.1001/archinternmed.2009.56] [PMID: 19433696]

[65] Champagne CM. Dietary interventions on blood pressure; the dietary approaches to stop hypertension (DASH) trials. Nutr Rev 2006; 64(2): S3-S56.

[66] Appel LJ, Moore TJ, Obarzanek E, *et al.* A clinical trial of the effects of dietary patterns on blood pressure. N Engl J Med 1997; 336(16): 1117-24.
[http://dx.doi.org/10.1056/NEJM199704173361601] [PMID: 9099655]

[67] Mellen PB, Gao SK, Vitolins MZ, Goff DC Jr. Deteriorating dietary habits among adults with hypertension: DASH dietary accordance, NHANES 1988-1994 and 1999-2004. Arch Intern Med 2008; 168(3): 308-14.
[http://dx.doi.org/10.1001/archinternmed.2007.119] [PMID: 18268173]

SUBJECT INDEX

A

ACE inhibitors 151, 160, 167
Active metabolite of vitamin D 307, 308, 312
Activity of RVLM 247
Adipocytes 285, 287, 288, 289, 292
Adipokines 283, 284, 285, 286, 287, 290, 294, 295
Adiponectin 241, 253, 284, 285, 286, 292
Adipose tissue 283, 285, 286, 287, 288, 289, 290, 291, 294, 317
Adrenal Cushing's syndrome 216, 217, 218
Adrenal gland 202, 212, 218, 293
Adrenomedullin 145, 149, 152
Aircraft noise 1, 16, 20, 21, 22
Air 1, 2, 5, 10, 11, 22, 23, 24, 28, 31, 32, 33, 34, 35, 36
  pollutants 28, 31, 33, 36
  pollution 1, 2, 5, 10, 11, 22, 23, 24, 32, 33, 34, 35, 36
  pollution and hypertension 24, 34
  pollution-related hypertension 24, 35, 36
Albuminuria 160, 167, 168, 334
Alcohol consumption 20, 21, 60, 80, 88, 339, 348
Aldosterone 148, 160, 219, 220, 221, 293
  antagonists therapy 160
  production 148, 219, 220, 221, 293
Ambulatory blood pressure 3, 5, 25, 38, 39, 66, 67, 68, 69, 71, 72, 73, 76, 82, 83, 86, 88, 90, 102, 103
  monitoring 3, 25, 39, 67, 68, 71, 73, 76, 82, 83, 88, 90, 102, 103
Androstenedione 210, 211, 212
Angiotensin 120, 148, 164, 183, 234, 235, 261, 265, 267, 315, 316, 346
  converting enzyme (ACE) 120, 148, 234, 235, 261, 315, 346
Angiotensin 37, 39, 40, 120, 145, 148, 152, 160, 164, 167, 168, 169, 241, 253, 260, 287
  II (ATII) 120, 145, 148, 152, 164, 226, 241, 253, 260, 287

receptor blockade (ARBs) 37, 39, 40, 160, 167, 168, 169, 226, 227, 235
Anthropometry 26, 43, 81, 83, 84, 89, 90, 91, 92, 93
Antidiarrhoeals 115, 116
Antihypertensive 115, 118, 119, 120, 167, 168, 173, 191, 201, 233, 235, 340, 342, 350
  agents 115, 167, 168
  drugs 115, 118, 119, 120, 167, 168, 173, 191, 201, 233, 235, 340, 342, 350
Antihypertensive treatment 151, 165, 167, 168, 190, 191, 228
  multiple 167
Aortic arch 248, 251, 254
Apoptosis 179, 188, 209, 226, 232, 233, 236, 288, 303, 317
ARB blockers 160
Arrhythmia 119, 226, 230, 307
Arterial blood gas (ABG) 130
Arterial hypertension 62, 77, 78, 87, 160, 258, 343
Arterial pressure 16, 190, 243, 248, 249, 251, 262
Arterial stiffness 36, 146
Arterial wall 124, 128, 146, 258, 317
Artery pressure 124, 125
Receptors 260, 261, 262, 313, 314
  AT1 260, 261, 262, 313, 314
  AT2 313, 314
Atrial natriuretic peptide (ANP) 130, 146, 148, 185

B

Baroreceptors 245, 248, 249, 250, 251, 254, 255, 256, 261
  activity 254, 255, 256
  cardiopulmonary 245, 248, 250
  reflexes 248, 249, 250, 251
  type II 256
Baroreceptor sensitivity 241, 254, 255
Behavioral risk factors surveillance system (BRFSS) 79

www.ingramcontent.com/pod-product-compliance
Lightning Source LLC
Chambersburg PA
CBHW050802220326
41598CB00006B/96